AN INTRODUCTION TO EGYPTIAN COLLOQUIAL ARABIC

BY

T. F. MITCHELL

Professor of Linguistics
University of Leeds

CLARENDON PRESS · OXFORD

Oxford University Press, Walton Street, Oxford OX2 6DP

OXFORD LONDON GLASGOW
NEW YORK TORONTO MELBOURNE WELLINGTON
IBADAN NAIROBI DAR ES SALAAM CAPE TOWN
KUALA LUMPUR SINGAPORE JAKARTA HONG KONG TOKYO
DELHI BOMBAY CALCUTTA MADRAS KARACHI

———

First published 1956
Second impression 1960
Reprinted and first issued in paperback 1978

CASEBOUND ISBN 0 19 815149 7
PAPERBACK ISBN 0 19 815148 9

Printed in Great Britain by
REDWOOD BURN LIMITED
Trowbridge & Esher

FOREWORD

STUDENTS of literary Arabic are already in Mr. Mitchell's debt for his earlier book on *Writing Arabic*. No one will be inclined to underestimate the cultural importance of the Arabic script, both for the eye and for the hand. The obligations of speech are no less compelling and Mr. Mitchell, who has had field experience in Cyrenaica and North Africa, naturally turned to the spoken Arabic of Cairo as a leading cultural and political centre.

As a result of the interest and support of the then Shell companies in Egypt, Mr. Mitchell has been able to cast his description of this Colloquial in the form of lessons with exercises and texts, accompanied by grammatical guidance and a practical glossary. The book provides as good a guide to learners of the spoken language as the printed page can give them. The reading transcription, though not a rigid system of spelling, is thoroughly Arabic and is designed to help the student to acquire an early fluency in speaking and comprehension. The material to some extent caters for those engaged in the petroleum industry but it maintains a general interest and covers the main features of the language.

It is with great pleasure that I commend this instructive book to all those who may be in a position to begin the study of spoken Arabic through the medium of English.

J. R. FIRTH
Professor of General Linguistics
in the University of London

June, 1956

ACKNOWLEDGEMENTS

THAT this book appears at all is due to the initiative and encouragement of Anglo-Egyptian Oilfields Limited and the Shell Company of Egypt Limited, nationalized in 1956 and 1964 respectively, and to their generous financial assistance.

The book was first produced in draft form and issued to teachers and students at the several study centres of the Companies in Egypt. Sincere thanks are due to all—not least the students—who faced the difficulties of the experimental book, and to Dr. Harrel F. Beck, late Dean of the American University in Cairo, and other members of the staff of that University, without whose wholehearted co-operation the draft could never have been used. As a result of the experience gained, considerable changes were suggested and have been incorporated in the book as it now appears.

I am especially indebted to Mr. D. L. Hunt, formerly of Anglo-Egyptian Oilfields Ltd. Throughout the long period of preparation, Mr. Hunt spared himself no effort in making and collecting suggestions for the improvement of the book; more particularly, most of Part II is owed to him.

The Arabic material has been checked and rechecked with so many willing Egyptian helpers that it is impossible to acknowledge them all individually. I should like, however, to thank particularly Sheikh Ahmed Abdel Aziz, late of the Shell Company of Egypt, and Mr. Mohamed Ramadan Ali of that Company, and also Mr. K. Bishr and Mr. M. Hamad, for their devoted work in the selection and editing of material. I am likewise extremely grateful, for their constructive criticism and comment, to Miss Gamalat Shoukry, late of Anglo-Egyptian Oilfields Limited, to Mr. Boulos Abdel Messih, Mr. Nessim Habib, and Sheikh Fahmy Mansour of the School of Oriental Studies, American University, Cairo, to Mr. Mansour Hussein El Sawwah and Mr. Alfred Deeb of the British School at Suez, and to Mr. Saleh Sayed Ahmed and Mr. El Sayed Yousef Ahmed of the Egyptian Ministry of Education.

To Mr. David Cowan I am much indebted for reading the manuscript and making many valuable suggestions.

Finally, may I sincerely thank Professor J. R. Firth, not only for his guidance and encouragement academically, but also for the benefit of his wisdom and experience in practical matters of presentation. The roman system of writing employed in the book is owed almost entirely to Professor Firth.

T. F. M.

School of Oriental and African Studies
London

NOTE

This book was written over twenty years ago and one's thinking has naturally changed in some respects over this period. These are not, however, sufficiently great to merit the large increase in cost that incorporating them in the reprint would entail. It might be said, however, in relation to the transcription, that it would probably be improved by not using **q** with the value of the glottal stop and by introducing a distinction between front and back open vowels **a** and **ɑ**. This would enable, for instance, a transcribed difference of vowel, to be made between, say, **raagiȶ** 'returning' and **rɑɑgil** 'man', while **ʕinnaharḍa** 'today' could be written more realistically as **ʕinnɑhɑrḍɑ**. Such changes, however, would in any case have been of only minor importance.

T.F.M.

CONTENTS

FOREWORD *by* J. R. FIRTH v

ACKNOWLEDGEMENTS vii

PART I. INTRODUCTION AND GRAMMAR

Introduction 1

LESSON

1. The article; nominal sentences; the construct . . 15
2. Particles; bitaaç 17
3. Gender 19
4. Number 21
5. Plural noun-adjective agreement; pronouns . . 24
6. Pronouns (*cont.*): fiih and çand- . . 27
7. Verbs 30
8. Verbs (*cont.*): the imperfect and imperative . . 33
9. bi- and ḥa-; kaan, yikúun . . . 35
10. kaan, yikúun (*cont.*); anomalous verbs . . 38
11. Suffixation; the particle Çinn . . . 40
12. Negation 43
13. Negation (*cont.*) 46
14. Interrogation 49
15. Interrogation (*cont.*) 51
16. Demonstratives: Çaho, Çahe, Çahum . . 54
17. The relative Çílli 57
18. Numerals 59
19. Numerals (*cont.*) 62
20. Time; fractions; days and dates . . 64
21. Hollow and doubled verbs . . . 67
22. Weak verbs 69
23. Derived forms of the verb . . . 71
24. Derived forms of the verb (prefix Çit-) . . 75
25. Derived forms of the verb (*concluded*); quadriliteral verbs 77
26. The imperfect without prefix . . . 80

27. The imperfect without prefix (*cont.*) . . . 83
28. Conditional sentences; verbal sequences; qaam . 86
29. Comparison of adjectives; colours and physical defects 89
30. Numerals (*concluded*) 91
31. Collectives and units 94
32. Number (broken plural patterns) . . . 96
33. Participles 100
34. Use of the (active) participle 104
35. The verbal noun; nouns of place and instrument . 107

APPENDIX A. Prominence or Accentuation . . 110
          B. Long vowels 111
          C. Elision 113

PART II. TEXTS 117

Text No.
  1. tawbíix bi Sádab 120
     (*A polite rebuke*)
  2. Sittáꭓlab ilmakkáar 120
     (*The cunning fox*)
  3. Siṭṭámaꭓ yiqíllï ma gámaꭓ 120
     (*The best-laid schemes of mice and men . . .*)
  4. Sinnaggáar ilkasláan 122
     (*The lazy carpenter*)
  5. Silyaʃíim w-innaṣṣáab 122
     (*The simpleton and the cheat*)
  6. muḥáwra ben ṣáaḥib béet wi xaddáamu(h) . . 124
     (*Conversation between a man and his servant*)
  7. muḥáwra ben ꭓáamil w-ilmúʃrif ꭓaléeh . . 126
     (*Exchange between a workman and his supervisor*)
  8. muḥáwra ben síttï-w xaddámha . . . 128
     (*Dialogue between a woman and her servant*)
  9. listiꭓdáad lissáfar min máṣrï li-ʃbíin ilqanáaṭir . . 130
     (*Setting-out from Cairo for Shibin el Qanatir*)
 10. máktab ilbúṣṭa 132
     (*The Post Office*)

CONTENTS   xi

11. muḥáwra ben síttĭ-w gózha   134
    (*Dialogue between a woman and her husband*)
12. muḥáwra ben ʕagnábi-w máṣri   .   .   . 138
    (*Conversation between a foreigner and an Egyptian*)
13. xáan ilxalíili 140
    (*The Muski*)
14. muḥáwra ben wáḥda síttĭ maṣríyya w-iṭṭabbáax bitáɣha   142
    (*Dialogue between an Egyptian woman and her cook*)
15. takmílit ilmuḥáwra-ssábqa   .   .   . 146
    (*Conclusion of the preceding dialogue*)
16. fiṣáal ben táagir wi-zbúun   .   .   . 148
    (*Bargaining between a shopkeeper and a customer*)
17. ʕilḥaʃʃáaʃ wi-ḥmíiru(h)   .   .   . 150
    (*The hashish smoker and his donkeys*)
18. gúḥa filmáṭɣam   152
    (*Guha in the restaurant*)
19. ʕilfalláaḥ w-ilɣarḍiḥálgi   .   .   . 154
    (*The peasant and the scribe*)
20. ʕidáarit ilḥukúuma-f máṣr   .   .   . 156
    (*Government administration in Egypt*)
21. ʕiṭṭáqsĭ-f máṣr   158
    (*The weather in Egypt*)
22. ʕaháali-lqúṭr ilmáṣri 160
    (*The people[s] of Egypt*)
23. ʕiddíin ilʕisláami   160
    (*The Muslim religion*)
24. ʕilmuwaṣaláat fi máṣr 162
    (*Communications in Egypt*)
25. ʕistixráag izzéet ilxáam   .   .   . 164
    (*The production of crude oil*)
26. takríir izzéet ilxáam 166
    (*Refining the crude oil*)
27. tawzíiɣ wi béeɣ ilmuntagáat ilbitrolíyya   . 168
    (*The distribution and marketing of petroleum products*)
28. ḥuqúul ʕabáar izziyúut   .   .   . 170
    (*The oilfields*)

CONTENTS

29. ʕizzetíyya 172
    (*The Refinery*)
30. furúuʒ ʃírkit ʃíllĭ-l máṣr 174
    (*The branches of the Shell Company of Egypt*)
31. ʕidáarit iʃʃarikáat fi máṣr 176
    (*The administration of the companies in Egypt*)
32. ʕistiʒmáal ilmuntagáat ilbitrolíyya . . . 178
    (*The use of petroleum products*)
33. máktab ilmustaxdimíin 180
    (*The Personnel Department*)

Appendix A. Greetings (taḥiyyáat) . . . 184

Appendix B. Exclamations and 'Oaths' . . . 190

PART III. VOCABULARY

Arabic–English 195
English–Arabic 235

PART IV. KEY TO EXERCISES . . . 273

INTRODUCTION

A. *The colloquial language*

In this book we are not at all concerned with *Classical* Arabic nor with the language as *written in the Arabic script*. Rather is the aim to introduce the student to the *colloquial* language of everyday life.

There are numerous forms of Egyptian colloquial Arabic, just as there are many dialects of English. Divergence may be considerable, as for example between Cairo, Qena in Upper Egypt, and the Bedouin area west of Alexandria, or it may be less marked, as, say, between the towns and villages of the Delta. In addition, differences of educational standard and class correspond to speech differences in a single district. It is clearly impossible to account for all varieties in a book of this nature. Fortunately, however, they do not all enjoy the same prestige among Egyptians, and we are able to select as most suitable for our needs the colloquial Arabic of the educated, and especially that spoken by educated people in Cairo. It may be added that this form of Arabic offers little difficulty nowadays to sophisticated speakers from other countries.

An educated Egyptian has very definite ideas on what constitutes a 'prestige' pronunciation, turn of phrase, &c., and the dominance of Cairo need not surprise us, since the part played by capital cities in establishing a norm is well known. In England, London as the centre of government, commerce, literature, law, &c., attracted in the past people from many parts of the country who helped fashion the dialect of English which was to become so widespread, and which, in its modern form, is spoken by most educated Englishmen today. At this point, however, any resemblance between the situation in England and that in Egypt, ends. So-called 'Standard' English is recognized and maintained by authority, and systematically taught; moreover, although there are differences between literary and colloquial English, nevertheless the spoken language has preserved its bonds with the written. This is not so in Egypt, nor indeed in the Arabic-speaking world as a whole.

In spite of their recognition of a colloquial norm, the majority of Egyptians view any form of colloquial Arabic with something like contempt and may even consider it—quite erroneously—as a degenerate form of Classical Arabic. The Classical language of the Koran and early literature, and the grammatically similar neo-Classical or 'Modern' Arabic of contemporary literature, journalism, broadcasting, and public address, are alone regarded as worthy objects of study, while, with rare exceptions, it is this 'Classical' Arabic only which is written in the Arabic script. The student must be prepared, therefore, to hear—and generally to ignore—the dogmatic expression of views which, based usually on obsession with 'Classical' and written forms, run counter to the statements of grammar and pronunciation made in this book.

B. *The system of writing and hints on pronunciation*

(i) We shall use the following 26 consonant- and 5 vowel-letters:

    (*a*) **b, d, ḍ, f, g, h, ḥ, k, l, m, n, q, r, s, ṣ, t, ṭ, w, x, y, z, ẓ, ʕ, ʃ, ɛ, ɣ.**

    (*b*) **a, e, i, o, u.**

There is an easily observed correspondence between the majority of the above and the letters of ordinary English orthography. In the case of **ḍ, ḥ, ṣ, ṭ, ẓ, ʕ, ʃ, ɛ,** and **ɣ,** however, the letter shape is strange and its strangeness usually betokens special pronunciation difficulty. In the case of **q** and **x,** the letters are used with very different values from those associated with them in English spelling.

Vowels occur both short and long. Long vowels are shown by doubling the letter, i.e. long **a** by **aa,** long **i** by **ii,** &c.

Capital letters are not used.

(ii) It is most important for both student and teacher to realize that our writing is based on colloquial *pronunciation*; we are concerned neither with a transliteration of Arabic written forms nor with an orthography, which would require a constant shape for a given word, whatever its pronunciation. Nor is our writing that kind of phonetic transcription which aims at representing as many features of consonant- and vowel-sound as possible, but rather one whose object is to suggest an acceptable pronunciation, with as few frills as possible and without losing sight of the grammar and lexicon.

The lack of rigid correspondence between Arabic letters and the roman ones we use cannot be too strongly stressed, especially perhaps for the benefit of Egyptian teachers using the book. For example, **sanduuq** *box* begins in Arabic writing with a letter which usually corresponds to roman **ṣ**; Egyptian pronunciation nevertheless requires the first letter to be written **s**: conversely, **ṣufra** *dining-table* is written in Arabic with the normal counterpart of **s**. Similarly, when we write **ʕinnaharḍa** *today*, **lukanḍa** *hotel*, **ḥiḍaaʃar** *eleven*, we do not claim that the letter written **ḍ** necessarily corresponds in sound to the usual Arabic equivalent, but simply that writing the words in this way suggests the pronunciation more satisfactorily than **ʕinnaharda, lukanda, ḥidaaʃar**: indeed, those who would prefer **lukanda** on the basis of Arabic writing, may be asked why they would not rather have **luukaandah** which faithfully transliterates the Arabic written form. Other examples are **buliiṣ** *police* (not **buliis**), **mutawaṣṣiṭ** *medium, average* (not **mutawassiṭ**), **ṭarabeeẓa** *table* (not **ṭarabeeza**), **gaẓẓaar** *butcher* (not **gazzaar**), &c. The fact is that vowel- and consonant-quality belong as often as not to the word as a whole and, as will be seen below, the use of **ẓ** in **gaẓẓaar**, for example, immediately indicates the manner in which the vowels of the word should be pronounced.

Using the name of an Arabic letter to identify a given sound, and asking an Egyptian, for example, 'Is it **daal** (usually = **d**) or **ḍaad** (usually = **ḍ**)?' is, therefore, fallacious, but once the danger has been realized, this kind of question is nevertheless useful as a short-cut to identification. For this reason, the Egyptian names for the Arabic letters most frequently corresponding to our own are given below. To pronounce the names it will be necessary to refer to the pronunciation hints given subsequently.

b — bee	ḥ — ḥaa	r — ree	x — xaa	ع — ʕeen
d — daal	k — kaaf	s — siin	y — yee	ɣ — ɣeen
ḍ — ḍaad	l — laam	ṣ — ṣaad	z — zeen	
f — fee	m — miim	t — tee	ẓ — ẓaa	
g — giim	n — nuun	ṭ — ṭaa	ʔ — hamza	
h — hee	q — qaaf	w — waaw	ʃ — ʃiin	

For the vowels, the names **fatḥa (a)**, **kasra (i)**, and **ḍamma (u)** may also prove useful. There are no Arabic names corresponding to **e** and **o**.

It will be seen, therefore, that although the roman writing of Arabic words in the book does not bear a one-to-one relation to the spelling of cognate forms in Classical, nevertheless it may be considered a transliteration in this sense, that the number of letters used corresponds closely to the number used in the Arabic script. A bridge is thus provided from roman to Arabic writing. If this principle were abandoned, then presentation would be 'illiterate' or, at best, made solely from a European point of view.

(iii) There is a minimum of phonetic courtesy to be achieved in learning any language; moreover, the advantages that proficiency in pronouncing Arabic confer on the English speaker are self-evident: among them, the respect of the Egyptian is not the least. A book of this kind can only supply general hints but they suffice for practical purposes, providing at the same time a sound foundation on which a more detailed study of Egyptian pronunciation can be built.

(a) *Pronunciation of consonants*

Certain consonant sounds offer little difficulty to English speakers. These are the sounds we write with

f	Arabic	**filfil**	*pepper*	English	'film'
b	,,	**baab**	*door*	,,	'bad'
t	,,	**taag**	*crown*	,,	'tag'
d	,,	**damm**	*blood*	,,	'dam'

Note

For **t** and **d**, ensure that the tongue is in contact with the teeth and not the ridge behind the teeth as generally in English. **t** and **d** must always be distinguished from **ṭ** and **ḍ** (see below).

s	Arabic	**sitt**	*lady*	English	'sit'
z	,,	**zeet**	*oil*	,,	'zebra'
ʃ	,,	**ʃams**	*sun*	,,	'*sh*am'
k	,,	**kibiir**	*big*	,,	'kipper'
g	,,	**guwwa**	*inside*	,,	'goose'
m	,,	**maat**	*he died*	,,	'mad'

n	„	**naam**	*he slept*	„	'nap'
w	„	**walla**	*or*	„	'wallet'
y	„	**yiktib**	*he writes*	„	'yes'

The following require more careful attention:

ʕ. This symbol stands for the glottal stop or catch. It is the sound which occurs commonly in English between words ending and beginning with a vowel, e.g. 'Jaffa ʕorange', 'sea ʕeagle', or when we wish to stress a word beginning with a vowel as in 'it's ʕawful'. It is frequent, too, in English dialects: listen to the Cockney or Glaswegian pronunciation of 't' in such words as 'water', 'bottle', &c. In Egyptian Arabic, no word or sentence begins with a vowel-sound and it is, therefore, important to take care that you pronounce **ʕiktib** *write!* or **ʕumm** *mother* with the glottal stop and not as **iktib** or **umm**.

q. This usually stands for the same sound as **ʕ**, i.e. the glottal stop. You may wonder why two letters are necessary. The answer is that, unlike **q**, **ʕ** is often not a radical (see C on p. 14) and in certain conditions (see Appendix C) is elided. In most other forms of Arabic, **ʕ** and **q** would represent different sounds. Examples of **q** are **qult** *I/you said*, **daqiiqa** *minute*, **ḥaqq** *right*.

Keeping the tongue flat in the mouth, look into a mirror and you will see *the uvula* hanging down at the extreme back of the mouth. If you articulate **k** as far back as you can, i.e. at the uvula, the distinctive sound produced is that of a 'Classical' pronunciation of **q**. This sound is used by educated speakers for 'classicisms' in the colloquial, e.g. **qarya** *village*, **ʕilqurʕaan** *the Koran*. The use of this sound—in the right places—is probably the most important single phonetic feature distinguishing educated speech.

h. **h** will not be found difficult when it begins a word or syllable. Pronounce it in **haat** *bring!* and **muhimm** *important* as you do in English 'ham' and 'behind'. Be careful, however, to produce the same kind of sound when **h** ends a syllable or word, e.g. **ʕabuuh** *his father*, **qahwa** *coffee*. Above all, don't

make it sound like **x** (see below). If you have difficulty, it will
help early on to put in an extra vowel following **h,** i.e. **qaḥawa**
(for **qaḥwa**) and to aim at eliminating it gradually.

l. Imagine you are going to pronounce the English word 'leave'
but keep the tongue in the 'l'-position, prolonging the sound
and without uttering the '-eave' portion. You will realize that
this is a very different 'l'-sound from that of, say, 'feel'. It is
the 'l' of 'leave' that you want almost at all times in Arabic.
There is the world of difference between the 'l' s of English
'milk' and Arabic **milk** *property* or English 'feel' and Arabic
fiil *elephant.* An important exception to the rule is that you
must use the 'l' of 'feel' in **ʕallaah** *God* and derivative forms,
as **ʕinʃalla** *I hope.* **ʕa** of **ʕallaah** is elided if preceded by a
vowel, and if this vowel is **i,** then **ll** is pronounced with the 'l'
of 'leave', e.g. **ʕilḥamdu lillaah** *Praise be to God.* Most Irish-
men use the right kind of 'l' in 'milk' and 'feel': listen to them.
Most Scots and Americans use the wrong kind even in 'leave'.

r. The English 'r' of 'red' or 'road' will never do. The rolled
Scottish 'r' or 'burn' is what is wanted. Many English people
make this kind of 'r' in words such as 'very', 'thorough', &c.;
if you don't, try to make a very quick 'd' in place of 'r' in these
words. Don't forget to pronounce Arabic **r** when final:
ʕamiir *prince* sounds nothing like 'a mere'. If you cannot roll
or trill an **r,** this will require more practice: Arabic **r** when
doubled (written **rr**) is always strongly rolled. Examples are
raml *sand*, **bard** *cold*, **barra** *outside.*

ʕ, ẓ, ṭ, ḍ. These are the so-called 'emphatic' consonants, always
to be distinguished from **s, z, t,** and **d** respectively. For all
the emphatics, the tongue must be broad and 'thick', filling the
mouth: for **s, z, t,** and **d,** on the other hand, the tongue is
narrow and 'thin'. You can practise the lateral contraction
and expansion of the tongue when looking in a mirror. At the
same time, the front of the tongue is very much lower in the
mouth for the emphatics: you should feel this if you move
from, say, the **t**-position to the **ṭ**-position and vice versa while
maintaining the necessary contact at the teeth or junction of
teeth and gums. Using the mirror again, practise hollowing

the tongue from front to rear, and retain the hollowing when pronouncing the emphatics. The position of the lips is also important: for the emphatics, they are held neutral or slightly rounded and protruded; for **s, z, t,** and **d,** they are spread. These factors combine in the emphatics to produce a characteristically 'hollow' resonance: for example, the hiss of **ṣ** is much more indeterminate than the clear-cut sibilance of **s.** In the case of the **s-ṣ** distinction, it is also helpful to pronounce **s** with considerably greater tension in the tongue and lips. Examples are:

tiin	*figs*	**ṭiin**	*mud.*
baat	*he spent the night*	**baaṭ**	*armpit.*
seef	*sword*	**ṣeef**	*summer.*
bass	*only*	**baṣṣ**	*he looked.*
dall	*he directed*	**ḍall**	*he lost (his way).*
baɛd	*after*	**baɛḍ**	*some.*
zaayir	*visitor*	**ẓaahir**	*clear.*
mafruuz	*selected*	**maḥfuuẓ**	*learnt by heart.*

x. This is not a difficult sound. Feel back along the roof of the mouth with your tongue until you come to *the soft palate*; the soft palate and the uvula (see under **q** above) must be made to vibrate for **x** as, for example, when breathing out heavily during snoring. It is much the same sound as in Scottish 'lo*ch*' or 'o*ch* aye' and German a*ch*tung. Examples are **xaʃab** *wood*, **muxx** *brains*. More practice is required with this sound before and after the **i** (or **ii**) vowel, e.g. **baxiil** *miser, miserly*.

ɣ. This is **x** with the vocal cords vibrating. This means that you must introduce into **x** the buzzing you make when passing, e.g. from **s** to **z**, i.e. **sss-zzz, xxx-ɣɣɣ.** If you find difficulty, try 'dry gargling'. **ɣ** is also the sound of the French **r** in Paris and Northern France. Examples are **ɣafiir** *watchman*, **ṣuɣayyar** *small*.

ḥ. In order to master **ḥ** (and **ɛ**), you must 'get the feel' of the throat area above the windpipe. Try swallowing; you will see the Adam's apple rise considerably; now try keeping it at the top of its run instead of allowing it to descend as you do when swallowing—the discomfort you feel is in the region where you must make ḥ. To pronounce ḥ, adopt a posture as if you are about to retch, then release the tension just enough to allow egress of air from the lungs. The result should be an acceptable ḥ. Try to make the root of the tongue fill the throat for ḥ which, remember, is not in the least like x or h. Examples are ḥaalan *immediately, soon,* malḥ *salt.*

ع. This is ḥ with the vocal cords vibrating (see ɣ above). Do not confuse it with ʕ (or q). Examples: عeen *eye,* niعnaaع *mint,* rabiiع *spring.*

Doubled consonants

Any of the Arabic consonants may be doubled. A doubled consonant must be pronounced approximately twice as long as a single one. Consonants which are pronounced long occur in English at the junction of words or of affixes and words; for example, 'bla*ck k*ing', 'mis*s*pelt', 'u*nn*ecessary'; contrast 'black king' and 'blacking'. On the other hand, the written double **tt** of English words like 'better' and 'butter' are pronounced as single sounds. The **ss** of Arabic **kassar** *he smashed,* however, must be pronounced double: contrast **kasar** *he broke.* Pay special attention to this feature at the end of words, e.g. ḥabb *he liked,* **muhimm** *important.*

Addenda

1. The sounds written **p** and **v** in English do not occur regularly in Arabic. In loan-words they appear—at least with less sophisticated speakers—as **b** and **f**, e.g. **biiba** *pipe,* **balf** *valve.*

2. The letter **j** is used in the loan-word **jaketta** *jacket* and a few learned words occurring in Part II, e.g. **juluuji** *geologist.* **j** should be pronounced as the English 'j' in 'jeep'.

(b) Pronunciation of vowels

There are five vowels in Egyptian Arabic, each of them occurring both long and short. When pronouncing a vowel long, give it twice the length you give its single counterpart. You can practise this between, say, **ṣadaf** *sea-shells* and **ṣaadif** *he chanced upon.* Let us now take each vowel in turn.

a. This vowel has two very different sounds. The sound which you use depends mainly on the neighbouring consonants.

(i) 'front' **a**:

Between the vowel sounds of 'Standard' English 'hat' and 'hurt' or 'had' and 'herd'. This is the most difficult vowel sound you have to face and a very common one. To practise it, start from the English vowel in, say, 'hat' and try to make it sound a little like the vowel in 'hurt' or, better still, take the complete word 'hat' and make it sound something like 'hurt' without going the whole way. If you have also made the vowel sufficiently long, the result should be an acceptable pronunciation of Arabic **haat** *bring!* Examples: **katab** *he wrote,* **daras** *he studied,* **baab** *door.*

(ii) 'back' **a**:

Between the 'Standard' English vowel sounds in 'hurt' and 'hot'. The vowel of 'heart' is for practical purposes adequate. 'Back' **a** occurs as follows:

(*a*) invariably after and before the emphatics, e.g. **ṣabr** *patience,* **ḍarab** *he hit,* **faḍḍa** *he emptied,* **ḥaaḍir** *certainly,* **maṭbax** *kitchen.* It is not necessary that the vowel should immediately follow or precede the emphatic, e.g. **xaaliṣ** *completely, very,* **lafẓ** *pronunciation*;

(*b*) very commonly preceding and following **r,** e.g. **raff** *shelf,* **raaḥ** *he went,* **raagil** *man,* **ḥufra** *hole,* **barra** *outside,* **barraad** *fitter,* **naar** *fire.* It is, however, 'front' **a** in **raayiḥ** *going,* **raagiɛ** *returning,* **bard** *cold,* **xaarig** *going out,* **warra** *he showed,* **firaan** *mice.* There is much to be said for using two **r**'s (**r** and **ṛ**) or two vowel letters (**a** and **ɑ**) and writing, e.g. **ṛaagil** but **raagiɛ**, or **rɑɑgil** but **raagiɛ**. For a number of reasons, however, this has not been done and the student should note for himself the pronunciation of **a** in association with **r** as examples occur, and then check his observations against the indications given in the Vocabulary;

(c) after and before **q** in its 'Classical' pronunciation.

This distinction between the two qualities of **a** is important and the student should pay particular attention to it. It must be realized that the above summary presentation of the facts applies only to Cairene colloquial, and from one part of the country to another or even within one area considerable divergence may be observed: for example, **xaaf** is usually pronounced with 'back' **a** in Upper Egypt but with 'front' **a** in Cairo, while 'Classical' pronunciation anywhere requires 'back' **a** in this word as well as in **qaal** *he said*, **ɣaayib** *absent*, **xaal** (*maternal*) *uncle*, **fiiraan** *mice*, &c.; similarly, in parts of the Delta, **maḍraṣa** indicates local pronunciation more accurately than **madrasa** (Cairene) *school*.

In some cases the hints given above will not supply the right quality: ask an Egyptian to pronounce, for example, **ʕilqurʕaan** *the Koran*, **habhab** *it barked*, **mayya** *water*, and make up your mind about the quality of the a's. **ʕallaah** *God* is pronounced with 'back' **a** throughout, but if the vowel **i** precedes then **aa** is 'front', e.g. **lillaah** *to God*; contrast **walla** ('back') *by God* and **walla** ('front') *or*.

e. This is a sound approximately mid-way between the vowels in 'bet' and 'beet'. If you pronounce the vowel sound in English 'bit' energetically, at the same time spreading the lips, you will be very near what is wanted. The sound occurs in many dialects of English, for example, in southern Ireland. The Devonian pronunciation of 'made' provides a vowel closely resembling **e**, but should be made to sound a little more like 'mead'. Beware of any tendency to pronounce **e** like the 'ay' sound in 'day' or 'bait'. Examples: **beet** *house*, **beeḍ** *eggs*.

i. As in English 'bit', e.g. **bint** *girl*. This vowel has a different sound when long or when occurring final. Pronounce **ii** and final **i** approximately as the vowel in English 'beet' but with more tension in the tongue and greater spreading of the lips, e.g. **ʃiil** *remove*, **tamalli** *always*.

ii is regularly shortened in certain contexts, e.g. **ʃilhum**

remove them !, but the sound of the vowel remains as for **ii** (see Appendix B).

o. This is a sound between the English vowels in 'hawk' and 'hook'. Try pronouncing the vowel of 'hawk' with stronger rounding and protrusion of the lips: an acceptable **o** should result. The sound is common in certain English dialects, but the usual 'o' of English 'no' will not do at all; nor will the sound of 'ow' in 'now'. Examples: **fooq** *above, on top*, **miṣoogar** *registered*.

u. As in English 'put', e.g. **kutub** *books*. Like **i,** this vowel has a somewhat different sound when long or final, approximating to that of 'oo' in English 'food' but pronounced with greater tension and with strong rounding and protrusion of the lips: e.g. **ʃuuf** *see*, **duxuul** *entrance, entry*, **yinsu** *they forget*.

Diphthongs

A diphthong is a combination of two vowel sounds in the same syllable. This may occur in Egyptian Arabic when, following a vowel, **y** and **w** are either final or precede another consonant. In these circumstances **y** and **w** are often pronounced as **i** and **u** respectively. Examples are **ṭayyaara** *aeroplane*, **ʃaay** *tea*, **law** *if*, **mawguud** *present*, **yiwṣal** *he arrives*.

> N.B. In English we 'slur' the vowel-sounds in the majority of syllables which are unstressed. Consider the vowels of 'the', 'of', and '-land' in 'the Queen of England', or of 'from' and 'to' in 'from head to foot'. This must be avoided at all costs in Arabic and the vowels clearly pronounced whenever they occur. For this among other reasons, do not try to speak too rapidly at first—the formation of good habits early on will save a lot of trouble later.

(c) Other features of pronunciation

The pronunciation of isolated sounds and words, however important, is only half the battle. The stringing together of words and phrases into the sentences required for speech purposes needs constant practice from the outset. Moreover, the sentence brings out features of pronunciation not apparent with the word in isolation but which must be observed if accuracy and fluency are to be achieved.

The method of writing employed in this book is basically a 'reading transcription', designed to assist the student to read and utter Arabic accurately and with as little delay as possible. To achieve the latter object, it has been necessary to avoid any cluttering of the writing with additional symbols and diacritics aimed at giving a more detailed phonetic rendering of the material. Such additions would, moreover, hinder rather than assist the learning of grammar and lexicon. Nevertheless, the writing throughout the book is 'narrowly phonetic' in five respects:

(i) If a vowel is pronounced short, then it is written short, even where grammar and lexicon would suggest a long vowel. For example, the student will be told to form the feminine of **faahim** *understanding* by adding **-a,** but the pronunciation of the feminine form will be taken into account when we write **fa̲hma,** not **fa̲ahima.**

(ii) Elided vowels are not written, cf. the elision of **i** in **fahma** above. The feature of vowel-elision often occurs also in the first syllable of a word. The junction of **ʕana** *I* and **fihimt** *understood* must be pronounced with **i** elided and the syllable division **ʕanaf-himt.** The linking in one syllable of the end of one word and the beginning of the next—usually as a result of elision—is an important step towards fluency and is marked in our writing by the hyphen, i.e. **ʕana-fhimt.** The hyphen may also mark the elision of a final or initial vowel (see Appendix C).

(iii) Initial **ʕ** of the word in isolation is also frequently elided when something precedes, e.g. **ʕabuuk** *your father* but **ʃuft abuuk** *I saw your father.*

(iv) Every polysyllabic word in Arabic has a prominent syllable which stands out to the ear above the others, and it is most important for pronunciation purposes that the student should pick the right one. Just as the *-ra-* syllable is prominent in the English word 'pano*ra*ma', so **-giin** is prominent in Arabic **fanagiin** *cups* and **ḍa-** in **ḍarab** *he hit.* We shall henceforth indicate prominence by the accent mark on the vowel of the appropriate syllable, thus **fanagíin, ḍárab.**

It must be remembered that in phrases and sentences it frequently happens that a word is pronounced without prominence in relation to adjoining words. Thus, standing alone, both **kitáab** and **faríid** have their prominent syllable, but in **kitab faríid** *Fareed's book* it is possible for the prominent syllable of the second word only to stand out. Notice, too, how **kitáab** in the example is pronounced with a short vowel in the second syllable (see (i) above).

Note

Prominence, vowel-length, and elision ?re not arbitrary, haphazard features. On the contrary, certain definite rules can be stated about them. This is done in Appendixes A, B, and C of Part I. The student may refer to these Appendixes at any stage of progress, including the present one.

(v) Three consonants do not occur in succession in Egyptian Arabic. Such a cluster could potentially occur when a word ending in two consonants is followed by a word or suffix beginning with a consonant. To avoid such a sequence, a short vowel is introduced; in typically Cairene speech this vowel appears between the second and third consonant. The 'extra' vowel—often pronounced very short—will be indicated by the diacritic ˘ above the appropriate letter, e.g. **bíntĭ maḥmúud** *Mahmoud's daughter* (contrast **béet maḥmúud** *Mahmoud's house*), **ma fiʃ ḥáddĭ-hnáak** *there is no one there*, **ma rúḥtĭʃ** *I didn't go*. In suffixed words, this vowel may occur in the prominent syllable, e.g. **qult** *I/you said*+**lu(h)** *to him* = **qultĭlu(h)**, **ʃuft**+**ha** = **ʃuftăha** *I/you saw her*, **ḥaqq**+ **hum** = **ḥaqqŭhum** *their right*. Notice that the vowel is usually **ĭ** but may also be **ă** or **ŭ** with the pronominal suffixes (see Lesson 6, 1, note (2)).

The secret of success is constant practice. Learning by heart, with the aid of an Egyptian, some of the sentences in the Lessons and a few of the dialogues in Part II will help considerably, since it is surprising how little material is necessary to exhaust most of the difficult sequences which can occur in a language. Instil into your Arabic speaker the need for patience and careful correction, then listen to and repeat each phrase and sentence over and over again, trying to remember every detail, including the rise and fall of the speaker's voice. Imitate him slavishly and don't feel too embarrassed about it: the chances are that the more outlandish you sound to yourself, the nearer you are to the mark. Practice must also include as much listening for the sake of listening as possible, for you must train not only your tongue to utter Arabic but also your ear to catch what is going on in the language.

C. *Roots and radicals*

Perhaps the most striking characteristic of all forms of Arabic is that the great majority of words are built on a framework of three consonants. By ringing the changes with affixes, vowel differences, &c., on a given base, e.g. **k-t-b,** we obtain a series of related words, e.g. **kátab** *he wrote*, **káatib** *clerk*, **maktába** *library*, **máktab** *office, desk*, &c. The base, e.g. **k-t-b,** is called the *root* and each consonant of the root a *radical*. The terminology is equally applicable when bases are of less or more than three consonants.

PART I

GRAMMAR

LESSON 1

The article; nominal sentences; the construct

1. (a) béet kibíir   *a big house*
   (b) ʕilbéet ilkibíir   *the big house*
   (c) ʕilbéet kibíir   *the house is big*

Notes

1. beet *house* is a noun and kibíir *big* an adjective. Note the adjective follows the noun.
2. The article in Arabic is ʕil. Compare the noun-adjective phrases (a) and (b) and observe that, if the noun has the article, then so also has the adjective. Proper nouns also require the article prefixed to an accompanying adjective, e.g. máṣr ilqadíima *old Cairo*.
3. (c) differs from (b) in that the noun has the article but the adjective has not. This is an example of the very common pattern of the nominal sentence. Nominal sentences contain no verbal forms. Notice that *is* is required in the English translation.

2. Before certain consonants, the *l* of the article is pronounced, not as **l**, but as the following consonant. These consonants are: **t, d, s, z, ṭ, ḍ, ṣ, ẓ, n, r, ʃ**, and usually **k** and **g**. Before other consonants, **l** remains.

Examples:

ʕil*r*aagil *the man* pronounced ʕirráagil
ʕil*ṣ*ufra[1] *the dining-table* pronounced ʕiṣṣúfra
but ʕilmáktab *the office*, ʕilfilúus *the money*, &c.

Note

The pronunciation of *l* as **k** before **k** and **g** before **g** is common in Cairo, e.g. ʕikkitáab *the book*, ʕiggurnáal *the newspaper*.

3. ʕissámak ɣáali *fish is dear*
   ʕissuwées *Suez*
   ʕilfayyúum *Fayoum*

   [1] See Introduction, B (ii).

Notice that the article is often used where no article appears in the corresponding English translation. This is frequently the case with names of towns and countries.

4. **béet ilmudíir**   *the house of the manager, the manager's house*
   fárʒi bursaʒíid   *the Port Said branch*
   béet míin?   *whose house,* lit. *the house of whom?*

Notes

1. These are examples of the common pattern of the so-called 'construct', in which two or more nouns are closely linked (*of* or *'s* usually appears in translation). Notice that although the second noun may or may not have the article, the first can *never* be prefixed with it. Contrast, therefore, **béet ilmudíir** with **ʕilbéet ilkibíir** under 1 above.

2. A sequence of constructs is possible. For example, **báab ilbéet** *the door of the house* and **béet ilmudíir** may be combined to give **báab béet ilmudíir** *the door of the manager's house* in which neither **baab** nor **beet** can have the article.

EXERCISES

A

1. xaddáam kuwáyyis.
2. dúrg idduláab.
3. mudíir iʃʃírka.
4. ʕiʃʃúylĭ-ktíir.
5. béet ilmudíir kibíir.
6. híyya bĭnt ilfarráaʃ.

B

1. A bad road.
2. A cigarette box (*or* box of cigarettes).
3. Today's papers.
4. The price is too high.
5. The office door is open.
6. Bab el Hadiid Square.

LESSON 2

Particles; bitaaȝ

1. **húwwa min issuwées** *He is from Suez.*
ȝilbaʃkáatib filmáktab *The chief clerk is in the office.*
ȝilhudúum fóoq idduláab *The clothes are on top of the cupboard.*
ȝissandúuq taħt issiríir *The box is under the bed.*
ȝilfilúus ȝandĭ ȝáli *Ali has the money* (lit. *the money is with Ali*).
ȝilħisáab ȝala míin *Who is (going) to pay ?* (lit. *the account is on whom ?*)

Notes

1. The above nominal sentences contain prepositional particles. Most of them do not occur standing alone but always precede a noun or a pronoun suffix. Pronoun suffixes are not dealt with before Lesson 5 and will not, therefore, be illustrated here.

2. Some particles occur in isolation and may be termed adverbial. For instance, in answer to the question **ȝúmar féen?** *Where is Omar?*, we may say **fooq** *above, upstairs*, **taħt** *below, downstairs*, **gúwwa** *inside*, **bárra** *outside*, **quddáam** *in front*. Certain of these often appear with **min** to form a complex prepositional particle, e.g. **bárra min** *outside*. Corresponding adjectives are formed with the addition of a suffix **aani** (masc. sing.), e.g. **guwwáani** *inner*, **barráani** *outer*, **taħtáani** *lower*, **foqáani** *upper*, **quddamáani** *front*.

3. The particle **bi** *by, with* most frequently appears in verbal sentences, e.g. **míʃi bilȝágal** or **míʃi-b súrȝa** *he went quickly* (lit. *with speed*). Observe that when **ȝ** or the vowel **i** is elided in the junction of a particle and the following noun, we write the two elements as one, cp. **bilȝágal** and also **filmáktab** in the second sentence above (= **fi**+**ȝilmáktab**). **min** and **ȝala** require special notice in this respect since **in** and **la** respectively are usually omitted, e.g. **milmáktab** for **min ilmáktab** and **ȝaṭṭarabéeẕa** for **ȝala-ṭṭarabéeẕa** *on the table*.

4. Note the common word **baȝḍ** which frequently follows a particle as in **fóoq báȝḍ** *on top of each other*, **záyyĭ báȝḍ** *like each other, the same*, **gámbĭ báȝḍ** *beside each other*, **wáyya báȝḍ** *with each other, in each other's company*.

5. Adverbs differ from adverbial particles (note 2) in that they never appear in association with a following noun or suffix. Examples are the 'time-words' **dilwáqti** *now*, **baȝdéen** *later*, **ȝimbáariħ** *yesterday*, **ȝinnahárḍa**[1] *today*, **búkra** *tomorrow*, &c.

6. **sáaħil xalíig issuwées** *the coast of the Gulf of Suez* is an example of a sequence of constructs (see Lesson 1, 4, note (2)), but notice the introduction of the particle **min** when **sáaħil** is followed by an adjective in **ȝissáaħil ilɣárbi min xalíig issuwées** *the west coast of the Gulf of Suez*. Notice also that since

[1] See Introduction, B (ii).

sáaḥil is no longer in construct with xalíig, it may, of course, take the article. An alternative form is sáaḥil xalíig issuwées ilɣárbi. The particle li *to, for* is often used in a similar way, e.g. ˁissáaḥil ittáani lilbáḥr (or milbáḥr) ilˁáḥmar *the other shore of the Red Sea.*

2. bitáaɛ

(a) ˁilmuftáaḥ da-btaɛ[1] ilqíflī da   *this key belongs to this lock.*

(b) ˁilbéet bitaɛ ilmudíir   *the manager's house.*

(c) ˁilbéet ilkibíir bitaɛ ilmudíir   *the manager's big house.*

Notes

1. In (a) bitáaɛ behaves in the same way as the prepositional particles in 1 above.

2. (b) illustrates the common use of bitáaɛ as an alternativè to the use of the construct. ˁilbéet bitaɛ ilmudíir and béet ilmudíir are variánts, but note that when bitáaɛ is used, the first noun has the article.

3. In (c) the first noun *is followed by an adjective* and in consequence bitáaɛ is no longer optional but essential.

4. bitáaɛ (masculine singular) is inflected for gender and number. Examples of the feminine singular and the plural form will be given in their appropriate places below (Lessons 3 and 5).

EXERCISES

A

1. ˁinnahárḍa[2] zayy irrabíiɛ.
2. ˁilbálṭu ɛaʃʃammáaɛa wara-lbáab.
3. maḥáṭṭit ilˁizáaɛa-f ʃáariɛ ɛílwi-f máṣr.
4. ˁilqamíiṣ bitaɛ ilwálad ɛand ilmakwági min imbáariḥ.
5. háat idduséeh min ɛalmáktab!
6. ˁilbáar táḥt wilmaktába fiddóor ilfoqáani.

B

1. The money's in the trouser pocket.
2. The airfield is outside the town.
3. The sheets are next to the towels in the clothes cupboard.
4. Fetch the mistress's coat from behind the door!
5. He's downstairs with the manager.
6. They're on top of each other in the drawer.

[1] See Introduction, B (c), (i) and (ii), p. 12.
[2] See Introduction, B (ii).

LESSON 3

Gender

1. (*a*) Masculine. **béet kibíir**   *a big house*
   (*b*) Feminine. **ginéena-kbíira**   *a big garden*
   (*c*) Masculine. **qamíiṣ wísix**   *a dirty shirt*
   (*d*) Feminine. **maɣláqa wísxa**   *a dirty spoon*
   (*e*) Masculine. **ʕilwálad iṭṭawíil irrufáyyaɣ**   *the tall, thin boy*
   (*f*) Feminine. **ʕissítt iṭṭawíila irrufayyáɣa** *the tall, thin woman*

Notes

1. Two genders, masculine and feminine, are formally distinguished. This lesson deals with nouns and adjectives only, but gender differences are also made in many other parts of speech, e.g. verbs, pronouns, and demonstratives, which we shall deal with in their turn. Gender is, of course, important because on it depends not so much the form of individual nouns, adjectives, &c., as their agreement when occurring together.

2. Gender distinction in Egyptian Arabic is made *in the singular only*. The feminine ending is **-a**, cf. **rufáyyaɣ** (masc. sing.) and **rufayyáɣa** (fem. sing.) in the examples; but, to anticipate Lessons 4 and 5, there is only one common plural form **rufayyaɣíin**. When the feminine ending occurs before a pause, it is usually pronounced with a weak final **h**.

3. Whether or not there exists a corresponding masculine form, the ending **-a** is, with few exceptions, the sign of a feminine noun, e.g. **ḥáaga** *thing*, **ʃírka** *company*, **ɣarabíyya** *car*. Exceptions are **xalíifa** *caliph*, **xawáaga** *gentleman*, **ɣúmda** *headman of village or town-quarter*, **dáwa** *medicine*, and some plurals referring to human beings, e.g. **riggáala** *men*, **rúyasa** *supervisors*, **makanikíyya** *mechanics*.

4. As with the adjectives **kibíir**, **wísix**, &c., above, **-a** is often suffixed to the corresponding masculine form of a noun, e.g. **málik** *king*—**málika** *queen*, **xaddáam** *servant*—**xaddáama** *maidservant*. If the masculine form ends in **-i**, then the feminine ends in **-ya** or **-yya**, e.g. **ɣáali** *dear*—**ɣálya**, **ʕagnábi** *foreign, foreigner*—**ʕagnabíyya**.

5. Do not confuse gender with sex. There are certain special words for sex-reference which are masculine or feminine as the case may be, e.g. **wálad** and **sitt** in examples (*e*) and (*f*). This, however, is as far as the relation between grammatical gender and sex goes.

6. Some words *which do not end in* **-a** are nevertheless feminine. They include
   (i) **ʕarḍ** *earth, floor*, **naar** *fire*, **ʃams** *sun*, **márkib** *ship*, **bálad** *town*, **filúus** *money*;
   (ii) some parts of the body, e.g. **ʕiid** *hand*, **rigl** *leg*, **widn** *ear*, **ɣeen** *eye*, **raas** *head*, **daqn** *chin*, **baṭn** *stomach*;
   (iii) names of towns and countries, e.g. **maṣr** *Cairo*, **ʕissuwées** *Suez*, **libnáan** *Lebanon*.

7. Adjectives of origin and nationality—ending in -i—are generally invariable unless the noun they accompany is of personal reference, e.g. **qáhwa faransáawi** (not **faransawíyya**) *French coffee*, **siggáada ʒágami** *a Persian carpet*, **gíbna báladi** *local cheese*, but **sitt ingilizíyya** *an English lady*.

2. Feminine nouns in construct (see Lesson 1, 4).

Feminine nouns in the construct have the ending **-(i)t**, not **-a**. Thus, **ʕilginéena** *the garden* but **ginént ilbéet** *the garden of the house*, **ʕiʃʃírka** *the company* but **ʃírkit ʃíll** *the Shell Company*. The vowel **i** occurs before **t** to obviate the impossible pattern of three or more successive consonants.

bitáaʒ (see Lesson 2, 2) agrees in gender with the preceding noun but is always in construct with a following noun. Thus, as an alternative to **ginént ilbéet,** we may say **ʕilginéena-btaʒt ilbéet.** Since **bitáaʒ** is always in construct, a feminine form **bitaaʒa** never occurs.

Note

ʕilginéena-btaʒt ilbéet may also mean *the garden belongs to the house* (see Lesson 1, 4).

EXERCISES

A

1. ráas ilwálad súxna.
2. ʒarabíyyit ilmufáttiʃ gamíila xáaliṣ.
3. ʕilbínt ilkibíira taʒbáana-nnaharḍa.
4. maḥáṭṭit ilbanzíin ʒalyimíin.
5. ʕárḍ ilmáṭbax wísxa qáwi.
6. ʕiʃʃáqqa-btaʒt iʃʃéex ḥílwa-w wásʒa.

B

1. A large packet of cigarettes.
2. The fingers of the left hand.
3. She's a very pretty girl.
4. The bus stop is very near the house.
5. She's not feeling very well (*tr.* she's rather unwell) today.
6. Zamalek is quite a long way from the centre of the city.

LESSON 4

Number

1. The unfamiliar use of **ʒand** and the suffixes **-i** and **-hum** in the following examples will be explained in Lessons 5 and 6. Meanwhile attention is directed to the suffixes **-een, -iin, -aat,** and **-iyya.**

(a) **ʒándi yoméen ſagáaza**   *I have two days' leave.*

(b) **kullŭhum kuwayyisíin qáwi**   *They are all very good.*

(c) **ʒandŭhum ſahadáat**   *They have certificates.*

(d) **ſilmuwaʒʒafíin kullŭhum maʂriyyíin**   *The staff* (lit. *officials*) *are all Egyptian.*

(e) **ſinnaggaríin ʒarfíin ſuɣlŭhum kuwáyyis**   *The carpenters know their job well.*

(f) **dáragit ilmakanikíyya ʒálya**   *The mechanics' standard is high.*

Notes

1. Disregarding collectives (see Lesson 31), distinction has to be made between singular, dual, and plural. The dual concerns nouns only. Once again, number is important since there are patterns of agreement between nouns, pronouns, adjectives, verbs, &c. Agreement between nouns and adjectives is given in the following lesson.

2. The dual is formed by suffixing **-een** to the singular noun (example (a)). Whenever a suffix is added to a feminine noun in **-a**, then **t** appears as in the construct, e.g. **ṭarabéeʒa**[1]—**ṭarabeʒtéen** *two tables.* Some nouns do not occur in the dual form but appear with the numeral **ſitnéen** *two* (see Lesson 18, 1, note (3)).

3. There are two types of plural formation for nouns and adjectives:
   (i) straightforward addition of certain suffixes to the singular and
   (ii) *internal* difference in relation to the singular, e.g. **beet—biyúut** *house/s.* Plurals under (ii) are very common and are termed 'broken' plurals. They are examined in some detail in Lesson 32. In the meantime, nouns of which the plural is 'broken' are included in the lessons and exercises and should be learned as they are met. In the present lesson, we shall deal under 2 with suffixed plurals only.

2. The plural suffixes are **-iin, -aat,** and **-iyya,** the last being relatively rare.

(a) **-iin** is used for the plural of
   (i) (examples 1 (d) and 1 (e)), nouns and adjectives of the

---

[1] See Introduction, B (ii).

patterns **sawwáaq**/pl. **sawwaqíin** *driver/s* and **muɤállim**/**muɤallimíin** *teacher/s*. Other examples are **kaddáab**/fem. sing. **kaddáaba**/pl. **kaddabíin** *liar/s*, **malyáan/malyáana/malyaníin** *full*. Nouns of these patterns are usually occupational.

Note

   muɤállim and **muwázẓaf** are strictly participial forms (see (ii) following and Lesson 33).

   (ii) (example (*e*)), the active and passive participles of verbs (see Lesson 33), e.g.

masc. sing.	**ɤáarif**	*knowing*	**maftúuḫ**	*open*
fem. sing.	**ɤárfa**		**maftúuḫa**	
common pl.	**ɤarfíin**		**maftuḫíin**	

   (iii) (example (*b*)), adjectives of the pattern **kuwáyyis** *good, nice*, **ṣuɤáyyar** *small*, **quṣáyyar** *short*, **rufáyyaɤ** *thin, flimsy*, **quráyyib** *near*:

masc. sing.	**kuwáyyis**	**quṣáyyar**
fem. sing.	**kuwayyísa**	**quṣayyára**
common pl.	**kuwayyisíin**	**quṣayyaríin**

   (iv) (example (*d*)), most derivative nouns and adjectives of which the singular is formed with a suffix **-i** or **-aani**, e.g. **maṣr** *Cairo, Egypt*—**máṣri** *Cairene, Egyptian*, **diin** *religion*—**díini** *religious*, **bárra** *outside*—**barráani** *outer*. In the plural, **-yy-** is inserted between **i** and the plural **-iin** suffix (cf. the feminine **-yya** ending in Lesson 3, 1, note (4)):

masc. sing.	**máṣri**	**ʕingilíizi** *English(man)*
fem. sing.	**maṣríyya**	**ʕingilizíyya**
common pl.	**maṣriyyíin**	**ʕingiliziyyíin**[1]

---

[1] More commonly **ʕingilíiz** (see Lesson 5, 1, note (3)).

Note

Some singulars of this type have no corresponding plural form, e.g.
fayyúumi, fayyumíyya *one from Fayoum*; there is no form **fayyumiyyíin.**

(*b*) **-aat** (example (*c*)), suffixed to nouns having only one form in
the singular, is used

(i) with a number of patterns in which the final radical is
preceded in the singular by the long vowel **aa.** The singular is frequently feminine, ending in **-a.** Examples are
ḥáaga/ḥagáat *thing/s,* **ḥisáab/ḥisabáat** *account/s,*
maqáas/maqasáat *size/s,* **ʃaháada/ʃahadáat** *certifi-
cate/s,* **talláaga/tallagáat** *refrigerator/s,* **ṭayyáara/ṭay-
yaráat** *aeroplane/s;*

(ii) with many loan-words, with or without **-a** in the singular,
e.g. **duséeh/dusehháat** *file/s, dossier/s,* **ʕutubíis/
ʕutubisáat** *bus/es,* **baskalítta/baskalittáat** *bicycle/s,*
ʕistíbna/ʕistibnáat *spare wheel/s;*

(iii) with nouns of the pattern **dáraga/daragáat** *class/es,
rank/s, step/s,* **ḥáʃara/ḥaʃaráat** *insect/s,* **bádana/
badanáat** *tribe/s;*

(iv) with a number of nouns which in the singular end **-iyya,**
e.g. **ḥanafíyya/ḥanafiyyáat** *tap/s,* **masʕulíyya/
masʕuliyyáat** *responsibility/ies;*

(v) in certain **m**-prefixed patterns, e.g. **mixádda/
mixaddáat** *pillow/s,* **magálla/magalláat** *magazine/s,*
mufakkíra/mufakkiráat *diary/ies,* **muɣáskar/
muɣaskaráat** *(military) camp/s;*

(vi) in the 'counted' form of collective nouns (see Lesson 31);

(vii) in verbal noun plurals (see Lesson 35).

(*c*) **-iyya** (example (*f*)). A number of nouns of trade or occupation are found with the suffix **-gi,** or less often, with **-i.** The
plural of these nouns is in **-iyya.** So, too, are the plurals of
most military and police ranks. Examples are **makwági/
makwagíyya** *laundryman/-men,* **ɣarbágii/ɣarbagíyya**
gharry-driver/s, **gazmági/gazmagíyya** *shoemaker/s,*
makaníiki/makanikíyya *mechanic/s,* **ʃawíiʃ/ʃawiʃíyya**
policeman/-men, sergeant/s.

EXERCISES

A

1. ςissawwáaq wáaqif quráyyib milmaḥátṭa.
2. ginént ilḥayawanáat filgíiza.
3. ςilbarradíin mawgudíin filwárʃa.
4. ςilʒummáal ʒayzíin ziyáada filςúgra.
5. ςiṣṣufragíyya maʃʒulíin dilwaqti.
6. ʒasáakir ilbulíiṣ[1] labsíin zayyï báʒḍ.

B

1. Two hours ago.
2. Their customs are similar.
3. The majority of Egyptians are Muslims.
4. They are going this afternoon.
5. It's only a market for tourists.
6. I (fem.) know all tradesmen (*tr.* the tradesmen) are profiteers.

LESSON 5

Plural noun-adjective agreement; pronouns

1. *Plural noun-adjective agreement*

The following are the corresponding plural forms of the examples at the head of Lesson 3:

(*a*) **biyúut kibíira** or **kubáar**   *big houses*
(*b*) **ganáayin kibíira** or **kubáar**   *big gardens*
(*c*) **qumṣáan wísxa**   *dirty shirts*
(*d*) **maʒáaliq wísxa**   *dirty spoons*
(*e*) **ςilwiláad iṭṭuwáal irrufayyaʒíin**   *the tall, thin boys*
(*f*) **ςissittáat iṭṭuwáal irrufayyaʒíin**   *the tall, thin women*

Notes

1. The adjective accompanying plural nouns—other than those referring to human beings (exx. (*e*) and (*f*))—is almost always in the feminine singular (cf. (*c*) and (*d*)). Those adjectives having a broken plural, however, may be in either the

[1] See Introduction, B (ii).

plural or, more commonly, the feminine singular (cf. (a) and (b)). Notice, therefore, that

(a) plural adjectives in **-iin**, e.g. **wisxíin** *dirty*, are generally used with nouns of personal reference only (but see also note (2));

(b) some adjectives which never accompany such nouns, rarely occur in a plural form, e.g. **matíin, matíina** *durable, strong,* **baṣíiṭ, baṣíiṭa** *small, trifling*;

(c) the vast majority of noun plurals which are 'broken' or in **-aat** usually require a feminine singular adjective;

(d) gender and number agreement in Arabic is quite unlike that in, say, French, or other languages with which the student may be familiar; it might perhaps be said of such an Arabic noun as **qamíiṣ** *shirt* that it is masculine in the singular but feminine in the plural.

2.ֱ The plural adjective is essential with the dual form of the noun, e.g. **betéen kubáar** *two big houses,* **qamiṣéen wisxíin** *two dirty shirts.* Even the rare plural of **matíin**, for example, is essential in this context, e.g. **qamiṣéen mutáan** (cf. note (1), (b)). The plural is necessary, too, in agreement with a succession of singular nouns, e.g. **sikkíina-w ʃóoka wisxíin** *a dirty knife and fork.*

ₐ 3. As a general rule adjectives ending in **-i** behave as with a singular noun (see Lesson 3, 1, note (7)) and are invariable, e.g. **sagáayir ingilíizi** *English cigarettes,* **ʕinnáas dóol báladi qáwi** *those people are decidedly low-class,* but an exception is **magáalis baladíyya** *local councils,* while both **ʕingilíizi** and **ʕingilizíyya** may be used with, for example, **badʾáayiꭓ** *goods.*

Adjectives of nationality following nouns of personal reference do not behave in the same way, nor indeed in the same way as each other: e.g.

naas (*people*)	maṣriyyíin BUT n.	ʕingilíiz (NOT ʕingiliziyyíin)
wiláad (*boys*)	„	w. „
banáat (*girls*)	„	b. „
waladéen (*two boys*)	„	w. „

ʕasbaniyyíin *Spanish* is like **maṣriyyíin** and **ʕalmáan** *German* like **ʕingilíiz.**

Following a dual feminine noun, adjectives in **-i** sometimes themselves occur in a dual feminine form with the ending **-teen**, e.g. **sanatéen ʃamsiyyitéen** *two sunny years*: contrast **ʃahréen ʃamsiyyíin** *two sunny months.*

4. Notice once more that in the plural there is no gender distinction (cf. (e) and (f) above and contrast (e) and (f) at the head of Lesson 3).

5. The plural form of **bitáaꭓ** (see Lessons 2 and 3) is **bitúuꭓ**, e.g. **ʕilbiyúut bituꭓ** (or **bitaꭓt**) **iʃʃírka** *the company's houses.*

2. *Pronouns*

A. **míin inta?** B. **ʕana ꭓáli maḥmúud.** A. **wi míin illi wayyáak?** B. **ʕaxúuya muṣṭáfa.** A. **bitiʃtáꭰal féen?** B. **baʃtáꭰal fi ʃírkit ʃíll.** A. **w-axúuk biyiʃtáꭰal féen?** B. **huwwa-mꭓállim fi madrása sanawíyya.** A. **ʕintu sakníin féen?** B. **ʕiḥna múʃ sakníin wayya báꭰd.** **ʕana sáakin filbálad, ʕána w-issítti-btáꭓti**[1] **wi-wláadi, w-axúuya filʕaryáaf wayya-(u)xtína.**

---

[1] Note **ʕissítti-btáꭓti** 'my wife', **sítti** 'my grandmother'.

A. *Who are you?* B. *(I am) Ali Mahmoud.* A. *And who is that (who is) with you?* B. *My brother Mustapha.* A. *Where do you work?* B. *I work for* (lit. *in*) *Shell.* A. *And where does your brother work?* B. *He's a secondary school teacher.* A. *Where do you* (pl.) *live?* B. *We don't live together. I live in the town with my wife and children, and my brother lives in the country with our sister.*

There are two classes of pronoun: (1) independent and (2) suffixed. Notice from the following lists that, as with the adjective, there is gender distinction in the singular (2nd and 3rd persons) only. This is true of Egyptian Arabic in general and will be found again in the verb and elsewhere.

		Singular	Plural
(1) *Independent*			
1st person		ʕána *I*	ʕíḥna *we*
2nd person (masc.)		ʕínta *you* ⎫	ʕíntu *you*
„ (fem.)		ʕínti „ ⎭	
3rd person(masc.)		húwwa *he, it* ⎫	húmma *they*
„ (fem.)		híyya *she, it* ⎭	
(2) *Suffixed*			

Note

Pronominal suffixes are added to nouns, verbs, and particles. The part of speech does not affect the suffix with the one exception that, added to a *verb*, the 1st pers. sing. suffix is **-ni**, not **-i** or **-ya** as elsewhere. Singular suffixes except **-ni** and **-ha** differ in form according to whether the noun, verb, or particle ends in a consonant or in a vowel.

	Singular			Plural	
	After consonant	*After vowel*			
1st person	**-i** (**-ni** after verb)	**-ya**	*my/me*	**-na**	*our/us*
2nd person (masc.)	**-ak**	**-k**	*your/you* ⎫	**-ku** or **-kum** *your/you*	
„ (fem.)	**-ik**	**-ki**	„ ⎭		
3rd person (masc.)	**-u(h)**[1]	**-h**	*his, its/him, it* ⎫	**-hum**	*their/them*
„ (fem.)	**-ha**	**-ha**	*her, its/her, it* ⎭		

N.B. The nouns ʕaxx *brother* and ʕabb *father* must be specially noticed. They are of the forms ʕaxu and ʕabu respectively when occurring (*a*) with a pronominal suffix and (*b*) in construct; e.g. ʕaxúuh *his brother* (for long vowel see following lesson), ʕáxu-brahíim *Abraham's brother*: contrast ʕáxxi múslim *a Muslim brother*, ʕaxxéen *two brothers* and compare also ʕaxúuh ibrahíim *his brother Abraham*, ʕáxu ʕabúuh *his father's brother*.

Further notes on the pronouns will be given in the following lesson. Notice in the meantime that not only adjectives but also pronouns, verbs, &c., of the 3rd person are commonly in the sin-

[1] Usually pronounced with a weak final *h* before a pause. We indicate this by writing (*h*) where appropriate.

gular feminine form in agreement with a preceding plural noun
(see 1, note (1) and Exercise B 6 below).

EXERCISES

A

1. muntagáat izzéet muxtálifa.
2. ʕinta fáahim kaláami biẓẓábʈ?
3. húmma mittifqíin wayya báɣd.
4. bétna[1]-bɣíid ʃuwayya min hína.
5. ʕaxúuya quddáamak.
6. ʕilfilúus ɣandu húwwa.

B

1. We're going to their house for dinner.
2. They have two Nubian servants.[2]
3. They've known[3] my father for a long time.
4. He has some very attractive brassware (*tr.* things made from
   brass) for sale.
5. Where's my box of matches? This is yours.
6. There are some very nice things in the bazaar but they're
   dear.

LESSON 6

Pronouns (*cont.*): fiih and ɣand-

1. *Notes on the pronouns*

1. Final vowels are lengthened when suffixes are added, e.g.
wáyya *with*—**wayyáaki** *with you* (fem.), **wayyáah** *with him*.

2. The 'extra' vowel (see Introduction, p. 13) which, taking
the language as a whole, is usually **ĭ**, is more frequently **ă** or **ŭ** with
the suffixes. With one exception, the vowel is the same as the
vowel of the suffix; the exception is with **-na** before which **ĭ** is
regular: e.g. **ʕuxtáha** *her sister*, **ʕuxtŭku(m)** *your* (pl.) *sister*,
ʕuxtína *our sister*.

---

[1] See Introduction B (*c*), (i) and Appendix B.
[2] Use ʕitnéen xaddamíin.   [3] ɣarfíin.

3. Remember that when a suffix is added to a noun in -a, then t appears, e.g. ҙarabíyya + na = ҙarabiyyítna *our car*, riggáala + u(h) = riggáltu(h) *his men*.

4. The independent and suffixed pronouns are often used together for emphasis, cf. Exercise A, ex. 6, in Lesson 5. Another example is da-btáaҙu húwwa, múʃ bitaҙak ínta *this is* HIS, *not* YOURS.

5. A suffixed noun cannot take the article, but in the noun-adjective phrase, the following adjective requires it, e.g. béetu-lkibíir *his big house*. Contrast béetu-kbíir *his house is big*.

6. The dual of certain parts of the body occurring in pairs (e.g. rigléen *legs*, ʕidéen *hands*, ҙenéen *eyes*) requires special notice when suffixes are added. Final n of -een is dropped throughout, and with the suffix -ya, the ee of the dual appears as ay, e.g. rigláyya *my legs*, ҙenéeh *his eyes*, ʕidéeki *your* (fem.) *hands*, ʃuftŭhum maʃyíin ҙala rigléehum *I saw them walking* (lit. *going on their legs*).

7. The suffixed forms of some common particles need special attention. Inspect the following table and note particularly the italicized features.[1]

fi	*bi*	*li*[2]	*wayya*
fíyya	bíyya	líyya	wayyáaya
fiik	biik	liik, l*a*k, or l*i*k	wayyáak
fíiki	bíiki	líiki or l*í*ki	wayyáaki
fiih	biih or b*u*(h)	l*u*(h) or liih	wayyáah
fíiha	bíiha	l*á*ha, l*í*ha, or líiha	wayyáaha
fíina	bíina	l*í*na or líina	wayyáana
fíiku(m)	bíiku(m)	l*ú*ku(m) or líiku(m)	wayyáaku(m)
fíihum	bíihum	l*ú*hum or líihum	wayyáahum

ҙala	*ҙand*	*min*
ҙaláyya	ҙándi	mínni
ҙaléek	ҙándak	mínnak
ҙaléeki	ҙándik	mínnik
ҙaléeh	ҙándu(h)	mínnu(h)
ҙaléeha	ҙandăha	mínha or minnăha
ҙaléena	ҙandína	mínna or minnína
ҙaléeku(m)	ҙandŭku(m)	mínku(m) or minnŭku(m)
ҙaléehum	ҙandŭhum	mínhum or minnŭhum

[1] Alternative forms are given in the order corresponding to estimated frequency of their occurrence in educated speech.

[2] Suffixed to verbs, there is a different system of *li*- forms which is given in Lesson 11, 1.

8. The adverbial particles of Lesson 2, 1, note (2) often occur with the pronominal suffixes, e.g. **waráah** *behind him*, **quṣádha** *opposite her*, **ʕiddulááb táḥtu-tráab** *there's dust under the cupboard* (lit. *the cupboard under it (is) dust*). In most cases they may optionally be compounded with **min**, i.e. **ʕiddulááb taḥtĭ mínnu-tráab**; in the case of **bárra** *outside*, **min** is essential: you cannot say **barraaha** but must use **bárra mínha** *outside it* (fem.).

2. **fiih** and **ʒand-**

   (a) A. **fih¹ ḥáddĭ mawgúud?** B. **ʕáywa, fíih.** A. *Is there anyone there?* B. *Yes, there is.*
   (b) **fih ʕáyyĭ ḥáaga ʒaʃáanu?** *Is there any message* (lit. *thing*) *for him?*
   (c) **fih ʕéeh lilʕákl?** *What is there to eat?*
   (d) **ʒándu ḥáqq.** *He is* (lit. *has*) *right.*
   (e) **ʒándik gawáab líyya?** *Have you* (fem.) *a letter for me?*
   (f) A. **ʒándak sagáayir?** B. **láʕ, maʒa-lʕásaf, ma ʒandíiʃ.** A. *Have you any cigarettes?* B. *No, I'm sorry, I haven't.*

Notes

  1. The sentence patterns consisting of suffixed **fi** or **ʒand** with or without a following noun are extremely common. In this use **fi** appears only with a 3rd person suffix, generally **-h**. Translate **fiih** by *there is/are* and **ʒand-** by the appropriate form of the verb *to have*.
  2. If the order of the sentence **fih náas kitíir filʕóoḍa** *there are a lot of people in the room* is changed and **ʕilʕóoḍa** put at the head, then the suffix with **fi** must agree with **ʕóoḍa**, i.e. **ʕilʕóoḍa fíiha náas kitíir.** The first order is more usual but remember the second for the use of the suffix referring to a preceding noun, since you will meet this feature elsewhere. A similar example is **kúllĭ ráff fóoqu ḥagáat** *there are things on every shelf*, or more commonly, **fih ḥagáat foq kúllĭ ráff.**
  3. The particles **li**, **wáyya**, and **máʒa** are often used in a similar way to **ʒand**, e.g. **lák ḥáqq** *you are right*, **wayyáaya** (or **maʒáaya**)-**flúus** *I have money on* (or *with*) *me*. **li** is generally used with reference to property and translated by *to own, possess*, e.g. **líyya ʒízba** *I own a farm*; with **wayya** and **maʒa**, reference is usually to small portable objects carried on the person. Note the use of **li** in **híyya filbéet laha sáaʒa** *she's been in the house for an hour*.

¹ See Introduction B (*c*) (i), and Appendix B.

EXERCISES

A

1. ʒenéeh taχbáana-ʃwayya-nnahárḍa.
2. xaddamíthum fissúuq laha saχtéen.
3. Ꜥana χaláyya xámsa-gnéeh li-mḥámmad.
4. χándak ẓárfï gawáab, ya χaadil?
5. χándak banzíin lilwallaχáat, wi-ḥyáatak?
6. fih xábar múdhiʃ innahárḍa filgaráayid.

B

1. They're going on foot.
2. Come with me to my room. I've something for you.
3. I don't understand the problem.[1] It's too difficult for me.
4. I have an appointment with the dentist tomorrow afternoon.
5. Are there any other special travel[2] regulations?
6. There's someone outside with a complaint (to make) (*tr.* he has a complaint).

LESSON 7

Verbs

1. *Introductory notes*

1. The forms of the Arabic verb are primarily divisible into (i) the *simple* form and (ii) a number of forms which may be derived from the simple one in various ways: for example, doubling the 2nd radical[3] as in **dárris** (or **dárras**) *he taught* (cf. **dáras** *he studied*), or prefixing **Ꜥista-** as in **Ꜥistáχmil** *he used* (cf. **χámal** *he did, made*).

2. In addition, there are differences of conjugation corresponding to differences in the pattern of the radicals. Thus, considering simple forms only, **kátab** *he wrote* has the 'expected' 3 radicals, but **qaal** *he said* has **aa** in place of a 2nd radical, **ráma** *he threw* has **a** and **míʃi** *he went* has **i** in place of a 3rd radical, and

---

[1] Translate ꜤilmasꜤaláadi (lit. 'this problem').
[2] xáṣṣa bissáfar.
[3] See Introduction, C.

ḥabb *he liked, wanted* has the same consonant as 2nd and 3rd radicals and no vowel separating them. We shall call the **kátab-** type *regular*, **qaal** *hollow*, **ráma** and **míʃi** *weak*, and **ḥabb** *doubled*.

3. For the present we shall consider regular verbs of the simple form only, deferring until Lessons 21–25 consideration of the derived forms and of hollow, weak, and doubled verbs. Common examples of the latter types as well as of derived forms (all types) will nevertheless be included in the grammar and exercises of earlier lessons and should be learned as they are met.

4. For all forms and types of the verb, we have to distinguish two tenses, perfect and imperfect, and an imperative. In this lesson, we shall deal only with the perfect, which is generally to be translated in English by the past or the form with *have*, e.g. **kátab** *he wrote, has written*. Distinctions of person, gender, and number parallel those of the independent pronouns of Lesson 5.

5. For reasons which will appear below, a verb is always quoted in the shape of the 3rd pers. sing. masc.

2. *Perfect tense (regular verb)*

(*a*) **xárag min ilbéet bádri-w rígiɛ wáxri.** *He left the house early and returned late.*

(*b*) **simíɛt innŭkum ṭalábtu ṭarabéeẓa-zyáada lilmáktab.** *I hear* (lit. *heard*) *that you* (pl.) *have asked for an extra table for the office.*

The 3rd pers. sing. masc. is taken as the 'basic' shape from which the other persons may be formed by the addition of suffixes as follows:

			kátab	*he wrote*	fíhim	*he understood*
Sing.	3rd pers. masc.	-	kátab	*he wrote*	fíhim	*he understood*
	3rd pers. fem.	-it	kátabit	*she wrote*	fíhmit	*she understood*
	2nd pers. masc.	-t	katábt	*you* (m.) *wrote*	fihímt	*you* (m.) *understood*
	2nd pers. fem.	-ti	katábti	*you* (f.) *wrote*	fihímti	*you* (f.) *understood*
	1st pers.	-t	katábt	*I wrote*	fihímt	*I understood*
Pl.	3rd pers.	-u	kátabu	*they wrote*	fíhmu	*they wrote*
	2nd pers.	-tu	katábtu	*you wrote*	fihímtu	*you understood*
	1st pers.	-na	katábna	*we wrote*	fihímna	*we understood*

Notes

1. Notice that the 1st pers. sing. and the 2nd pers. sing. masc. have the same form.

2. The vowel sequences a–a (*katab*) and i–i (*fihim*) correspond to a rough division of transitive and intransitive verbs. Exceptions, however, are fairly numerous, e.g. símiᵹ *he heard*, mísik *he grasped*.

3. Notice the elision of the second i in the 3rd pers. sing. fem. and 3rd pers. pl. of i–i verbs, cf. fihmit and fihmu above.

4. The sequence u–u occurs for i–i with some speakers, e.g. xúruṣ *he was struck dumb*. i–i (xíriṣ), however, is much commoner and may always be used.

EXERCISES

A

1. xáragit min ɣéer barníiṭa (*or* burnéeṭa).
2. wiqíᵹtï-w garáḥtï rígli.
3. ya dóobak wíqif dilwáqti quddam ilbéet.
4. ʃírib iddawa kúllu márra wáḥda.
5. maḥmúud baᵹat lína hadíyya gamíila.
6. ʕana katábtï gawabéen imbáariḥ li qaráybi[1] fingiltíra.

B

1. He asked me for money for his fare home.
2. My watch stopped without my realizing.[2]
3. We've just heard that they've arrived.
4. They opened the door and went straight in.
5. He lost his temper with me and made (*tr.* made for me) a scene.
6. He was paid (*tr.* he received his money) only two days ago, yet he's spent the lot.

[1] = *qardayib+i.*   [2] *w-ana muʃ wdaxid bdali.*

LESSON 8

Verbs (*cont.*): the imperfect and imperative

1. (*a*) **bitíᵹmil éeh?** *What are you doing?*

   (*b*) **filᵹáada báfṭar issaᵹa sábᵹa-w núṣṣ (ṣabáaḥan)** *I usually have breakfast at 7.30 (a.m.).*

   (*c*) **biyíwṣal ilmáktab issaᵹa tísᵹa** *He gets to the office at 9 o'clock.*

   (*d*) **ḥayuskúnu féen?** *Where are they going to live?*

   (*e*) **ḥayíktib taqríiru baᵹdï ma yírgaᵹ (missáfar)** *He will write his report after he returns (from the journey).*

   (*f*) **ᵹífham ʃákwit ilᵹáamil kuwáyyis wi balláɣha-l qálam ilmustaxdimíin** *Go into* (lit. *understand) the workman's complaint thoroughly and forward it to the Staff Department.*

Note

bállaɣ in ex. (f.) is the imperative of a derived form and will not, therefore, be considered at present.

2. *The imperfect (regular verb)*

The above examples illustrate the imperfect with the extremely common prefixes **bi-** and **ḥa-**. These do not, however, form part of the tense and are not considered specifically until the following lesson.

In contrast with the perfect, *prefixes* (not suffixes) characterize the imperfect, although three imperfect forms combine both a prefix and a suffix. Taking the typical example **yíktib** *he writes* add the affixes in the following table to the portion **-ktib**, which is constant. The alternative prefix vowels **i** or **u** in the table are explained by reference to the following vowel (between the 2nd and 3rd radicals): if this vowel is **i** or **a**, then the prefix vowel is **i**; if it is **u**, then the prefix vowel is usually **u** also.

Singular

	Affix	Example	
3rd pers. masc.	yi- or yu-	yíktib yífham yúṭlub	*he writes* *he understands* *he asks for*
3rd pers. fem.	ti- or tu-	tíktib tífham túṭlub	*she writes* *she understands* *she asks for*
2nd pers. masc.	ti- or tu-	tíktib tífham túṭlub	*you* (masc.) *write* *you understand* *you ask for*
2nd pers. fem.	ti-i or tu-i	tiktíbi tifhámi tuṭlúbi	*you* (fem.) *write* *you understand* *you ask for*
1st pers.	ɛa-	ɛáktib ɛáfham ɛáṭlub	*I write* *I understand* *I ask for*

Plural

	Affix	Example	
3rd pers.	yi-u or yu-u	yiktíbu yifhámu yuṭlúbu	*they write* *they understand* *they ask for*
2nd pers.	ti-u or tu-u	tiktíbu tifhámu tuṭlúbu	*you write* *you understand* *you ask for*
1st pers.	ni- or nu-	níktib nífham núṭlub	*we write* *we understand* *we ask for*

Notes

1. It is fairly common to hear i for u in the prefixes, i.e. yíṭlub for yúṭlub, yídxul for yúdxul *he enters*.

2. Notice that the 3rd pers. sing. fem. and 2nd pers. sing. masc. have the same form.

3. The second vowel may be a, i, or u. As a general rule, when the second vowel of the *perfect* is a, the corresponding imperfect vowel is i or u, whereas i in the perfect corresponds to a in the imperfect. Certain consonants, however, occurring as 2nd or 3rd radical, 'prefer' a in the imperfect even when the corresponding perfect vowel is also a. These consonants are x, ɣ, ḥ, ɛ, h, ṣ, ṭ, ḍ, ẓ, r, and, sometimes, q, e.g. fátaḥ, yíftaḥ *to open*, ḍárab, yíḍrab *to hit*.

4. The remarks at (3) may be taken as a general guide, but you should note and learn the imperfect with each perfect as you meet it. In the word-lists and vocabulary both tenses are given in the 3rd pers. sing. masc. and translated by the English infinitival form, e.g. fíhim, yífham *to understand*.

3. *The imperative*

The imperative offers no difficulty. Take the three 2nd person forms of the imperfect and substitute ɛ for t, i.e.

Masc. Sing.		Fem. Sing.		Plural	
Affix	*Example*	*Affix*	*Example*	*Affix*	*Example*
ʕi-	ʕíktib	ʕi-i	ʕiktíbi	ʕi-u	ʕiktíbu *write!*
or ʕi-	ʕídrab	or	ʕidrábi	or	ʕidrábu *hit!*
ʕu-	ʕúṭlub	ʕu-i	ʕuṭlúbi	ʕu-u	ʕuṭlúbu *ask!*

Notice the vowel difference between, e.g. **ʕíktib** and **ʕáktib** (1st pers. sing. imperfect).

EXERCISES

A

1. ʕíẓmil kída záyyĭ ma katabtílak.
2. ʕiktib lína ṭálab w-ibẓátu filbúṣṭa.
3. ḥaníḥḍar illéela ḥáflit tawdíiẓ ilʕustáaz maḥmúud.
4. ḥatilbísi fustáanik iggidíid búkra ẓaʃáan ilḥáfla?
5. ʕíḥna ya maṣriyyíin, biníʃrab ʃáay tiqíil qáwi.
6. ʕísʕal ilbaʃkáatib féen ilmudíir, ya ẓábdu!

B

1. He looks ill today. Ask him what's the matter!
2. Close the windows! There's dust everywhere (*tr.* the world is full of dust).
3. I don't know what to do. Shall I write to him or what?
4. I want to have breakfast early tomorrow because I'm going to Suez.
5. Be quiet (*pl.*) and get on with (*tr.* see) your work! Wash the car down for a start.[1]
6. Listen (fem.), I want you to do it like this.

LESSON 9

bi- and ḥa-; kaan, yikúun

1. (*Refer to examples at head of Lesson* 8)

yírgaẓ following **baẓdĭ ma** in example (*e*) illustrates the imperfect without **bi-** or **ḥa-**. Other examples will occur from time to

---

[1] **ʕáwwil ḥáaga** (*lit.* 'first thing'). . . .

time but detailed examination of the contexts in which examples
of the tense occur without prefix will be deferred until Lessons 26–
27. We may, however, observe in passing that in comparable
examples to those given with **bi-** and **ḥa-** above, the imperfect
used alone often has an imperative sense: **ʕínta tíktib ilgawáab
dilwáqti** *you will write the letter now* is said emphatically to someone unwilling to do as he is told.

bi- is used when reference is to continuative or habitual action,
e.g. **biyíktib ilgawáab dilwáqti** *he is writing the letter now*,
biyilɣábu tínis tálat marráat filʕusbúuɣ *they play tennis three
times a week*. For continuative action, the word **qáaɣid** (inflected
for gender and number) may precede the verb while a following
noun or pronoun may be preceded by **fi**, e.g. **huwwa qáaɣid
biyíɣmil fíih** *he is doing it*.

ḥa- is a future prefix, e.g. **ḥaktíblak baɣdï yoméen taláata**
I will write to you in a few days' time (lit. *after two days (or) three*).
The imperfect with **ḥa-** often has the sense of intention to do some-
thing or being about to do it (see examples in Lesson 8).

raḥ (invariable) may sometimes be heard for **ḥa-**, while **ráayiḥ**
(with corresponding feminine and plural forms **ráyḥa** and **rayḥíin**)
also occurs: **ḥayilɣábu, raḥyilɣábu, rayḥíin yilɣábu** *they are
going to play* are all possible but the student is advised to adopt **ḥa-**
exclusively.

Notice the elision of ʕ in the 1st pers. sing. when **bi-** and **ḥa-** are
prefixed, e.g. **bálɣab** *I play, am playing*, **ḥálɣab** *I will play*. The
vowel of **bi** is, of course, elided when a vowel precedes as in
huwwa-byilɣab.

2. **kaan, yikúun** *to be*

(a) **ʕissandúuq kan malyáan**   *The box was full.*

(b) **ʕilʕáklï ḥaykun gáahiz baɣdï-ʃwáyya**   *The meal will be
ready soon* (lit. *after a little*).

(c) **kúntï ɣayyáan imbáariḥ**   *I was ill yesterday.*

(d) **kan fíih ḥádsa fiʃʃáariɣ dilwaqti**   *There was an accident
in the street just now.*

(e) **kan ɣandína wáqtï-ktíir**   *We had plenty of time.*

Notes

1. **kaan, yikúun** is a hollow verb which, however, must be learned at this stage in view of the frequency of its occurrence.

2. The time-reference of any nominal sentence given so far is made past or future by the use of the appropriate tense and person of **kaan, yikúun** (exx. (*a*)–(*c*)).

3. In **fiih** and **ʒand-** sentences (exx. (*d*) and (*e*)), the verb is used only in the 3rd pers. sing. masc. forms (**kaan, yikúun**). **káanit** (3rd pers. sing. fem.) agrees with **ʕóoḍa** in **ʕilʕóoḍa káanit malyáana** *the room was full*, but **kaan** is invariable in **kan fih náas kitíir filʕóoḍa** *there were many people in the room* or in **ʕilʕóoḍa kan fíiha nas kitíir** which has the same meaning (see Lesson 6, 2).

4. The complete paradigm of the verb is as follows:

		Perfect	*Imperfect*	*Imperative*[1]
	3rd pers. masc.	kaan	yikúun	. .
	3rd pers. fem.	káanit	tikúun	. .
Sing.	2nd pers. masc.	kunt	tikúun	kuun
	2nd pers. fem.	kúnti	tikúuni	kúuni
	1st pers.	kunt	ʕakúun	. .
	3rd pers.	káanu	yikúunu	. .
Pl.	2nd pers.	kúntu	tikúunu	kúunu
	1st pers.	kúnna	nikúun	. .

Notice the elision of the vowel of the imperfect prefix when **ḥa-** precedes (cf. **ḥaykúun** in ex. (*b*)).

EXERCISES

A

1. ʕilmuwaẓẓafíin biyuxrúgu min ʃuɣlúhum bádri-f ramaḍáan.
2. ḥaykúun ʒandína-dyúuf búkra lilɣáda.
3. ʕana baɣráfu min múdda ṭawíila qáwi.
4. ḥayinzílu-f lukánḍit[2] máṣrï fissuwées.
5. ḥaykúun fih ʕagáaza yom litnéen iggáay ɣaʃan ilɣíid.
6. ʕana ɣáawiz áṣrif ʃíik biɣáʃara-gnéeh.

B

1. Hurry up! We're going out in ten minutes.
2. He spends a lot of money on amusements.
3. They generally arrive before now.[3] Shall we telephone (them)?
4. Two policemen were present at the time.
5. The sea was calm this morning but is rough now.

[1] The imperative is rare: cf. *xallík ráagil* 'be a man!'
[2] See Introduction, B (ii).
[3] *qábli kída.*

6. I'm going to divide it (fem.) between you so that there will be no quarrelling.

LESSON 10

kaan, yikúun (*cont.*); anomalous verbs

1. kaan, yikúun+*the tenses*

kaan, yikúun is also used as an auxiliary before the perfect and imperfect tenses with corresponding differences of time-reference, e.g.

(*a*) **kan ɣámal iʃʃúɣl lamma daxált** *He* HAD DONE *the job when I went in.*

(*b*) **kan biyíɣmil iʃʃúɣl lamma daxált** *He* WAS DOING *the job when I went in.*

(*c*) **filwáqtĭ dá-ykunu ɣámalu-ʃʃúɣl** *They* WILL HAVE DONE *the job by then.*

(*d*) **filwáqtĭ dá-ykunu-byiɣmílu-ʃʃúɣl** *They* WILL BE DOING *the job then.*

(*e*) **kuntĭ ḥáɣmil iʃʃúɣl wi baɣdéen nisíit** *I* WAS GOING TO DO *the job but then forgot.*

Note, then,

ɣamal *he did, has done*; **kaan ɣamal** *he had done*; **yikuun ɣamal** *he will have done.*

biyíɣmil *he does, is doing*; **kaan biyíɣmil** *he used to do, was doing*; **yikuun biyíɣmil** *he will be doing.*

ḥayíɣmil *he will do, is going to do*; **kaan ḥayíɣmil** *he was going to do.*

yikuun ḥa- does not occur. Notice the use of **qarrab**+imperfect in the following example:

law rúḥtĭ ɣandĭ midáan ilḥurríyya issaɣa taláata mazˌbúuṭ, ḥatʃúuf raɣíis ilwizˌáara,[1] yikun (*or* **ḥaykun**)

---

[1] See Introduction, B (ii).

qárrab yúxrug filwaqtída *If you go to Liberty Square at exactly 3 o'clock, you will see the Prime Minister.* He WILL BE ABOUT TO COME OUT *then.*

2. The following four verbs do not conform to the patterns of other verbs, but their occurrence is so frequent that they should be learned at an early stage.

	kal, yáakul *to eat*			xad, yáaxud *to take*		
	Perfect	*Imperfect*	*Impera- tive*	*Perfect*	*Imperfect*	*Impera- tive*
Sing.	kal (*he*)	yáakul		xad	yáaxud	
	kálit (*she*)	táakul		xadt	táaxud	
	kalt (*you* (m.s.))	táakul	kul	xadt	táaxud	xud
	kálti (*you* (f.s.))	tákli	kúli	xádti	táxdi	xúdi
	kalt (*I*)	ʕáakul		xadt	ʕáaxud	
Pl.	kálu (*they*)	yáklu		xádu	yáxdu	
	káltu (*you*)	táklu	kúlu	xádtu	táxdu	xúdu
	kálna (*we*)	náakul		xádna	náaxud	

Note

xadt, xádti, and xádtu are pronounced xatt, xátti, and xáttu. The implications of t in the perfect suffixes often demand special attention: cf. ʕinbaṣáṭt (pronounced ʕimbaṣáṭṭ) *I was/you were pleased,* qaɣádt (pronounced qaɣátt) *I/you sat down.*

	ʕídda, yíddi *to give*			geh, yíigi *to come*	
	Perfect	*Imperfect*	*Impera- tive*	*Perfect*	*Imperfect*
Sing.	ʕídda (*he*)	yíddi		geh	yíigi
	ʕíddit (*she*)	tíddi		gat	tíigi
	ʕiddéet (*you* (m.s.))	tíddi	ʕíddi	geet	tíigi
	ʕiddéeti (*you* (f.s.))	tíddi	ʕíddi	géeti	tíigi
	ʕiddéet (*I*)	ʕáddi		geet	ʕáagi
Pl.	ʕíddu (*they*)	yíddu		gum	yíigu
	ʕiddéetu (*you*)	tíddu	ʕíddu	géetu	tíigu
	ʕiddéena (*we*)	níddi		géena	níigi

Note. There is no imperative of **geh, yíigi.** Cf. **taɣáala** (masc. sing.)/**taɣáali** (fem. sing.)/**taɣáalu** (pl.) = *Come (here)!*

gaa and **guu,** not **geh** and **gum,** are used when a suffix follows, e.g. **gáani** (or **gáali**) *he came to me* (for the suffix **-li,** see the following lesson).

EXERCISES

A

1. ɣáamil ittilifóon kan bárra lamma-ttilifóon ḍárab.
2. Ṣinnaggáar kan biyíɣmil ʃúɣlu filmáktab wi baɣdéen báttal.
3. kan ɣáawiz yiddíini filkitáab sítta-qrúuʃ.
4. taɣáala hína, y-áḥmad, Ṣana ɣáyzak.
5. xud báalak! fih naʃʃalíin kitíir hináak.
6. di Ṣáaxir móoḍa, wí̬lit min faránsa.

B

1. He was cooking lunch when I last saw him (*tr.* the last time I saw, &c.)[1]
2. I left him asleep and found him still sleeping when I got back.
3. He was going out as we came in.[2]
4. They always take a long time to answer.
5. I'm very busy now. Can you come again in an hour's time?
6. We're very hungry, we ate very little[3] for breakfast.

LESSON 11

Suffixation; the particle Ṣinn

1. The addition of pronominal suffixes to verbs, as to other parts of speech, produces new syllable structures and hence differences in pronunciation affecting especially vowel-length and accentuation. Remember that final vowels are lengthened when a suffix is added, e.g. **fíhmu—fihmúuh** *they understood it/him*, **fihmúuha** *they understood it/her*, **fihímti—fihimtíina** *you* (f.s.) *understood us*. Remember also that the 'extra' vowel will vary with the suffix, e.g. **fihimtína** *you* (m.s.) *understood us*, **fihimtắha** *I/you* (m.s.) *understood her*, **fihimtŭhum** *I/you* (m.s.) *understood them*.

Notice the phonetic similarity between the verbal suffix **-u** (2nd and 3rd pers. pl.) and the pronominal suffix **-u** (3rd pers. sing.

---

[1] Ṣáaxir márra ʃúftu(h).   [2] w-íḥna daxlíin.
[3] kalna Ṣáklī baʂíṭ.

masc.): thus **kátabu** = either *they wrote* or *he wrote it*, **bitiɣráfu** =
either *you* (pl.) *know* or *you* (m.s.) *know him* or *she knows him*.

The particle **li** + pronominal suffix (see Lesson 6) is very frequently added to verbs and has implications similar to those of the
pronominal suffixes alone, e.g. **ʕísmaḥ** *excuse, forgive!*, **ʕismáḥli**
excuse me!, **ʕismaḥíili** *excuse* (f.s.) *me!* Suffixed to verbs, **li**- forms
differ from those given in Lesson 6, 1, note (7), and are as follows:

li, lak, lik, lu(h), líha, lína, lúku(m), lúhum.

If the '1-piece' is of two syllables, e.g. **lína, líha,** and if the verb
ends in a consonant, then **lína, líha,** &c., are treated as separate
words from the point of view of accentuation, e.g. **ʕísmaḥ lína**
excuse us! If, however, the verb ends in a vowel, then the short
vowel following **l** is elided and the whole complex treated as one
word, e.g. **ʕismaḥúlna** *excuse* (pl.) *us*, **ʕismaḥílha** *excuse* (f.s.)
her!

It is common for both a pronominal suffix and an '1-piece' to be
added in that order to one verb. This is especially frequent with
ʕídda, yíddi *to give.*

Examples are:

> **ʕiddiháali**   *Give it* (f.) *to me!*
> **ʕiddíhli**   *Give it* (m.) *to me!*
> **ʕiddetúlha** (i) *I/you* (m.s.) *gave it* (m.) *to her.* (ii) *You* (pl.)
>   *gave to her.*
> **ʕiddetháalu(h)**   *I/you* (m.s.) *gave it* (f.) *to him.*
> **ʕiddéthum lúhum**   *I/you* (m.s.) *gave them to them.*
> **hathálha**   *Bring it* (f.) *to her!*
> **ʕimlahúmlu(h)**   *Fill them for him!*
> **ʕimlahálhum**   *Fill it* (f.) *for them!*
> **ʕimláahum lúhum**   *Fill them for them!*

2. A number of verbs are commonly followed by the conjunctive
particle **ʕinn** introducing a verbal sentence, a nominal sentence,
or one with **fiih** or **ɣand-**. Such verbs, mostly of patterns not yet
examined, are **símiɣ, yísmaɣ** *to hear*, **ʕiftákar, yiftíkir** or **ʒann,**
yiʒúnn *to think, believe*, **ʃaaf, yiʃúuf** *to see*, **qaal, yiqúul** *to say.*

Examples are:

(a) ˤaftíkir inn ilwálad raḥ ilbéet   *I think (that) the boy went home.*

(b) ˤaftíkir innĭ ɡáli raḥ ilbéet   *I think Ali went home.*

(c) ˤaftíkir innu raḥ ilbéet   *I think he went home.*

(d) ˤaftíkir innăha maʃɣúula   *I think she is busy.*

(e) ˤaftíkir innĭ ɡandŭhum filúus kitíir   *I think they have a lot of money.*

Notice the use of the pronominal suffixes in (c) and (d) rather than ˤinnĭ huwwa, ˤinnĭ hiyya, &c. (see also Note below).

Other examples for practice are:

(f) ˤaz̧únn innu (ḥa)ykun ɡámalu dilwáqti   *I think he will have done it by now.*

(g) simíɡt innăha (ḥa)tíwṣal búkra   *I hear(d) she's arriving tomorrow.*

(h) nífriḍ innĭ fih fáyda mínnu(h)   *(Let us) suppose there is something to be gained from it.*

(i) biyqúulu[1]-nn iʃʃíta-f ɡurúbba bárdĭ-ktíir   *They say the winter in Europe is very cold.*

Note

ˤinn does not occur solely after verbs, cf. ˤana mabṣúuṭ innak géet *I am pleased you came*, la ʃákk innu biyqúul ilḥáqq *there is no doubt he is telling the truth*. Notice again the use of the pronominal suffix when ˤinn is not followed by a noun and contrast ˤinn ilwálad and ˤinnĭ ɡáli in (a) and (b) above. Note, too, that ˤinn is never suffixed when it introduces a sentence of the fiih or ɡand- type (see exx. (e) and (h)).

EXERCISES

A

1. ˤaz̧únn innu ḥaygíini búkra.
2. ˤaftíkir innína níqdar nixállaṣ illéela.
3. ɡandak máaniɡ inn-áagi-mɡáak?
4. máalak innaharḍa! báayin ɡaléek taɡbáan.
5. taxúdli gawáab wayyáak tiddíih labúuya min fáḍlak.
6. waɡádni-nnu ḥayiddíini-lkitáab baɡdĭ ma yíxlaṣ mínnu(h).

---

[1] Pronounce *biqúulu*.

`B`

1. Please excuse (pl.) us, it's late[1] and we're rather tired.
2. I asked for coffee but you've brought me tea.
3. Can I borrow it (fem.)? I'll return it to you in a couple of days.
4. I'm sorry, I think he's gone.
5. I think it's unlikely he'll be here before tomorrow.
6. They say the elections are coming off[2] in two months' time.

LESSON 12

Negation

1. (a) **muʃ (or miʃ) múmkin agíilak qabl issaɣa sítta** *It isn't possible for me to (or I cannot) come to you before 6 o'clock.*

   (b) **húmma muʃ mittifqíin wayya báɛḍ ɛaʃan kúllï wáaḥid muʃ fáahim masˁuliyyáatu-kwáyyis** *They don't get on well together since neither of them fully understands his responsibilities.*

   (c) **maniʃ gáyy (or gáay) innahárḍa baɛd iḍḍúhr** *I am not coming this afternoon.*

   (d) **ma fíiʃ luzúum tiʃtiríihum** *There is no need for you to buy them.*

   (e) **ma gatlúuʃ ɛiláawa ɛaʃan ma-byiʃtayálʃï-kwáyyis** *He hasn't had a rise because he doesn't work well.*

2. The two most frequent forms of negation are:

   (i) with the negative particle **muʃ,(or miʃ)**;[3]

   (ii) with **ma** preceding and **ʃ** following (suffixed to) the word negated.

Considering for the moment one-word sentences, (i) occurs with nouns, participles, adjectives, adverbs, &c., and (ii) with verbs and **fiih** and **ɛand-**, e.g.:

   (i) **muʃ ilwálad** *Not the boy*; **muʃ láazim** (*It is*) *not necessary*;

---

[1] *ˁilwáqtï mitˁáxxar.*   [2] *ḥatkúun.*
[3] Both alternatives are illustrated in the examples.

muʃ ínta *Not you*; muʃ kibíir *Not big*; muʃ dá *Not this*;
muʃ fóoq *Not on top*; muʃ bisúrɤa (kída) *Not (so) fast*.

(ii) ma-fhímtiʃ *I didn't understand*; ma-byiɤráfʃ *He doesn't
know*; ma-fíiʃ *There isn't (any)*; ma-ɤandíiʃ *I haven't (any)*.

3. muʃ is essential in the negative nominal sentence, e.g.

Ɂana múʃ xaddáamak *I am not your servant*.

humma múʃ mawgudíin *They are not present*.

dá muʃ minnína *We are not responsible for that* (lit. *that is
not from us*).

muʃ is also common with a following imperfect prefixed with
ḥa-, e.g. múʃ ḥaysáafir *he will not be making the journey*.

4. Although nowadays muʃ is generally used, you will still hear
instances of the 'split' negative (ma -ʃ) with the independent pronouns, e.g. mantíiʃ gáyya (or gáaya)-mɤáana? *Aren't you
(fem.) coming with us?* (or Ɂinti miʃ gáyya-mɤáana?); cf. also
1 (c) above.

The negative pronouns are as follows:

Singular	*Plural*
3rd pers. masc. **mahuwwáaʃ** (or **mahúuʃ**)	3rd person **mahummáaʃ**
3rd pers. fem. **mahiyyáaʃ** (or **mahíiʃ**)	
2nd pers. masc. **mantáaʃ**	2nd person **mantúuʃ**
2nd pers. fem. **mantíiʃ**	
1st pers. **maníiʃ**	1st person **maḥnáaʃ**

Notes

(i) We write **ma** prefixed to the pronoun.
(ii) Notice the **ii** vowel in the 1st pers. sing.

5. We have noted the occurrence of the particles **li**, **maɤa**, and
wayya with pronominal suffixes in sentences of the ɤand- type
(see Lesson 6, 2, note (3)). Negation of **wayya** is with **miʃ**, e.g.
miʃ wayyáaya *I haven't*, not ma wayyayáaʃ. With **li** and
maɤa, however, **ma -ʃ** is used, in addition to which two further
features must be noticed:

(i) **ii** is used in the 1st pers. sing., i.e. **ma líiʃ, ma-mɣíiʃ,** cf. **maníiʃ** above. **maliyyáaʃ** occurs but rarely;

(ii) the vowel of the particle is elided in **ma l(a)háaʃ, ma l(i)kíiʃ, ma l(u)húmʃ, ma l(u)kúmʃ, ma l(i)náaʃ, ma m(a)ɣíiʃ, ma m(a)ɣákʃ,** &c.

6. h of **fiih** is not pronounced in the corresponding negative form **ma fiiʃ** unless required by agreement with a preceding noun (see Lesson 6, 2, note (2)), i.e. **ma fíiʃ ḥáddï filbéet** but **ʕilbéet ma fíhʃï ḥádd** *there is nobody in the house.*

7. Notice that, in common with other suffixes, **ʃ** implies:

(i) occurrence of the 'extra' vowel to avoid a sequence of 3 consonants, e.g. **líssa ma rúḥtïʃ** *I haven't been yet;*

(ii) lengthening of a preceding vowel, e.g. **ma katabúuʃ** *they did not write* or *he did not write it.* Contrast **ma katabúuʃ** with **ma katabúhʃ** *they did not write it;*

(iii) the forms **gaa** and **guu** for **geh** and **gum** in **ma gáaʃ** *he didn't come, hasn't come,* **ma gúuʃ** *they didn't, haven't come.*

EXERCISES

A

1. miʃ ḥáqdar aʃúufak búkra.
2. ma-mɣanáaʃ sagáayir kifáaya-lleláadi.
3. líssa ma gáaʃ. yimkin ḥaṣállu ḥáaga fissíkka.
4. ma ɣandíiʃ fúrṣ(a)-aruḥ aqáblu ɣalmaḥáṭṭa.
5. ma-byismáɣʃï kaláami lamm-anṣáḥu(h).
6. húmma muʃ mitɣawwidíin ɣala ʃúrb ilxámra.

B

1. This isn't my responsibility. It comes under[1] the Accounts Department.
2. I know nothing about the (*tr.* that) matter.
3. This is yours, not mine.
4. It's no longer any use.
5. We haven't enough eggs for breakfast.
6. These shoes don't fit me.[2] They're rather tight.

[1] Use *tábaɣ.*   [2] Use *ɣala qdddi* lit. '(on) my size'.

LESSON 13

Negation (*cont.*)

1. (*a*) **ma tidxúlʃ** (or **tud-**); *Don't go in!*
   (*b*) **ma-trúḥʃï-hnáak** *Don't go there!*
   (*c*) **ma-txalliníiʃ** *Don't leave me!*
   (*d*) **ma-tzaɣɣáqʃï kída** *Don't shout (so)!*

Notice that in the negative imperative the 2nd person *imperfect* forms are used. See also below 2, note (i) and 3, note (iii).

Note

   tz- in (*d*) above is usually pronounced, as elsewhere, **dz-**.

2. (*a*) **láada waláada lakin dúkha** *Neither this nor this but that.*
   (*b*) **la-ɣáyyar wala-kbíir qáwi lakin mutawáṣṣiṭ**[1] *Neither small nor very big but average.*
   (*c*) **la ráaḥ wala ḥayrúuḥ** *He has neither been nor is he going.*
   (*d*) **ʕirráagil dá la-byíqra wala-byíktib** *That man neither reads nor writes.*
   (*e*) **la géh ɣandína filmáktab wala qáabil ilmudíir wala ḥáddï ʃáafu xáaliṣ** *He has neither come to us in the office, nor been to* (lit. *met*) *the manager, nor has anyone seen him at all.*

la ... wala corresponds to English *neither ... nor*. The negative particle in the construction is **la**— for the lengthening of the vowel in (*a*) see Lesson 16, 1, note (3). **wa** is prefixed to every **la** after the first. There is no limit to the number of component words or clauses which may be preceded by the particle, cf. (*e*).

Notice that the imperfect prefixes are often omitted with verbs other than the first as in **la ḥatʃúuf wala tísmaɣ** *You will neither see nor hear*. In (*d*) above, ... **la-byíqra wala yíktib** is a possibility.

[1] Or the 'more characteristically colloquial' *mitwáṣṣaṭ* used by less educated speakers.

It is possible for ʃ to be suffixed to a verbal form after the first, e.g. **la ráaḥ ilmáktab wala-ʃṭírʃ** *he has neither gone to the office nor even breakfasted.* It is also possible for the first negative to be of the **ma -ʃ** type as in **ma katábtïʃ filgaráayid wala ɣamáltïʃ xúṭab** *I have neither written for* (lit. *in*) *the press nor made (any) speeches.*

Notes

(i) **ya . . . ya** is used in the way of English *either . . . or*, e.g. **yáada yáada** or **ya dá ya dá** *either this or that*, **ya-trúuḥ ya tistánna** *either go or stay*. Notice again the imperfect verbal form in the last example.

(ii) The negative particle **la** may be compared with **laʕ** *no*. **laʕ**, when used for emphatic disagreement, often has the form **laa**, e.g. **láa, láa, ʕábadan** *no, no, never!*

(iii) Do not confuse **wala** with **walla** *or*.

(iv) Distinguish also negative **la** from the emphatic particle **la** in **ʕúskut, la-(ʕa)ḍrábak** *be quiet or I'll hit you!* This second **la** is rare.

3. *Emphatic negation*

The term emphatic negation is reserved for the use of **ma** without ʃ. This occurs (i) with a few words commonly associated with negation, e.g. **ɣumr, ḥadd**, and (ii) with the 'oaths'.

(i) **ɣumr** (lit. *life*) + pronominal suffix + **ma** = *never*, e.g. **ɣúmri ma ʃúftï wáaḥid záyyu** *I have never seen anyone like him*. ʃ may be included, with less emphasis, i.e. **ɣúmri ma ʃúftïʃ wáaḥid záyyu. ma -ʃ** may also be applied to **ɣumr** rather than the following verb, i.e. **ma ɣumríiʃ ʃúftï wáaḥid záyyu**. Cf. **ma ḥáddïʃ yíɣraf yiftáḥu** *Nobody knows how to open it*, alternative forms of which include the use of **fiih** in **ma fiʃ ḥáddï yíɣraf yiftáḥu.**[1]

(ii) The common 'oaths' are **walláahi** (lit. *and my God*), **winnábi** (*and the Prophet*), **wirabbína** (*and our Lord*), to which may be added **ʕinʃalla** (derived from the divine name) in the specialized use with a following perfect shown below:

láa walláahi m-áqdar (= **ma** + **ʕáqdar**)   } *No, by heaven,*
láa winnábi m-áqdar.   } *I cannot* (see
láa wirabbína m-áqdar.   } Note (ii) below).

ʕinʃálla ma ḥáddï kál   *May nobody ever eat, then!*
ʕinʃálla ma rúḥt   *Go or not, as you please.*

---

[1] In the examples given under (i), *záyyu* and *yiftáḥu* may, of course, be pronounced with final *h*.

Notes

(i) **la wálla** is a very common alternative to **láa walláahi.**

(ii) The 'oaths' have greater variety, power, and binding force outside the towns and among less sophisticated townsmen. For sophisticated speakers, the above examples with **walláahi,** &c., mean little more than *I really cannot.* The above use of **ʕinʃálla,** always associated with considerable displeasure, is more frequent in the speech of women.

(iii) Do not confuse negative **ma** with a relatively rare particle **ma** used with an imperative sense as in **ma titkállim** *Speak up! say something!*

EXERCISES

A

1. ma-trúhʃĭ lilfakaháani-nnahárḍa.¹ ʕihna miʃ ɣawzíin ḥáaga.
2. ma-tsíbʃ iʃʃibbáak maftúuḥ táani, baqúllak.
3. la-byíɣraf yíqra wala yíktib ɣárabi.
4. ya réetu ma ráaḥ.
5. la wálla, ma ɣandíiʃ ʃahíyya.²
6. la baṭṭáal qáwi wala-kwáyyis qáwi lakin béen litnéen.

B

1. Don't forget to bargain with the shopkeeper. Otherwise he'll have you for certain.
2. Please be quiet (pl.). I can't hear what is being said (*tr.* can't hear a thing) on the phone.
3. Don't bite it or chew it, swallow it straight away!
4. Haven't I seen that man before?³ Didn't he used to work for us?⁴
5. He's never mentioned that to me. I wonder (*tr.* I don't know) why not.
6. I've left my cigarettes at home. I haven't a single one on me.

---

¹ After verbs of motion the particle *li* is used with nouns of personal reference. Contrast, for example, *ʕana ráayiḥ issúuq* 'I am going to the market'.
² *ʕáakul* may be added.
³ *qábli kída.*
⁴ *ɣandína.*

LESSON 14

Interrogation

1. An Arabic sentence, affirmative or negative, may also be used as a question by changing the intonation. Compare the way you say in English, 'He's the man I saw yesterday' and 'Is he the man I saw yesterday?' A questioning rise of the voice on 'yesterday' corresponds to a similar feature at the end of Arabic interrogative sentences. Get an Egyptian to say to you, both as statements and as questions, **biyitkállim ɣárabi-kwáyyis** (*he speaks Arabic well*) and the corresponding negative **ma-byitkallímʃï ɣárabi-kwáyyis,** and notice particularly what happens to **kwáyyis**: then, as always, mimic your informant.

2. We can put the English question another way and say 'He's the man I saw yesterday, isn't he?' in which the first part (up to 'yesterday') is commonly said as a statement, the rise of the voice taking place in 'isn't he?' Egyptian Arabic does the same thing with the very common **muʃ kída** (lit. *not so?*) and says **biyitkállim ɣárabi kwáyyis, muʃ kída?** *He speaks Arabic well, doesn't he?* The formula is reminiscent of others in European languages, cf. French 'n'est-ce pas', German 'nicht wahr', Spanish '(no es) verdad'. In English the device varies with the sentence, e.g. 'doesn't he, aren't you, haven't they, &c.'

There is little difference of meaning between this use of **muʃ kída** and the less common device of prefixing **muʃ** to the sentence, e.g. **muʃ húwwa ragil¹ ṭáyyib?** *Isn't he a good man?* (cf. French 'n'est-ce pas que . . .').

3. Another very common interrogative construction is with **walla** *or* either in the fixed formula **walla laʕ** *or not* or used to introduce an alternative. The sentence up to **walla** has the interrogative

---

¹ See Introduction, B (*c*), (i), and Appendix B.

(rising) intonation while from **walla** on, it has the typically affirmative (falling) tone. This is again paralleled in English:

(a) **húwwa-lli** (= **huwwa ſilli**) **ſúftu-mbáariḥ walla láſ?**
Is he the one I/you saw yesterday or not?

(b) **húwwa-lli ſúftu-mbáariḥ walla káan fih waḥid táani?**
Is he the one I/you saw yesterday or was it someone else?

(c) **géh walla líssa?**   *Has he come yet or not* (lit. *has he come or not yet*)?

4. The above questions generally seek information but there is also the type which is rather more of an exclamation, involving surprise or even indignation, as when you say to someone who contradicts you 'He isn't the man I saw yesterday!' Once again, the grammatical structure of the sentence is as that of the affirmative form and it is the intonation, with a more marked final rise, that helps to mark the 'interrogation'. The Arabic sentence **biyitkállim ҁárabi kwáyyis?** (*Do you mean to tell me*) *he speaks Arabic well!?* can be uttered in a similar way.

5. In answer to negative questions, you will sometimes hear **ſáywa** *yes* and **laſ** *no* used in a way misleading to English speakers. For example, in reply to **ma rúḥtĭʃ?** *Didn't you go?* you may hear **ſáywa, ma rúḥtĭʃ** *No, I didn't* or **láſ, rúḥt** *Yes, I did.* **laſ** for **ſáywa** and vice versa is, however, possible.

6. You will sometimes but rarely, hear **ʃ** (not to be confused with **ʃ** of the negative) following verbs or **fiih** or **ҁand-** in interrogative sentences: e.g. **ʃúftĭʃ duséeh ҁalmáktab?** *Did you see a file on the desk?*, **ҁandákʃĭ sagáayir?** *Have you any cigarettes?*

EXERCISES

A

1. ҁáayiz qáhwa sáada walla-b súkkar?
2. rúḥtĭ-hnáak qablĭ kída? da makáan gamíil gíddan.
3. tiftíkir fih fárqĭ ben láḥgit máṣrĭ wi-skindiríyya?
4. tíqdar tifukkíli-gnéeh min fáḍlak?
5. fih súrҁa maḥdúuda lilҁarabiyyáat fi máṣr?
6. ҁandak xíbra sábqa fiṭṭábx?

B

1. The letter's finished. Shall I bring it in for your signature (*tr.* for you to sign it)?
2. Are you free or busy now?
3. Is there a taxi-rank anywhere near here?[1]
4. Is this for me? Thank you very much, but are you sure[2] you don't want it?
5. Aren't you going to come with us? It's only a little way, isn't it?
6. Are we going to play or not? You don't really[3] want to, do you?

LESSON 15

Interrogation (*cont.*)

1. (*a*) **bitíჳmil éeh dilwáqti?** *What are you doing now?*
   (*b*) **ḥatúxrug ímta?** *When are you leaving, going out?*
   (*c*) **ʕinta ráayiḥ féen?** *Where are you going?*
   (*d*) **ʃúfti míin?** *Whom did you see?*
   (*e*) **míin illi wayyáak?** *Who is that with you?*
   (*f*) **ḥatgáhhiz iṣṣúfra issaჳa káam?** *At what time are you going to lay* (lit. *prepare*) *the table?*

The specifically interrogative words are as follows: **ʕeeh** *what*, **leeh** *why*, **miin** *who*, **feen** *where*, **ʕímta** *when*, **ʕayy** *which*, **ʕizzáay** *how*, **kaam** *how much, many*, **qáddi ʕéeh** *how far, how much, to what extent*.

2. Notice that the typical unemphatic order of the sentence containing one of the above words is an inverted one in relation to English. Other examples are:

---

[1] *fi ʕáyyi ḥitta hina-qráyyib.*
[2] Use *mutaʕákkid* (or *mitʕákkid*) *inn* . . .
[3] Use *law* (or *ʕin*) *géet lilḥáqq* lit. 'if you come to the truth'.

húwwa féen? *Where is he* (lit. *he* (*is*) *where*)?
ráʕyak éeh finnáas dóol? *What do you think* (lit. *what is your opinion*) *of those people?*
ḥatrúuḥ izzáay? *How are you going?*
ʕiʃtaréetu-b káam? *How much did you buy it for?*

The reverse order, e.g. **féen huwwa?**, often gives an emphatic turn to the sentence. If **ʕeeh** is placed first in a verbal (or **fiih** or **ʒand-**) sentence, then it is followed by **ʕilli** (see Lesson 17), e.g. **ʕéeh illi btiʒmílu(h)?** *What are you doing* (lit. *what are you doing* IT)?

3. Sentences with the specifically interrogative words usually have the (falling) intonation of the affirmative sentence. This is also the case in English: contrast 'When did he come?' and 'Did he come?' Surprise, indignation, anger, &c., will, of course, introduce intonational differences which it is impossible to account for here. Quite commonly, however, one hears examples of a pattern sounding very foreign to English ears. In it the final interrogative word is pronounced on a monotone (no rise or fall) and on a higher pitch than the preceding syllable. **bitiʒmil éeh?** *What are you doing?* uttered in this way, may be represented graphically ‐ ‾ ₋ ‐.

4. leeh = li + ʕeeh, feen = fi + ʕeen. You will hear **ʕeen** preceded by **min** in, e.g. **ʒirífti-mnéen** *How* (lit. *from where*) *did you know?*

The interrogative is commonly preceded by a preposition, e.g. **ʒamálti kída ʒalaʃan éeh?** *Why* (lit. *for the purpose of what*) *did you do so?*, **bitittíkil ʒala míin?** *Whom do you rely on?*

5. In colloquial Arabic word-order is fixed in noun-verb-noun sentences: **ʒáli ḍarab maḥámmad** *Ali hit Muhammad* but **maḥámmad ḍarab ʒáli** *Muhammad hit Ali.* Similarly with **miin**, **ʃáaf míin?** means *Whom did he see?* not *Who saw?* (= **míin ʃáaf?**). **ʃáaf míin** may be inverted but if so, then **miin**, like **ʕeeh** above, is followed by **ʕilli**, i.e. **míin illi ʃáafu(h)?** *Whom did he see* (lit. *see* HIM)? Contrast, however, **ʃáafu míin?** *Who saw him?*

6. kaam requires a following noun in the singular, e.g. **ḥatistánna kam yóom**? *How many days are you going to stay?*

7. The form **ʕizzáyy**, not **ʕizzáay**, is used in the greetings formulae **ʕizzáyyak, ʕizzáyy iṣṣíḥḥa, ʕizzáyy ilḥáal**, &c., *How are you?*

8. ʕánhu (masc. sing.)/**ʕánhi** (fem. sing.)/**ʕánhum** (pl.) *which* is an alternative to the commoner **ʕayy** (invariable). **ʕánhu** may accompany a noun which it either precedes or follows: if it precedes, the noun has no article; if it follows, the noun takes the article, i.e. **ʕánhu-ktáab** or **ʕilkitáab ánhu** *which book?* If the sentence is extended, then the second pattern requires **ʕilli**, the first does not, i.e.

> **ʕánhu-ktáab ɤáyzu(h)?**
> or
> **ʕilkitáab anhú-lli-nta (= ʕánhu +**
> **ʕílli + ʕínta) ɤáyzu(h)?**

} *Which book do you want (lit. want it)?*

ʕánhu, therefore, behaves exactly as the ordinal numerals (see Lesson 30, 2),

cf.

> **táalit kitáab fi dóol**
> or
> **ʕilkitáab ittáalit illi-f dóol**

} *the third among those books.*

EXERCISES

A

1. míin qállak inn-ána miʃ ráayiḥ?
2. ʕéeh izzáḥma-lli-hnáak di? fíih ʕéeh?
3. kúntĭ féen? ma ʃuftákʃĭ min zamáan.
4. ṣabáaḥ ilxéer, ʕitfáḍḍal úqɤud, ʕáyyĭ xídma?
5. ʕíntu, ya-lli waqfíin hináak! ma-btiʃtaɤalúuʃ léeh?
6. qaddĭ ʕéeh ilmasáafa ben máṣrĭ w-issuwées?

B
1. Shall I throw it away or what?
2. Who wrote this report? It doesn't make sense at all.[1]
3. How do you say it (fem.) in Arabic?
4. What kind (*tr.* kinds) of meat is there[2] in the market today?
5. Where's he put the book I gave him?
6. How much would it cost me to stay[3] in a hotel?

LESSON 16

Demonstratives: ʕaho, ʕahe, ʕahum

1. (*a*) ʕilfingáan dá ɣalaʃáan ilqáhwa w-ilfanagíin dóol ɣalaʃáan iʃʃáay *This cup is for coffee and these cups for tea.*

(*b*) ʕiʃʃánṭa dí ʕátqal min díkha *This bag is heavier than that.*

(*c*) da-lmuftáaḥ bitaɣ ilbáab *This is the key of the door.*

Restriction of the gender distinction to the singular applies also to the two demonstrative series:

masc. sing.	*fem. sing.*	*plural*	
da[4]	di	dool	*this/that, these/those*
dúkha	díkha	dúkham	*that, those*

Of the two, the **da**-series is more frequent and **dúkha,** &c., is rarely heard in typically Cairene speech, **da** corresponding to both *this* and *that* in English. **dúkha** is perhaps most frequent when a specific contrast is made as in (*b*) above or in, e.g. **múʃ dá lakin dúkha** *not this but that.*

Notes

1. These forms are used as pronouns (cf. (*c*) above) or adjectives (cf. (*a*) and (*b*)). Notice that the noun preceding adjectival **da** must take the article. If

---

[1] *xáaliṣ.*   [2] Use *mawgúud* 'present'.
[3] Translate *lamm-ánzil.*
[4] Usually pronounced with weak final *h* when the word is in isolation or in final position.

another adjective accompanies the noun, then **da** may follow either noun or adjective, e.g. **ʕilḥáaga dí-lkuwayyísa** or **ʕilḥáaga-lkuwayyísa di** *this nice thing.*

2. **díyya** and **díyyat** are alternative forms of adjectival **di** following the noun.

3. **da** and **di** are often suffixed to the noun. Notice the accentuation difference between **ʕilqálam dá** and **ʕilqalámda** *this/that pencil* both of which occur. Also **ʕissána dí** (or **díyya** or **díyyat**) or **ʕissanáadi** *this year.* As a general rule the first of these alternatives is more emphatic.

4. Remember the possible use of the feminine singular accompanying plural forms, e.g. **ʕilkútub dóol** or **ʕilkútub dí** *these/those books.*

5. Do not confuse **da** with the first **d** in the common interjection **déhda!** *What!, What is this?*

2. (*a*) **ʕaho géh**   *Here he is* (lit. *has come*)!

   (*b*) **ʕahe-lwáraqa**   *Here/There is the sheet* (*paper*).

   (*c*) **ʕahum** (or **ʕahe**) **ilkútub**   *Here/There are the books.*

Similar gender and number distinctions operate in the series **ʕaho** (masc. sing.), **ʕahe** (fem. sing.), **ʕahum** (pl.), usually to be translated *here/there is/are.*

These forms may be used with a noun or verb, or in isolation. With nouns they may precede or follow, i.e. **ʕahum ilkútub** or **ʕilkútub ahúm.** Following a noun, or in isolation, a variety of related forms occur as alternatives: e.g.

Q. **ʕilkitáab féen?**   A. **ʕahóh**[1] or **ʕahúwwa** (or, rarely, **ʕahúwwat**)

   ʕilɣílba féen?   **ʕahéh**[1] or **ʕahíyya** (or, rarely, **ʕahíyyat**)

   ʕilkútub féen?   **ʕahúm** or **ʕahúmma** (or, rarely, **ʕahúmmat**)

With a following verb of persons other than the 3rd sing. fem. and 3rd pl., **ʕaho** is used as an invariable form together with the appropriate independent pronoun, e.g. **ʕahó-na** (= **ʕana**) **géet!** *Here I am!*, **ʕahó-nti** (= **ʕinti**) **géeti!** *There you* (fem. sing.) *are!*[2] (Cf. **ʕahe** and **ʕahum** with the 3rd pers. fem. sing. and 3rd pl. in **ʕahe gát!, ʕahum gúm!**)

---

[1] Before pause, *ʕaho* and *ʕahe* are pronounced with final *h*.

[2] *ʕahúwwa* is sometimes used for *ʕaho* in these contexts, e.g. *ʕahuww-ána géet* 'Here I am!', *ʕahuwwá-nti géeti* 'There you (fem. sing.) are!'

The invariable ſáadi can be substituted for ſaho, ſahe, &c.,
with the reservations

(i) that it must always precede the noun or verb, e.g. ſáadi
maḥaṭṭítna *this is our stop*, not maḥaṭṭitna ſaadi;

(ii) that it requires the suffixed, not the independent pronoun.
Note, too, that the suffix of the 1st pers. sing. is (the verbal
suffix) **-ni,** e.g.

> ſadíini géet = ſahó-na géet   *Here I am!*
>
> ſadíiku géetu = ſahó-ntu géetu   *There you* (pl.) *are!*

ſaadi and ſaho, &c., may combine, or ſaho may be repeated, e.g.
ſadi (or ſaho)-ſſéex ɣazíiz ahóh! *There's Sheikh Aziz!*

EXERCISES

A

1. ſilmaɣíiſa ɣálya liyyámdi xáaliṣ.
2. da ráagil ſáaṭir, yágib innu (*or* láazim) yitráqqa.
3. dol náas nubiyyíin, ɣandŭhum lúɣa xáṣṣa bíihum.
4. tiqdar táaxud ikkitáab iṣṣuɣáyyar da baláaſ.
5. ſáadi-lmudárris bitáaɣi gáyyï-hnáak ahoh!
6. ſahe-ṣṣuffáara ḍárabit! yálla bíina!

B

1. What does that word mean (*tr.* what is the meaning of that
   word)?
2. I saw that man in Suez last week.
3. There they are over there, sitting next to each other.
4. There you are at last! You've kept me waiting (*tr.* you have
   delayed me) a long time.
5. Here it is! I've found it! It was in this drawer under the
   papers.
6. Here's a pound for you! Give it back to me[1] later.

---

[1] Translate *w-ibqa raggaɣúuli*, or *wi tíbqa-traggaɣúuli.* See also Lesson 20,
Exercise B, 2.

LESSON 17

The relative ſílli

1. If we take either of the sentences **biyízɣal bi súrɣa** *he loses his temper quickly* or **yistaḥáqq ittarqíya** *he deserves promotion* and join it to **huwwa ráagil** *he is a man*, we get the new sentences **huwwa ráagil biyízɣal bi súrɣa** *he is a man* WHO *loses his temper quickly* and **huwwa ráagil yistaḥáqq ittarqíya** *he is a man* WHO *deserves promotion.* Notice that there is no specific equivalent of English 'who'.

If, however, we take the same original sentences **biyízɣal**, &c., and join them to **huwwa-rráagil** *he is* THE *man*, then the relative **ſílli** is necessary in Arabic, i.e. **huwwa-rráagil illi-byízɣal bi súrɣa** *he's* THE *man* WHO *loses his temper quickly.*

ſílli is necessary, therefore, if the preceding noun is defined. This is reminiscent of noun-adjective agreement with the article. We have seen that if the noun has the article, then so, too, has the adjective, e.g. **ráagil ṭawíil** but **ſirráagil iṭṭawíil** *the tall man*. In our present example, the clause **biyízɣal bi súrɣa** corresponds to **ṭawíil** and **ſílli** to the article **ſil.**

2. The use of the article is not the only way of 'defining' a noun in Arabic. Another most important way is to add a pronominal suffix. **ſílli** is, therefore, essential in, e.g. **ṣaḥíbna-lli** (= **ṣaḥibna+ſílli**) **tiɣrafúuh** *our friend whom you know* (lit. *who you know him*).

3. The last example contains an important feature which has occurred in previous examples and to which particular attention should be paid. Such distinctions as 'who, whom, whose, which, of which', &c., in English correspond in Arabic to the use of a pronominal suffix referring back to an earlier noun. For example, **ɣágabak ilqálam illi warretúulak imbáariḥ?** *Did you like the pen* WHICH *I showed you* (IT) *yesterday?* It may help to realize that the sentence may be split up as above into **ɣágabak ilqálam?** *Did you like the pen?* and **warretúulak imbáariḥ** *I showed you it yesterday.*

This feature is especially common with **ʕílli**, but cf. also **ʕánhu-ktáab ɣáyzu(h) ?** *which book do you want (it)?* in Lesson 15. Other examples for practice with **ʕílli** are:

> **ʕilbínt ill-axúuha ṣáḥbi**   *the girl whose brother is my friend.*
>
> **ʕilbanáat ill-axúuhum ṣáḥbi**   *the girls whose brother is my friend.*
>
> **ṣáḥbi-lli béetu filḥáyy iggidíid**   *my friend whose house is in the new quarter.*
>
> **ṣáḥbi-lli ɣarfíinu-nnáas kullǔhum**   *my friend whom everybody knows*
>
> **ʕaho-rráagil illi qultílak ɣaléeh**   *There is the man I told you about* (lit. *who I told you about him*)!

4. Corresponding to English 'he who, those who, that which, &c.', **ʕílli** is used without a preceding noun and may be preceded by a prepositional particle, e.g.

> **ʕilli ɣandǔhum filúus ɣandǔhum nufúuz**   *People with money have influence.*
>
> **háat illi fíih, ma ɣaléhʃ**   *Never mind* (**ma ɣaléhʃ**), *fetch what there is!*
>
> **háat wáaḥid milli** (= **min + ʕilli**) **fóoq iṭṭarabéeẓa**   *Bring one of those (which are) on the table!*

EXERCISES

A

1. ʕilli-byiʃtáɣal kitíir, biyíksab kitíir.
2. ʃúftĭ ya síidi-lkaláam illi biyqulúuh[1] filgaráayid?
3. fáakir ilḥikáaya-lli qultílak ɣaléeha-mbáariḥ?
4. ʕiddíini wáaḥid milli ɣándak.
5. ʕiʃʃúɣl illi zayyída, yiḥtáag li tafkíir kitíir.
6. ʕísmaɣ, ya-lli-hnáak! min fáḍlak taɣáala hína!

B

1. Take what you want!
2. We've a lot of work to do (*tr.* it is necessary we do it).
3. Is the car I asked for ready (*tr.* present)?

---

[1] Pronounce *biqulúuh*.

4. Who's that standing there near the door?
5. That's the man you want, over there beside the taxi.
6. I think you know what I'm going to say to you.

LESSON 18

Numerals

1. *1–10*

(a) ɣandu bíntï wáḥda w-ána ɣandi-tnéen (= ɣandi +
ʕitneen) *He has* ONE *daughter and I have* TWO.

(b) ʕana báxdim fiʃʃírka min ɣáʃar siníin *I have been
working for* (lit. *in*) *the Company for* TEN *years.*

(c) A. ɣándak ʕawláad? B. ʕáywa, xámsa. bintéen wi
tálat wiláad A. *Have you any children?* B. *Yes*, FIVE.
Two girls and THREE *boys.*

Numerals from 1 to 10 are as follows:

wáaḥid, wáḥda *1*; ʕitnéen *2*; tálat, taláata *3*; ʕárbaɣ,
ʕarbáɣa *4*; xámas, xámsa *5*; sitt, sítta *6*; sábaɣ, sábɣa
7; táman, tamánya *8*; tísaɣ, tísɣa *9*; ɣáʃar, ɣáʃara *10*.

Notes

1. With the exception of **ʕitnéen,** these numerals have two forms, the second
of which we may regard as being derived from the first by the addition of **-a.**
We will call these forms masculine and feminine respectively. Notice the elision
of the second vowel of the masculine form in **wáḥda, xámsa, sábɣa, tísɣa,** its
retention in **ɣáʃara,** and its lengthening in **taláata.** Note, too, the **y** in **tamánya.**

2. **wáaḥid** is most frequently used as an adjective, e.g. **béet wáaḥid** *one
house,* **sítti wáḥda** *one woman.* Like other numerals, however, **wáaḥid** can
precede a noun; for example, in the story-telling formula **kan fïh wáaḥid
ṣulṭáan** *there was* (*once*) *a* (*certain*) *Sultan.*

For the use of **wáaḥid** in 'tens and units' numbers, see 3 below.

3. **ʕitnéen** (invariable) is used comparatively rarely with a following noun,
the dual form of the latter being preferred (cf. **bintéen** in (c) above). It is, however, regularly used before nouns referring to human beings with the exception
of nouns of relationship: e.g. **ʕitnéen sawwaqíin/ɣasáakir/muɣallimíin/
ɣarbagíyya/ɣummáal/ʃúraka** *two   drivers/soldiers/teachers/gharry-drivers/
workmen/partners,* but **bintéen/ʕaxxéen/ʕuxtéen** *two daughters* (or *girls*)/
brothers/sisters, also **maratéen/ragléen/waladéen** *two women* (or *wives*)/*men*
(or *husbands*)/*boys* (or *sons*). Those nouns with which **ʕitnéen** is used do not, of
course, occur in a dual form.

ʕitnéen is also used with certain nouns of value and measurement (having no dual form and usually loan-words), e.g. ʕitnéen ginéeh £2, ʕitnéen mítr (or mitréen) 2 metres, ʕitnéen kíilu (or kéelu) 2 kilograms or kilometres. Notice the singular form of the noun in these cases.

Like wáaḥid, ʕitnéen may be used for emphasis and contrast (cf. (a) above). Like other numerals, it may be prefixed with the article and behave either as noun or adjective (see Lesson 30), e.g. ɣandŭhum litnéen (= ʕil+ʕitneen) they both have (or they have both), ʕiddíini-lkitabéen litnéen Give me both books!

4. Numerals from 3 to 10 behave differently from all other numerals in a variety of ways. This fact will appear again elsewhere below.

The 'masculine' form is used for enumerating a following noun, cf. ɣáʃar and tálat in (b) and (c) above. An exception to this is provided by certain nouns of value and measurement which, themselves in the singular, require the 'feminine' numeral, e.g. sábɣa-gnéeh £7, xámsa taɣríifa 5 half-piastres, taláata mallíim 3 millemes, xámsa kíilu 5 kilograms. Notice in passing that taɣríifa is only used with reference to the numbers 1, 3, and 5.

The 'feminine' form is used whenever the numeral does not enumerate a following noun, e.g. when the numeral occurs in isolation, finally in the sentence (cf. xámsa in (c) above), or in 'tens and units' numbers (see 3 below).

2. 11–19

ḥiḍáaʃar 11; ʕiṭnáaʃar 12; talaṭṭáaʃar 13; ʕarbaɣṭáaʃar 14; xamasṭáaʃar 15; siṭṭáaʃar 16; sabaɣṭáaʃar 17; tamanṭáaʃar 18; tisaɣṭáaʃar 19.

Learn ḥiḍáaʃar and ʕiṭnáaʃar separately. For the rest, add ṭáaʃar to the 'masculine' form of the corresponding unit. Note ṭṭ in talaṭṭáaʃar and siṭṭáaʃar.

3. 20, 30, 40, &c.

ɣiʃríin 20; talatíin 30; ʕarbiɣíin 40; xamsíin 50; sittíin 60; sabɣíin 70; tamaníin 80; tisɣíin 90.

Tens can be formed by suffixing -iin to the 'masculine' unit with vowel-elision in ɣiʃríin, xamsíin, sabɣíin, and tisɣíin. Note the vowel i, not a, in ɣiʃríin and ʕarbiɣíin.

In 'tens and units' numbers, the unit is placed first and followed by wi and. For numbers involving '1', the 'masculine' form wáaḥid is used, e.g. wáaḥid wi tisɣíin 91 (lit. 1 and 90). In contrast, for 3 to 9 the 'feminine' form is used, e.g. xámsa-w xamsíin 55. ʕitnéen is, of course, regularly used for 2, e.g. ʕitnéen wi talatíin 32.

4. *Number of the noun*

    (i) 3–10 require the following noun in the plural (with the exception of certain nouns of value and measurement—see above); e.g. **xámas riggáala/qurúuʃ/banáat** 5 *men/ piastres/girls*, but **xámsa-gnéeh** £5.

    (ii) 11 and above require the noun in the singular, e.g. **ḥiḍáaʃar/ talatíin ráagil/qírʃ/bínt** *11/30 men/piastres/girls*.

EXERCISES

A

1. béetu-f ʃáariɣ ɣábdu báaʃa, nímra xamasṭáaʃar.
2. ʕiddíini ɣáʃar ṭawáabiɣ búʃṭa min ábu qirʃéen.
3. ʕilbadláadi-b tisaɣṭáaʃar ginéeh. ɣálya-ʃwayya lakin ilqumáaʃ matíin.
4. huwwa ráyyis ɣala siṭṭáaʃar ráagil.
5. ʕilwáaḥid mínhum biyíksab xámsa-gnéeh filʕusbúuɣ ɣalʕaqáll.
6. ʕiṭṭarííq wíḥiʃ. ma-tsúqʃi ʕáktar min arbiɣíin kíilu fissáaɣa.

B

1. They went on leave three weeks ago.
2. My contract is for¹ five years subject to renewal.
3. The company awards (*tr.* gives) badges for service (*tr.* to those who serve in it) from ten to thirty years.
4. He is repaying the loan at the rate of £4 a month (*tr.* he is paying £4 a month in order to, &c.).
5. He first of all asked £18 for this suit but I finally bought it for £15.
6. Come back in ten minutes or quarter of an hour!

¹ Use *bi.*

LESSON 19

Numerals (*cont.*)

1. (*a*) raˤíis ilqálam mahiyyítu míit ginéeh ʃahríyyan *The head of the department's salary is £100 a month.*

   (*b*) sanat ˤálfï tusʒumíyya taláata-w xamsíin *The year 1953.*

   (*c*) tiʒdáad ilmaʂriyyíin ˤázyad min ʒiʃríin milyóon *The census of Egyptians totals* (lit. *is) more than 20,000,000.*

   (*d*) ʒummálna w-ilmuwaẓẓafíin bitúʒna ʒadádhum tísaʒt aláaf taqríiban *Our workmen and staff amount to* (lit. *their number is) approximately 9,000.*

2. *100, 200, 300, &c.*

   míyya *100* is a feminine noun with the dual form mitéen *200* and plural miyyáat.

   From 300 to 900 there is a special regular pattern:

   tultumíyya *300*; rubʒumíyya *400*; xumsumíyya *500*; suttumíyya *600*; subʒumíyya *700*; tumnumíyya *800*; tusʒumíyya *900*.

   Notice the contracted form miit and the final **t** of the construct in 1 (*a*) above; rubʒumíit sána *400 years* is another example.

3. *1,000, 2,000, 3,000, &c.*; *1, 2, 3,000,000, &c.*

   ˤalf *1,000* and milyóon *1,000,000* are nouns with dual and plural forms ˤalféen and milyonéen, ˤaláaf and malayíin. They differ, however, in the manner of their combination with a preceding numeral (cf. Notes (i) and (iii) following).

Notes

   (i) Notice the regular plural form ˤaláaf following a numeral from 3–10 (cf. 1 (*d*) above) and the singular ˤalf following 11 and over (see Lesson 18, 4).

   (ii) You would have expected in 1 (*d*) the form tísaʒ (ˤ)aláaf rather than tísaʒt aláaf (see Lesson 18, 2, note (4)). Final **t**, however, is commonly used with 3–10 numerals when the following noun elsewhere begins with ˤ. Contrast xámast iyyáam *5 days* with xámas qurúuʃ *5 piastres,* also tálatt aláaf *3,000,* and **tálatt iṣnáaf** *3 kinds* with **tálat banáat** *3 girls.* Notice also **tálatt úʃhur** or **tálat ʃuhúur** or **(ʕáʃhur)** *3 months.*

There are three main features to notice in, for example, **xámast iyyáam**: firstly, the form of the numeral, which is not **xámsit**, as might have been expected from the form of feminine *nouns* in construct; secondly, the elision of ʕ; thirdly, **i,** not **a,** in the first syllable of **iyyáam.** There are, however, reservations to be made as follows:

(*a*) **xámsit ʕayyáam** or **xámas ʕayyáam** are on the whole more usual among educated speakers;

(*b*) with nouns of certain other patterns, in which as a general rule there are only two other consonants, educated speakers *never* elide initial ʕ, and any preceding 3–10 numeral is used as elsewhere in the 'masculine' form, e.g. **tálat ʕuzúun baríid** *three postal orders.* This applies also to such a quadriliteral form as **ʕaráanib** (sing. **ʕárnab**) *rabbits,* in which initial ʕ is a radical, e.g. **tálat ʕaráanib** (see also Appendix C, 2).

(iii) **milyóon** (sometimes **malyóon**) is a loan-word and behaves accordingly (see Lesson 18, 1, notes (3) and (4)), e.g. **ʕitnéen milyóon (milyonéen** occurs but is rare) *2,000,000,* **xámsa milyóon** (not **xamas malayiin**) *5,000,000.* **malayíin** is only commonly used when reference is not to the specific number of millions (cf. below Exercise A, 5).

4. *Compound numerals*

The order of compound numerals corresponds to the English order with the important exception that units always precede tens (cf. 1 (*b*) above). The particle **wi** *and* always precedes the final numeral. Other examples for practice are:

sítta-w talatíin *36,* **míyya w-itnéen** *102,* **ʕálfï-w míyya** *1,100,* **míyya taláata-w sittíin** *163,* **ʕalféen míyya-tnéen wi tisɣíin** *2,192,* **xámast aláaf xumsumíyya-w sabɣíin** *5,570.*

'3–10' numerals in compounds are always in the 'feminine' form with a following noun in the singular, e.g. **míyya-w xámsa qírʃ** *105 piastres,* for which **míit qírʃï-w xámsa** is a commoner alternative.

EXERCISES

A

1. nímrit ittilifóon máṣr mitéen arbáɣa-w talatíin.
2. ʕana ɣúmri sítta-w talatíin sána w-íbni ɣúmru tísaɣ siníin.
3. ráaḥ bursaɣíid min múddit tálatt úʃhur.
4. fi máṣrï xámsa milyóon faddáan ṣalḥíin lizziráaɣa.
5. ʕittáagir da ɣáni gíddan, ɣandu malayíin.
6. fi gámɣit ilqahíra ḥawáali-ḥdáaʃar álfï ṭáalib.

B

1. Give me Cairo 563 please.
2. Ras Gharib is 150 miles (*tr.* at a distance of 150 miles) south of Suez.
3. Yesterday's temperature was 43° Centigrade, that's roughly 109° Fahrenheit.
4. He is due to retire in 1962.
5. I've taken out a life insurance policy for £1,000 (*tr.* I have insured my life for, &c.).
6. It's a big firm, employing not one or two men but hundreds.

LESSON 20

Time; fractions; days and dates

1. The essentials for telling the time are contained in the following:

A. **ſissáaɤa káam?** *What time is it?*

B. **ſissáaɤa tísɤa-w ɤáʃara** *It is 9.10.*

„	„	**-w rúbɤ**	*It is 9.15* (lit. $9\frac{1}{4}$).
„	„	**-w tílt**	*It is 9.20* (lit. $9\frac{1}{3}$).
„	„	**-w nú§§**	*It is 9.30* (lit. $9\frac{1}{2}$).
„	„	**-w nú§§ĭ-w xámsa**	*It is 9.35* (lit. $9\frac{1}{2}+5$).
„	„	**-(ſi)lla rúbɤ**	*It is 8.45* (lit. $9-\frac{1}{4}$).
„	„	**-(ſi)lla tílt**	*It is 8.40* (lit. $9-\frac{1}{3}$).
„	„	**-w nú§§ illa xámsa**	*It is 9.25* (lit. $9\frac{1}{2}-5$).

2. *Fractions*

rubɤ, tilt, and **nu§§** above are examples of a pattern for fractions from one-half to one-tenth. These are:

> **nu§§** (pl. **ſan§áa§** or **ſin§áa§**) $\frac{1}{2}$
> **tilt** (pl. **ſat-** or **ſitláat**) $\frac{1}{3}$
> **rubɤ** (pl. **ſar-** or **ſirbáaɤ**) $\frac{1}{4}$
> **xums** (pl. **ſax-** or **ſixmáas**) $\frac{1}{5}$
> **suds** (pl. **ſas-** or **ſisdáas**) $\frac{1}{6}$

subƹ (pl. **ʕasbáaƹ** or **ʕisbáaƹ**) $\frac{1}{7}$
tumn (pl. **ʕat-** or **ʕitmáan**) $\frac{1}{8}$
tusƹ (pl. **ʕat-** or **ʕitsáaƹ**) $\frac{1}{9}$
ƹuʃr (pl. **ʕaƹ-** or **ʕiƹʃáar**) $\frac{1}{10}$

Notes

(i) With the exceptions of **nuṣṣ** and **suds,** the fractions are directly relatable to the other numeral forms.
(ii) The vowel of the singular is **u** with the exception of **tilt.**
(iii) Notice the regular use of the dual, e.g. **tiltéen** $\frac{2}{3}$, **xumséen** $\frac{2}{5}$, &c.
(iv) Junctions of numeral (3–10)+fraction behave as indicated in Lesson 19, 3, note (ii). Educated speakers tend to prefer, for example, **xámsit ʕasdáas** or **xámas ʕasdáas** $\frac{5}{6}$ to the 'more colloquial' **xámast isdáas.** These forms may be used to illustrate an important principle: what a man says will depend a great deal on the situation in which he says it; the educated Egyptian will most certainly use the form **xámast isdáas** when addressing, say, a fitter.
In numeral + fraction junctions notice the form **írbaƹ** (NOT **irbaaƹ**) in, for example, **tálatt írbaƹ** $\frac{3}{4}$.
(v) When the denominator exceeds 10, the cardinal form is used, preceded by **ƹala,** e.g. **wáaḫid ƹala-ḫḍáaʃar** $\frac{1}{11}$ (lit. 1 on 11), **taláata ƹala ƹiʃriin** $\frac{3}{20}$, **sítta-w xámsa ƹala-ṭnáaʃar** $6\frac{5}{12}$, **ṣantimítr wáaḫid ƹala míyya milmítr** *a centimetre is one hundredth of a metre.*
(vi) Notice the use of the word **qism/ʕaq-** or **ʕiqsáam,** or **guzʕ/ʕagzáaʕ,** *part, portion,* e.g. **ʕilxáṭṭi mitqássim iṭnáaʃar qism** *the line is divided into twelfths,* **qassímu sítt iqsáam** (or **síttit ʕaqsáam**)[1] *Divide it into sixths.*
In similar contexts the plural of **míyya** and **ʕalf** may be used, e.g. **ʕilmaṣṭára mitqassíma-l miyyáat/ʕaláaf** *The ruler is divided into hundredths/thousandths.*

3. *Days and dates*

Notice the special numeral forms in the first five days of the week:

yóom ilḫádd *Sunday*; **yóom litnéen** *Monday*; **yóom ittaláat** *Tuesday*; **yóom lárbaƹ** *Wednesday*; **yóom ilxamíis** *Thursday*; **yóom iggúmƹa** *Friday*; **yóom issábt** *Saturday.*

Note

The article is omitted after **kull** *every,* e.g. **kúlli yóom gúmƹa** *every Friday.*

Practice the use of dates, as **yóom issábt, ʕarbáƹa-w ƹiʃríin**

[1] The bracketed form is more usual in educated speech in which *q* is here pronounced as in 'Classical' Arabic.

máaris, sanat ʕálfï tusǥumíyya wáaḫid wi xamsíin *Saturday,
24th March 1951*. The names of the months which we shall use
are

> **yanáayir** *January*; **fibráayir** *February*; **máaris** *March*;
> **ʕabríil** *April*; **máayu** *May*; **yúnya** *June*; **yúlya** *July*;
> **ʕaγúṣṭuṣ** *August*; **sibtímbir** *September*; **ʕuktóobar** *October*; **nufímbir** *November*; **disímbir** *December*.

You will find a good deal of individual variation in the pronunciation of these names.

EXERCISES

A

1. maqáas issiggáada tálatt imtáar fitnéen wi núṣṣ.
2. ʕiʃʃáhr illi fáat kan baqáali tálat siníin miggáwwiz.
3. ʕilmaṣáaliḫ ilḫukumíyya-btibtídi ǥamálha-ssaǥa tamánya-w núṣṣ.
4. ʕárbaǥt itmáan yisáawu núṣṣ ʕaw tamánya ǥala siṭṭáaʃar.
5. ʕiṭṭayyáara ḫatqúum yom lárbaǥ iggáay issaǥa ǥáʃara-lla rúbǥï masáaʕan.
6. ʃáqqa bilḫágmï da-tkállif ilwáaḫid miyyáat ǥaʃan yifríʃha.

B

1. I was born on 21st September 1921.
2. Wake me at 6.30 sharp and[1] bring me some hot water for shaving.
3. I'm going to the market. I shall be back in half an hour.
4. His pension will be two-thirds of his salary at the date of retirement.[2]
5. You change Centigrade into Fahrenheit by multiplying by[3] $1\frac{4}{5}$ and adding 32 (*tr.* in order to change . . . you multiply by . . . and add . . .).
6. To convert Fahrenheit into Centigrade, subtract 32 and divide by[4] $\frac{9}{5}$.

---

[1] Include *ʕibqa*, i.e. *w-ibqa hátli*, &c. *ʕibqa* is often so used in a succession of imperatives to mark future time; if it is omitted in the present example, then the water should be brought at once. See also Lesson 16, Exercise B, 6.

[2] Translate 'when he retires'.   [3] *fi*.   [4] *ǥala*.

LESSON

Hollow and doubled verbs

1. (a) ʕilkaláam illi qáalu-rráagil maẓbúuṭ   *What the man said is right.*

   (b) ʕiṭṭayyáara ḥatqúum issaɣa tamánya w-iḥna láazim nímʃi min ilbéet issaɣa sítta-w núṣṣ   *The plane is taking off at 8 o'clock and we must leave* (lit. *go from*) *the house at 6.30.*

   (c) nisíit aqúllak innu géh yom ittaláat illi fáat   *I forgot to tell you that he came last Tuesday* (lit. *Tuesday that passed*).

   (d) tiḥibbĭ tíigi wayyáana?   *Do you want to come with us?*

   (e) ḥaṭṭéet ilgawabáat féen?   *Where did you put the letters?*

   (f) fáḍḍi labríiq da-w baɣdéen ṣúbb iʃʃáay!   *Empty that jug and then pour out the tea!*

2. ## Hollow Verbs

ʃaal, yiʃíil *to carry, take away*[1]   raaḥ, yirúuḥ *to go*

		Perfect	Imperfect	Imperative	Perfect	Imperfect	Imperative
Sing.	3rd. pers. masc.	ʃaal	yiʃíil	..	raaḥ	yirúuḥ	..
	3rd. pers. fem.	ʃáalit	tiʃíil	..	ráaḥit	tirúuḥ	..
	2nd. pers. masc.	ʃilt	tiʃíil	ʃiil	ruḥt	tirúuḥ	ruuḥ
	2nd. pers. fem.	ʃílti	tiʃíili	ʃíili	rúḥti	tirúuḥi	rúuḥi
	1st pers.	ʃilt	ʕaʃíil	..	ruḥt	ʕarúuḥ	..
Pl.	3rd. pers.	ʃáalu	yiʃíilu	..	ráaḥu	yirúuḥu	..
	2nd. pers.	ʃíltu	tiʃíilu	ʃíilu	rúḥtu	tirúuḥu	rúuḥu
	1st pers.	ʃílna	niʃíil	..	rúḥna	nirúuḥ	..

naam, yináam *to sleep*   xaaf, yixáaf *to fear*

		Perfect	Imperfect	Imperative	Perfect	Imperfect	Imperative
Sing.	3rd. pers. masc.	naam	yináam	..	xaaf	yixáaf	..
	3rd. pers. fem.	náamit	tináam	..	xáafit	tixáaf	..
	2nd. pers. masc.	nimt	tináam	naam	xuft	tixáaf	xaaf
	2nd. pers. fem.	nímti	tináami	náami	xúfti	tixáafi	xáafi
	1st pers.	nimt	ʕanáam	..	xuft	ʕaxáaf	..
Pl.	3rd. pers.	náamu	yináamu	..	xáafu	yixáafu	..
	2nd. pers.	nímtu	tináamu	náamu	xúftu	tixáafu	xáafu
	1st pers.	nímna	nináam	..	xúfna	nixáaf	..

[1] For tense-affixes in this and following lessons, see Lessons 7 and 8, but disregard reference to the prefix-vowel *u* (Lesson 8).

Notes

1. Hollow verbs are characterized in the perfect (3rd pers. sing. masc.) by the vowel **aa** in lieu of a second radical consonant.
2. The corresponding vowel of the imperfect (and imperative) is usually **ii** (yiʃíil) or **uu** (yirúuḥ), less often **aa** (yináam).
3. When the *imperfect* vowel is **ii** or **uu**, the same vowel (**i** or **u**) appears instead of **aa** in those 5 forms of the *perfect* for which the suffix begins with a consonant,[1] e.g. ʃilt, ʃílti, &c. (cf. yiʃíil), ruḥt, rúḥti, &c. (cf. yirúuḥ). When, however, the imperfect vowel is **aa**, the perfect vowel in these 5 persons may be either **i** or **u** and there is no means of predicting which (cf. **nimt, nímti,** &c. but **xuft, xúfti,** &c., above).
4. Notice that the imperative, derivable as always from the imperfect, has no prefix.

3. Doubled Verbs

ḥabb, yiḥíbb *to like, want*

		Perfect	Imperfect	Imperative
	3rd pers. masc.	ḥabb	yiḥíbb	..
	3rd pers. fem.	ḥábbit	tiḥíbb	
Sing.	2nd pers. masc.	ḥabbéet	tiḥíbb	ḥibb
	2nd pers. fem.	ḥabbéeti	tiḥíbbi	ḥíbbi
	1st pers.	ḥabbéet	ʕaḥíbb	..
	3rd pers.	ḥábbu	yiḥíbbu	..
Pl.	2nd pers.	ḥabbéetu	tiḥíbbu	ḥíbbu
	1st pers.	ḥabbéena	niḥíbb	..

Notes

1. In those 5 forms of the perfect which have been noted above (2, note (3)), the vowel **ee** precedes the suffix consonant.
2. The vowel of the perfect is always **a**, e.g. **ḥabb, ḥaṭṭ** *he put*. The corresponding imperfect vowel may be **i**, e.g. **yiḥíbb**, or **u**, e.g. **yiḥúṭṭ**. If the vowel is **u**, one of the radicals is almost certain to belong to the list given in Lesson 8, 2, note (3).
3. Notice that, as with hollow verbs, the imperative has no prefix.
4. **-at**, not **-e(e)t**, is used in negative forms with the pronominal suffixes, e.g. **ʕana/ʕinta ma ḥabbatúuʃ** *I/you didn't like it.*

EXERCISES

A

1. ráaḥit mínni maḥfáẓti-w ḍayyáʒtï kúll ilmahíyya.
2. lamma tíigi, xúʃʃï ʒala ṭúul, ma-txabbáṭʃï ʒalbáab.
3. ma-tqúlʃï 'míin?' lamma-trúddï ʒattilifóon, qul ísmak ilʕáwwil, ʕáḥsan.
4. dáqq iggáras wilakin ilkahrába káanit maqṭúuʒa.

[1] See Lesson 7, 2.

5. Ṣana síbt issáaɣa-btáχti χalmáktab imbáariḫ, ya gamáaɣa. ma ḫáddïʃ ʃáfha?
6. Ṣilkitáab ráaḫ! Ṣana ḫaṭṭéetu hína-mbáariḫ, ma fíiʃ ʃákk.

B

1. What's the best (tr. most suitable) time to go and see them (tr. I can go, &c.)?
2. Say it slowly so that I can understand.
3. There's a plane leaving at 9.30, getting to Rome at 4.
4. They are very fond of politics and waste their time talking about it.
5. Call in and see[1] the Cashier on your way down.
6. Be quiet and don't answer me back! Go off and see to your work!

LESSON 22

Weak verbs

1. (a) **ma timʃíiʃ χalḫaʃíiʃ, ya wálad!** *Don't walk on the grass, boy!*

 (b) **nisíit afakkáru-nnak gáay innahárḍa** *I forgot to remind him that you were coming today.*

 (c) **laqéet ilwálad míʃi min ɣéer ma yíɣsil iṣṣuḫúun** *I found the boy had gone without washing the dishes.*

 (d) **χammáal aqúllu rúuḫ liggaẓẓáar bádri wi húwwa-byínsa** *I am continually telling him to go to the butcher's early, but he (always) forgets.*

2. **míʃi, yímʃi** *to walk, go*   **ráma, yírmi** *to throw*

		Perfect	Imperfect	Imperative	Perfect	Imperfect	Imperative
Sing.	3rd pers. masc.	míʃi	yímʃi	..	ráma	yírmi	..
	3rd pers. fem.	míʃyit	tímʃi	..	rámit	tírmi	..
	2nd pers. masc.	miʃíit	tímʃi	Ṣímʃi	raméet	tírmi	Ṣírmi
	2nd pers. fem.	miʃíiti	tímʃi	Ṣímʃi	raméeti	tírmi	Ṣírmi
	1st pers.	miʃíit	Ṣámʃi	..	raméet	Ṣármi	..
Pl.	3rd pers.	míʃyu	yímʃu	..	rámu	yírmu	..
	2nd pers.	miʃíitu	tímʃu	Ṣímʃu	raméetu	tírmu	Ṣírmu
	1st pers.	miʃíina	nímʃi	..	raméena	nírmi	..

[1] tr. *fúut χala.* . . .

nísi, yínsa *to forget*   **láqa, yílqa** *to find*

		nísi	yínsa		láqa	yílqa	
	3rd pers. masc.	nísi	yínsa	..	láqa	yílqa	..
	3rd pers. fem.	nísyit	tínsa	..	láqit	tílqa	..
Sing.	2nd pers. masc.	nisíit	tínsa	ʕínsa	laqéet	tílqa	ʕílqa
	2nd pers. fem.	nisíiti	tínsi	ʕínsi	laqéeti	tílqi	ʕílqi
	1st pers.	nisíit	ʕánsa	..	laqéet	ʕálqa	..
	3rd pers.	nísyu	yínsu	..	láqu	yílqu	..
Pl.	2nd pers.	nisíitu	tínsu	ʕínsu	laqéetu	tílqu	ʕílqu
	1st pers.	nisíina	nínsa	..	laqéena	nílqa	..

Notes

1. Verbs of which the 3rd pers. sing. masc. perfect ends in **i** or **a** will be termed 'weak'. Those ending in **-i**, we shall call type (*a*), e.g. **míʃi, nísi**, and those ending **-a** type (*b*), e.g. **ráma, láqa**. The first vowel of type (*a*) is always **i** (**míʃi**), and that of type (*b*) always **a** (**ráma**).

2. In perfect type (*a*), remember that the vowel (**i**) is lengthened when the suffix begins with a consonant. When the suffix begins with a vowel, notice the appearance of **y** (**míʃyit, míʃyu**).

3. The perfect suffixes for type (*b*) are as for the doubled verb (see Lesson 21, 3). Notice that final **-a** is dropped throughout, e.g. **ráma** but **rámit**, &c.

4. As a general rule, if the perfect ends in **-i**, the imperfect ends in **-a**, and vice versa, e.g. **nísi, yínsa, ráma, yírmi.** Learn both tenses together, however, since there are exceptions to the rule, e.g. **míʃi, yímʃi, láqa, yílqa.**

5. **-i** as the imperfect ending is constant throughout the tense with the exceptions of the 2nd and 3rd pers. pl., e.g. **tímʃu, yímʃu** (**-u** is, of course, always associated with these persons).

6. Similarly, **-a** is constant throughout the imperfect with the same exceptions, e.g. **tínsu, yínsu**, and the additional one of the 2nd pers. sing. fem., e.g. **tínsi** (**-i** is, of course, always associated with the 2nd pers. sing. fem.).

7. The imperative can be derived, as always, from the imperfect, this time with **ʕ** prefixed. Note in general that words cannot begin with two consonants in Egyptian Arabic. It is in order to avoid this pattern that **ʕ** + vowel is prefixed. The 'problem' does not arise in the case of hollow and doubled verbs, and **ʕ** is not required (see Lesson 21).

8. Again, as with the doubled verb, **-at**, not **-e(e)t**, appears in negative forms with the pronominal suffixes, e.g. **ʕinta ma kawatúuʃ** *you haven't ironed it.*

3. Etymologically, hollow and what we have called weak verbs are those with **y** or **w** as 2nd and 3rd radical respectively. Verbs with **y** as 1st radical do not occur, while those with **w**, e.g. **wíṣil, yíwṣal** *to arrive*, are regular with two exceptions, viz. **wíqif, yúqaf** *to stop* and **wíqiʒ, yúqaʒ** *to fall*, in which **w** is dropped in the imperfect: i.e.

Imperfect: **yúqaf, túqaf, túqaf, túqafi, ʕáqaf, yúqafu, túqafu, núqaf.**
Imperative: **ʕúqaf, ʕúqafi,   ʕúqafu.**

Note

u in the first syllable is also not according to rule. **i** is, in fact, sometimes heard for **u** in these verbs.

EXERCISES

A

1. baqúllak rúuḥ dilwáqti qabl iggaẓẓáar ma yíqfil.
2. ma tinsáaʃ tigi titɀáʃʃa-mɀáana búkra.
3. rúḥt aʃúufu-mbáariḥ, laqéetu ɀayyáan xáaliṣ.
4. ʕin ma-ʃríbtíʃ iddáwa, miʃ ḥatxíff.
5. baqáalak kam sána-f máṣr?
6. garálku ʕéeh bitzaɀɀáqu[1] wayya báɀḍ?

B

1. I don't think you'll find it (fem.) difficult.
2. Give me the duty slip to sign!
3. Iron this dress again! You haven't done it very well.
4. I can't read Arabic yet, I mean when it's written in the Arabic script (*tr.* with the Arabic letters).
5. He has been in hospital for some time but is getting better[2] now.
6. I'm afraid (*tr.* I'm sorry) I've forgotten to bring it. I must have left it at home.

LESSON 23
Derived forms of the verb

1. (*a*) **fahhímu kullï ḥáaga bittafṣíil qablï ma-tsallímu ʕáyyï ʃúɣl** *Explain everything to him in detail before you give* (lit. *deliver to*) *him any work.*

(*b*) **da suʕáal ana m-aqdárʃ agáawib ɀaléeh** *That is a question I cannot answer.*

(*c*) **ʕaftíkir innu-staqáal min ḥízb ilɀummáal issána-lli fáatit** *I think he resigned from the Labour Party last year.*

(*d*) **wíʃʃu-ḥmárrï milkusúuf** *He* (lit. *his face*) *went red with embarrassment.*

---

[1] Pronounce *bidz-*.
[2] Translate 'his condition is improving'.

2. It is convenient to consider the derived forms as derived from the simple form of the verb. There are essentially two methods of derivation for all verb-types: (i) *internal* modification and (ii) *prefixation*. Some forms show a combination of both. We shall deal with (i) in the present lesson and (ii) in Lessons 24 and 25.

The perfect and imperfect (also imperative) affixes are, of course, applied to all derived forms in the same way as to the simple form.

3. We have to distinguish between *internally* derived forms with

    (i) the 2nd radical doubled, cf. **fáhhim, yifáhhim,** and **sállim, yisállim** in 1 (*a*);

    (ii) **aa** infixed after the 1st radical, cf. **gáawib, yigáawib** in 1 (*b*);

    (iii) **t** infixed after the 1st radical, cf. **ſiftákar, yiftíkir** in 1 (*c*);

    (iv) the 3rd radical doubled, cf. **ſiḥmárr, yiḥmárr** in 1 (*d*).

For purposes of reference in this and the following two lessons, these forms will be labelled '**fáhhim** form', '**gáawib** form', &c.[1]

This preliminary classification does not take into account differences of vowel pattern between simple and derived forms. These differences will be described in detail below.

Notes

1. The **fáhhim** form is easily the commonest of the four.

2. In **ſiftákar** and **ſiḥmárr** forms, **ſi-** is prefixed to avoid the pattern of two consonants initial in the word (see Lesson 22, 2, note (7)), e.g. **ſiſtáɣal, yiſtáɣal** *to work,* **ſixtáar, yixtáar** *to choose, elect,* **ſiſtára, yiſtíri** *to buy,* **ſibyáḍḍ, yibyáḍḍ** *to turn white.*

To form the imperfect, replace **ſi-** by the appropriate imperfect affix (see table at Lesson 8, 2, but disregard reference to the vowel u).

3. The **ſiḥmárr** form is rare, concerns the regular verb only, and relates almost exclusively to colours (cf. however, **ſiḥláww, yiḥláww** *to become sweet*). The perfect suffixes associated with this form are as for the doubled verb (see Lesson 21, 3). Notice that there is no vowel difference between perfect and imperfect.

4. With **fáhhim** and **gáawib** forms, there is no imperative prefix with **ſ** for the reason given in Lesson 22, 2, note (7). For the imperative of the **ſiftákar** form, substitute **ſ** for the initial t of the 2nd pers. imperf., e.g. **ſiſtáɣal/ſiſtáɣali/ſiſtáɣalu** *work!*

5. With the **ſiftákar** form, when the 1st radical is **w, ſiwt-** is pronounced

---

[1] It is perhaps desirable to repeat here that we are only concerned in this book with Egyptian Colloquial Arabic. It should not be considered necessary to employ the traditional classification and nomenclature designed for the very different 'Classical' language (see Introduction).

Ṣitt-, e.g. Ṣittáṣaq, yittífiq *to agree*, Ṣittákal, yittíkil (ɣala) *to rely (on)*. Do not confuse the last example with Ṣittáakil, yittáakil *to be eaten, to be edible* (a derived form of kal, yáakul—see Lesson 10, 2), e.g. ṢilṢáklï dá ma-byittakílʃ *this food is uneatable*.

6. The remaining facts are summarized in the following table:

Regular	Hollow	Doubled	Weak
fáhhim form			
The first vowel is always a, e.g. lábbis, yilábbis *to dress, clothe*. The second vowel is either i or a, génerally a if preceded or followed by one of the consonants listed in Lesson 8, 2, note (3), e.g. náddaf, yináddaf *to clean*	w or y appear as the 2nd radical, and the forms are treated exactly as those of the regular verb, e.g. ḥáwwil, yiḥáwwil *to transfer*, ɣáyyin, yiɣáyyin *to engage, appoint*	Treated exactly as the regular verb, e.g. ḥáddid, yiḥáddid *to limit, fix (appointment)*	The perfect always ends in -a, the imperfect in -i, e.g. wádda, yiwáddi *to move, take away*, fádda, yifáddi *to empty* N.B. In *all* derived forms of the weak verb, the suffix of the 3rd pers. sing. fem. (perfect) is -at, not -it, e.g. wárrat *she showed*, Ṣiddínya ṭárrat *it has turned cool*, Ṣiʃtárat *she bought*
gáawib form			
The second vowel is i and there is again no vowel difference between perfect and imperfect, e.g. qáabil, yiqáabil *to meet*	As for the **fáhhim** form, e.g. gáawib, yigáawib *to answer*	Does not seem to occur	As for the **fáhhim** form, e.g. náada, yináadi *to call*
Ṣiftákar form			
The vowel sequence a–a occurs without exception in the perfect, e.g. Ṣiftákar, Ṣiʃtáɣal, and usually corresponds to i–i in the imperfect, e.g. yiftíkir; yiʃtáɣal is an exception	There is no vowel difference between perfect and imperfect, e.g. Ṣixtáar, yixtáar *to choose*. Unlike the simple form, the vowel. a remains throughout both tenses, e.g. Ṣixtárna *we chose*	As for the **gáawib** form	a–a always occurs for the perfect, invariably corresponding to i–i in the imperfect, e.g. Ṣiʃtára, yiʃtíri *to buy*, Ṣibtáda, yibtídi *to begin*

4. *General note*

Do not assume that the simple form corresponding to a derived form necessarily occurs, or vice versa. Moreover, you cannot take it that there is a foolproof correspondence of meaning between the simple and a derived form or between two derived forms. Thus, the **fáhhim** form above is often causative, e.g. **fáhhim** *he explained, made to understand* (cf. **fíhim** *he understood*), **náḍḍaf** *he cleaned, made clean* (cf. **niḍíif** *clean*), or intensive, e.g. **kássar** *he smashed* (cf. **kásar** *he broke*), but these are by no means the only possibilities and, with other derived forms, such relations are even more difficult to establish. In making your own word-list, therefore, keep as far as possible to the method of Arabic dictionaries, grouping your words according to the radicals of the root, but, as far as verbs are concerned, learn the meaning of each existing form separately. This is best done, moreover, by collecting your words in sentences rather than in isolation.

EXERCISES

A

1. ſilmurúur ɣaṭṭálni. ma-qdírtiſ áagi filmaɣáad.
2. ſana qabílt ilmudíir wi qultílu-lḥikáaya kulláha.
3. ſana-ſtaréetu-b xámas qurúuſ báss.
4. ruḥ wáddi-lwaraqáadi lilſafándi-lli filmáktab illi gámbi.
5. ya ſayyáal, tíqdar tiwaṣṣálni liḥadd irraſíif wi-ḥyáatak?
6. wíſſu-ɡmárrï baɣdï ma géh milbáḥr.

B

1. Smoking is expensive and bad for the health. Why not try to give it up?
2. Unload[1] those things from the lorry and put them in the store.
3. Give my regards to the family, and I hope to see you again soon.[2]
4. He doesn't want you to help him.
5. Do you think he'll show it (fem.) to me?
6. How do you expect them to work for so low a wage?

[1] *názzil.*   [2] Translate 'soon' by *quráyyib táani.*

LESSON 24

Derived forms of the verb (prefix ʕit-)

1. (a) **laqa kúll ilmirábba-tbáaɣit xaláaṣ** *He found all the jam had been sold out.*

(b) **ʕana batkállim ɣarabi-ʃwáyya báss** *I only speak a little Arabic.*

(c) **ma-ɣríftiʃ atnáaqiʃ wayyáah filmasʕála liʕannu káan munfáɣil** *I couldn't discuss the matter with him* (lit. *with him in the matter) since he was very angry.*

2. Derivation by prefix

The prefixes of the derived forms are **ʕit-, ʕin-,** and **ʕista-.** We shall consider **ʕin-** and **ʕista-** in the following lesson.

ʕit-, usually a passive, intransitive or reflexive sign, is prefixed to

(i) the simple form, e.g. **ʕitwágad, yitwígid** *to be found,* **ʕitbáaɣ, yitbáaɣ** *to be sold,* **ʕitɣádd, yitɣádd** *to be counted,* **ʕitnása, yitnísi** *to be forgotten.*

(ii) the **fáhhim** form (Lesson 23), e.g. **ʕitkállim, yitkállim** *to speak,* **ʕithʔáwwil, yithʔáwwil** *to be transferred,* **ʕitɣáyyin, yitɣáyyin** *to be appointed,* **ʕithʔáddid, yithʔáddid** *to be limited,* **ʕitqáwwa, yitqáwwa** *to become strong, improve.*

(iii) the **gáawib** form (Lesson 23), e.g. **ʕitnáaqiʃ, yitnáaqiʃ** *to discuss,* **ʕitgáawib, yitgáawib** *to be answered,* **ʕitráaḍa, yitráaḍa** *to agree, be reconciled.*

Notes

1. The prefix is essentially **t, ʕi-** being required to avoid the pattern of two initial consonants.

2. To form the imperfect, replace **ʕi-** by the appropriate imperfect affix (see table at Lesson 8, 2).

3. To form the imperative, substitute **ʕ** for initial **t** of the 2nd person imperfect forms, e.g. **ʕitkállim/ʕitkallími/ʕitkallímu** *speak!*

4. **ʕit-** forms frequently require an accompanying preposition. There is little difference in meaning between **ʕana kallímtu(h)** and **ʕana-tkallímtï wayyáah** *I spoke to him.*

5. As with *l* of the article, the junction of certain consonants with preceding *t* of the prefix has special implications as to pronunciation. These may be summarized as follows:

ʔit+d = ʔidd-, e.g. ʔiddálaq *it was spilt.*
ʔit+ṭ = ʔiṭṭ-, e.g. ʔiṭṭállaʕ *he peered through* (e.g. *window*).
ʔit+ḍ = ʔiḍḍ-, e.g. ʔiḍḍáffar *it was plaited.*
ʔit+ṣ = ʔiṣṣ-, e.g. ʔiṣṣáwwar *he was photographed.*
ʔit+ẓ = ʔiẓẓ-, e.g. ʔiẓẓábaṭ *he was caught out* (*in wrongdoing*).

ʔit+s = ʔits- or ʔiss-, e.g. ʔitsálax or ʔissálax *it was skinned.*
ʔit+k = ʔitk- or ʔikk-, e.g. ʔitkállim or ʔikkállim *he spoke.*
ʔit+ʃ = ʔitʃ- or ʔiʃʃ-, e.g. ʔitʃáʕlil or ʔiʃʃáʕlil *it flared up* (*fire*).

(*Note.* ʔitʃáʕlil is a quadriliteral verb—see Lesson 25, 5).

ʔit+z = ʔidz- or ʔizz-, e.g. ʔidzáyyit or ʔizzáyyit *it was oiled.*
ʔit+g = ʔidg- or ʔigg-, e.g. ʔidgárah or ʔiggárah *he was wounded.*

ʔit+ɣ = ʔidɣ-, e.g. ʔidɣálab *he was defeated.*

6. The remaining facts are summarized in the following table:

Regular	Hollow	Doubled	Weak
ʔit+simple form			
The vowelling of the perfect is invariably a–a, and that of the imperfect i–i, e.g. ʔitwágad, yitwígid	The vowel a(a) remains throughout the perfect and imperfect, e.g. ʔitbáaʕ, yitbáaʕ	As in the hollow verb, the vowel a remains throughout, e.g. ʔitʕádd, yitʕádd	As in the regular verb, perfect vowelling is always a–a with imperfect i–i, e.g. ʔitnása, yitnísi
ʔit+fáhhim form			
Vowelling is as for the **fáhhim** form (see Lesson 23), e.g. ʔitʕállim, yitʕállim *to learn*, ʔitkássar, yitkássar *to be smashed*			Unlike the **fáhhim** form, there is no vowel difference between perfect and imperfect, e.g. ʔitqáwwa, yitqáwwa *to become strong* (contrast qáwwa, yiqáwwi *to strengthen*)
ʔit+gáawib form			
Vowelling is as for the **gáawib** form (see Lesson 23), e.g. ʔitnáaqiʃ, yitnáaqiʃ, ʔiggáawib, yiggáawib			Unlike the **gáawib** form, there is again no perfect-imperfect vowel difference, e.g. ʔiddáawa, yiddáawa *to be treated, cured* (contrast dáawa, yidáawi *to treat, cure*)

EXERCISES

A

1. huwwa-tmásak w-itságan (or w-ithábas).
2. láazim tiṣṣáwwar ɣaʃan taḥqíiq iʃʃaxṣíyya.
3. Ꜥiddínya bitḍállim¹ bádri fiʃʃíta wi ɣaʃan kída lazim nixállaṣ bi súrɣa.
4. lamma titkállim ɣan ḥádd, xalli báalak, ma-tbalíyʃi filkaláam.
5. Ꜥiggawáab illi kuntĭ-btísꜥal ɣaléeh, Ꜥitwágad.
6. Ꜥilḥáaga-lli zayyídi ma-btitlaqáaʃ bi sahúula.

B

1. How long did it take you to learn this job?
2. He says he has been transferred but I think he has been discharged.
3. At what time do you (pl.) generally have dinner?
4. Do any of you² speak English?
5. Let's go out for a walk! We can talk as we go along.
6. Shall we meet (*tr.* do you like us to meet) on Wednesday morning and (*tr.* in order to) discuss the matter fully then?

LESSON 25

Derived forms of the verb (*concluded*); quadriliteral verbs

1. (*a*) **xud báalak! Ꜥilkubbáaya ḥatúqaɣ wi baɣdéen tinkísir!**
   Look out ! The glass is going to fall and (then) break !

   (*b*) **Ꜥistáfham minnŭhum in kanu gayyíin lilɣáʃa-lleláadi walla láꜥ** *Find out from them if they are coming to dinner tonight or not.*

2. *Prefix* **Ꜥin-**

   Ꜥin- (cf. 1 (*a*)) is prefixed to the simple form only. In theory, the prefixes **Ꜥin-** and **Ꜥit-** (Lesson 24) are interchangeable: thus, both

---

¹ Pronounced *biḍḍállim.*   ² *fiih ḥáddi mĭnku(m),* &c.

ʕitwágad and ʕinwágad, ʕitbáaʒ and ʕinbáaʒ are possible. In practice, however, ʕin- is usually associated with certain verbs and ʕit- with others, e.g. ʕinkásar rather than ʕitkásar and ʕitʒámal *it was done* rather than ʕinʒámal. Nevertheless, for a given verb, you will certainly hear both prefixes from different speakers: in general, it appears that ʕit- is commoner in Cairo than elsewhere.

The vowelling of both ʕin- and ʕit- forms is the same (see Lesson 24, 2, note (6)). Examples are ʕinbáṣaṭ, yinbíṣiṭ *to enjoy oneself*, ʕinbáll, yinbáll *to be wetted*, ʕinḥáka, yinḥíki *to be told, related*.

Note

n before **b** is pronounced **m**, e.g. ʕimbáṣaṭ.

3. *Prefix* ʕista-

ʕista- (cf. 1 (*b*)) is prefixed to the simple form with no vowel between the 1st and 2nd radicals, e.g. ʕistáfham, yistáfham *to inquire*, ʕistáʒmil, yistáʒmil *to use*.

Regular	Hollow	Doubled	Weak
As in the **fáhhim** form (with or without ʕit-), the vowel between the 2nd and 3rd radicals is either **i** or **a** depending on the consonants of the syllable (cf. ʕistáʒmil but ʕistáfham)[1] There is no vowel difference between the perfect and imperfect tenses	**aa** in the perfect corresponds to **ii** in the imperfect, e.g. ʕistaqáal, yistaqíil *to resign* Unlike the simple form, **a(a)** remains throughout the perfect, e.g. ʕistaqált *I/you resigned*	**a** in the perfect usually corresponds to **i** in the imperfect, e.g. ʕistamárr, yistamírr *to continue*, but cf. ʕistaḥáqq, yistaḥáqq *to deserve*	There is no vowel difference between perfect and imperfect, e.g. ʕistákfa, yistákfa *to have enough* It will be noticed that the perfect of *all* derived forms of weak verbs ends in **-a**

[1] ʕistáfhim is also used. ʕistáɣrab, yistáɣrab 'to be surprised' is an example in which *a* is *essential* in the final syllable.

The 'Classical' language distinguishes *a* in the final syllable of the perfect and *i* in the corresponding syllable of the imperfect. Some educated speakers in Cairo insist that they observe a similar distinction in day-to-day colloquial usage, i.e. ʕistáʒmal, yistáʒmil: this is extremely doubtful and may be ignored by the student. The distinction has certainly to be made in other dialects, for example, in the Qena area of Upper Egypt.

4. *Addenda*

(i) There is a prefix ʕa- occurring in a few 'learned' derived forms, e.g. ʕársal, yírsil *to send* (for the typically colloquial báɣat, yíbɣat), ʕafáad, yifíid *to be useful to, to inform*, ʕárḍa, yírḍi *to please, satisfy*. This form is so rare that for practical purposes it may be ignored.

(ii) ʕista- is prefixed to the **fáhhim** form in the common verb ʕistaráyyaḥ, yistaráyyaḥ *to rest*.

5. *Quadriliteral Verbs*

ʕírfaɣ ṣóotak ʃuwáyya, ma-twaʃwíʃʃi-f kaláamak *Speak up* (lit. *raise your voice a little*), *don't whisper* (*in your speech*) !

A large number of Arabic verbs have four radicals in the root: four different ones, e.g. xárbiʃ, yixárbiʃ *to scratch*, láxbaṭ, yiláxbaṭ *to confuse*; the 1st and 3rd, or 3rd and 4th the same, e.g. kárkib, yikárkib *to muddle*, ẓáqṭaṭ, yiẓáqṭaṭ *to be overjoyed*; the same two in the same order in both syllables, e.g. wáʃwiʃ, yiwáʃwiʃ *to whisper*, báṣbaṣ, yibáṣbaṣ *to ogle*.

These verbs follow exactly the pattern of the **fáhhim** form (Lesson 23), the vowel of the second syllable depending on the surrounding consonants.

The only derived form of quadriliteral verbs is with ʕit-, e.g. ʕitláxbaṭ, yitláxbaṭ *to be confused*, ʕitʃáɣlil, yitʃáɣlil *to flare up* (*fire*).

EXERCISES

A

1. ʕistánna! ʕana ɣáawiz atkállim wayyáak ʃuwáyya.
2. ʕiḥna láazim nistaɣíddi lissáfar, ma ɣandináaʃ wáqti-ktíir.
3. ma ḥáddïʃ yistáɣmil maktábi wᴵ-ana ɣáayib.
4. ʕilqáhwa-ndálaqit ɣaṭṭarabéeẓa. hat ḥíttit xírqa-w naʃʃífha.
5. ʕana-nbaṣáṭti gíddan lamma-smíɣt inni ṣiḥḥítu-tḥassínit.
6. ʕilkálbï biyhábhab. yíẓhar innï fih ḥáddï ɣaríib gáay.

ᴵ Notice this use of *wi* 'while'; it will occur again.

B

1. He's resigned because of ill health.[1]
2. How long do we have to wait for you?
3. We are invited out to friends (*tr.* to people our friends) every Friday evening.
4. Every letter is franked before it goes (*tr.* is sent) so that the stamp can't be used again (*tr.* so that no one uses, &c.).
5. Let the men have a rest! It's hot and they've worked hard.
6. Translate this letter into[2] English and let me have it back as soon as possible.

LESSON 26

The imperfect without prefix

1. It will have been noticed from examples in earlier lessons that the imperfect often occurs without the prefixes **bi** or **ḥa.** The most common contexts in which the prefixes are omitted are listed in this and the following lesson. In this lesson we shall deal only with a series of words which may be termed auxiliaries. These may be like

(i) **ɛáawiz** (*or* **ɛáayiz**) or **náawi,** i.e. inflected for gender and number, e.g.

 Sana ɛáawiz áakul   *I want to eat.*

Sissíttï ɛawzáak tirúuḥ lissúuq   *The lady wants you* (masc. sing.) *to go to the market.*

humma nawyíin yiʃúufu-lmudíir   *They intend to see the manager.*

or (ii) **nifs-, bidd-, qaṣd-,** and **ɣáraḍ,** which take a pronominal suffix, e.g.

Sana nífsi Sarúuḥ   *I very much want to go.*

ɛumar bíddu-yráwwaḥ   *Omar would like to go home.*

qaṣdǔhum or ɣaráḍhum yitkallímu-mɛáah   *They are determined to talk to him.*

---

[1] ʃaʃan ṣiḥḥïtu taɣbáana.   [2] li.

Notes

(a) Contrast **nifs-** above with (**bi**) **nafs-** in, e.g. **ʕana-b náfsi ḥarúuḥ** *I will go myself.*

(b) In the junction of **-i** and **ʕa-**, as in **nifsi ʕaruuḥ** above, i and ʕ are usually elided, i.e. **ʕana nífs-arúuḥ** (see Appendix C, 2 (*b*)).

or (iii) **láazim, múmkin,** and **gáayiz** which show a variety of possible forms from the same root in a variety of grammatical constructions.

láazim is an invariable form occurring with and without the pronominal suffixes, while **malzúum** (passive participle form—see Lesson 33) is inflected for gender and number, e.g.

> **láazim arúuḥ**   *I must, ought to go.*
> **lazímn-arúuḥ** (see (ii) note (*b*))   *I need to go.*
> **hiyya malzúuma-trúuḥ**   *She must, is obliged to go.*

Notes

(a) Cf. the impersonal verb **yílzam** *to need*, which in the invariable form of the 3rd pers. sing. masc. imperfect is also used with a following noun, e.g. **yilzámni-flúus** *I need money*, **yilzam káam ginéeh?** *How many pounds are necessary?*

(b) **ʕala** + pronominal suffix is sometimes used for **láazim**, e.g. **ʕaléek tirúuḥ** *You ought to go.* **la búdd,** to be translated *must*, is also frequent.

Both **múmkin** and the impersonal verbal form **yímkin** are invariable and occur with and without a pronominal suffix, e.g.

> **múmkin tiddíini qálamak ʃuwáyya?**   *Could you give me your pen for a moment?*
> **yímkin tiʃúfhum hináak**   *Perhaps you will see them there.*
> **yimkínni-nn-agíilak baʕd ilʕáʃa issaʕa tísʕa**   *I can come to you after dinner at 9 o'clock.*

gáayiz and the verbal form **yigúuz** are also invariable and both require the particle **li** + pronominal suffix, e.g.

> **gayízl-arúuḥ**   *I can (am allowed to) go.*
> **yigúzlak tirúuḥ?**   *Are you allowed to go?*

2. Any of these auxiliaries may be preceded by **kaan, yikúun,**

inflected before ǯáawiz, náawi, and **malzúum**, otherwise invariable, e.g.

> **kuntĭ ǯáawiz arúuḩ**   *I wanted to go.*
> **kuntĭ malzúum(a) arúuḩ**   *I had to go.*
> **kan bídd-arúuḩ**[1]   *I would have liked to go.*
> **kan múmkin(ni) arúuḩ**   *I could have gone.*
> **kan gayízl-arúuḩ**[1]   *I was allowed to go.*
> **kan láazim rúḩt**   *I ought to have gone.*

3. *Negative forms*

bidd-, nifs-, qaṣd-, and **ɣáraḑ** are treated like the verbal forms, taking the 'split' negative **ma -ʃ**, e.g.

> **ma biddúuʃ yiráwwaḩ**   *He would rather not go home.*
> **ma-yguzlákʃ**   *You may not.*

Contrast the use of **muʃ** (or **miʃ**) with the remaining auxiliaries, e.g.

> **muʃ ǯáawiz táakul?**   *Don't you want to eat?*
> **muʃ láazim tirúuḩ**   *You don't have to go.*
> **muʃ múmkin agíilak**   *I cannot come to you.*

When **kaan** is included, it is always **kaan** which takes **ma -ʃ**, e.g.

> **ma kúntĭʃ malzúum tirúuḩ**   *You were not obliged to go.*
> **ma kánʃĭ-ygúzlak**   *You were not able (permitted).*

EXERCISES

A

1. muʃ múmkin áṭlaǯ dilwáqti. lazim axállaṣ iʃʃuɣláadi qablĭ kúllĭ ʃéeʕ.
2. náaw-aṣáyyif fiskindiríyya-ssanáadi.
3. léeh baṭṭáltu-ʃʃúɣl? ɣaráḑku tiǯmílu ʕéeh?
4. ma yimkínʃĭ ḩáddĭ yúdxul min ɣéer tazkára.
5. yimkínn-addíilak xamsa-gnéeh báss.
6. la búddĭ náaxud bálna xáaliṣ.

B

1. I want to book two seats (*tr.* two places) on the first plane next Friday.

---
[1] See Appendix C, 2 (b).

2. Can you show me something different? This isn't quite what I want.

3. You need a really sharp knife to cut that string.

4. I don't want to buy anything, but may I take a look around?

5. I'm sorry I couldn't come yesterday but (*tr.* because) I had to visit my brother in hospital.

6. I should like to learn something of (*tr.* some) local customs. What's the way to go about it (*tr.* what shall I do to learn them)?

LESSON 27

The imperfect without prefix (*cont.*)

The imperfect is also used without prefix:

1. With an imperative sense, often corresponding to 'let . . .' in English (see Lesson 9, 1), e.g.

> **kullĭ wáaḥid yáaxud naṣíibu(h)**   *Let everyone* (or *everyone will*) *take his share.*
>
> **nífriḍ innĭ ɣándak filus kitíir**   (*Let us*) *suppose that you had a lot of money.*
>
> **níxlaṣ milkaláam ilfáariɣ**   *Let us stop talking nonsense* (lit. *let us finish with empty words*).

2. Commonly for verbal forms following the first in a series of imperfects linked by **wi** *and* (see also Lesson 13, 2). The prefix may, however, be included.

> e.g.   **ʕizzetíyya-btistílim izzéet milmaráakib wi (bi)txazzínu fittunúuk**   *The refinery receives the oil from ships and stores it in the tanks.*

3. After a number of common verbs including **qídir, yíqdar** *to be able to*, **ɣírif, yíɣraf** *to know how to*, **ḥabb, yiḥíbb** *to like to*, **xálla, yixálli** *to let, allow to*, **fíḍil, yífḍal** or **qáɣad, yúqɣud** *to continue to*, **ʕibtáda, yibtídi** *to begin to*. These verbs are often themselves used without prefix.

e.g. **(bi)yíɣraf yiɣúum** *He can swim.*

(b)aḩíbb álɣab ilkóora *I like playing football.*

xallíin-aráwwaḩ *Let me go home.*

ʕibtáda yiʃtímni *He started abusing me.*

ḩayifḍálu (or **ḩayuqɣúdu**) **yiʃtáɣalu liḩaddï núṣṣ illéel** *They will carry on working until midnight.*

Note

tann (invariable)+pronominal suffix is sometimes used for the perfect **fíḍil** or **qáɣad**, e.g. **tannŭhum** (or **fíḍlu** or **qáɣadu**) **yiʃtáɣalu liḩaddï núṣṣ illéel** *They carried on working until midnight.*

4. After verbs of motion when a following imperfect gives to the whole a purposive or continuative sense, e.g.

ráaḩ yiʃúuf ilmudíir *He went to see the manager.*

rúuḩ lidduktúur yíkʃif ɣaléek *Go to the doctor for an examination (for him to examine you).*

xárag yígri *He came out running.*

5. After **báɣdï ma** *after*, **qáblï ma** *before*, **lámma** *when*, **wáqtï ma** *at the time that*, **ɣándï ma** *while*, **bádal ma** *instead of*, **min ɣéer ma** *without*, and similar conjunctive particles in sentences containing more than one clause, e.g.

báɣdï ma nitɣáʃʃa, ḩanrúuḩ issínima *We are going to the cinema after having dinner.*

qáblï ma yíwṣal, ḩayiddílhum xábar *He will let them know* (lit. *give them news*) *before he arrives.*[1]

Note

If **ḩa-** is omitted in the last example, it can then be an instruction, i.e. 'he is to let them know, &c.' (see (1) above).

The common linking particle **ɣalaʃáan** or **ɣaʃáan** *in order to* may be included under the same heading, e.g.

bitrúuḩ ilmadrása ɣalaʃáan titɣállim *You go to school to learn.*

6. (*a*) in the 2nd pers. (sing. and pl.), after the 'exhortative'

---

[1] A noun may intervene before **ma**, which is always closely associated with the following verb. See, for example, Lesson 22, Ex. A 1.

particles ʕiyyáak (-ki, -kum), ʕíwɣa (-i, -u—an imperative form)
and ma (see Lesson 13, 3, note (iii)), e.g.

ʕiyyáak tigi wáxri!   *Mind you* (masc. sing.) *don't come late!*
ʕíwɣi-trúuḥi-hnáak!   *Mind you* (fem. sing.) *don't go there!*
ma-trúuḥu-hnáak!   *Why don't you go there, then!*

Notes

(i) Beware of the translation pitfall, cf. ʕíwɣa ma-tgíiʃ *Mind you come!* (not *Mind you don't come!*)
(ii) ʕiyyáak is also used like ʕinʃálla in the sense of *I hope* as in ʕiyyáak tilqáah hináak *I hope you will find him there.*
(iii) Do not confuse ma above with negative ma or the ma of the conjunctive particles in (5).

(*b*) generally in the 1st pers. pl. after yálla or yalla bíina, e.g.

yálla-nrúuḥ nitɣádda   *Let's go and have lunch.*

Note

yálla is used with other persons and is very frequent with a following imperative, e.g. yálla ráwwaḥ *Go home!*, yall-áʃrab *Drink up!*

(*c*) in the negative imperative and ya . . . ya . . . construction
(see Lesson 13).

7. In many greetings formulae (see Appendix A to Part II), e.g.
   ʕin ʃáaʕ alláah tikun ríḥla-kwayyísa   *Bon voyage!* (lit. *If God wills, it will be a pleasant journey*).
   rabbína yiʃfíilak íbnak   *I hope your son gets better* (lit. *may our Lord cure for you your son*).

8. In conjunction with ʕáḥsan and ʕilʕáḥsan *better*, e.g.
   ʕáʃrab máyy-áḥsan   *I would rather drink water* (lit. *I will drink water, (it is) better*).
   núqɣud hín-áḥsan   *We had better stay here.*

EXERCISES

A

1. ma qidrúuʃ yilḥáqu-lqáṭr. wíṣlu mitʕaxxaríin.
2. baɣáttu-ydáwwar ɣalfarráaʃ.
3. bádal ma tíṣrif filúusak ɣadduxxáan, ḥuṭṭáha-f ḥáaga tánya.

4. yalla bíina nitmáʃʃa, ҁawiz agárri dámmi.
5. rúuḩ lirráyyis yiҁarráfak kúllï ḩáaga. ҁána ma ҁandíiʃ ҁaxbáar.
6. xallíih, ҁáḩsan yikun li wáḩdu(h).

B

1. We'd just started working when they interrupted us (*tr.* came
   delayed us).
2. Don't keep on talking so much! Get on with the job!
3. That's enough! We can't possibly[1] use any more (*tr.* more
   than that).
4. Well,[2] if you'll (pl.) excuse me,[3] I must be getting home now.
5. Let's go fishing on Sunday.
6. You'd better go in the evening when it's cooler.

LESSON 28

Conditional sentences; verbal sequences; qaam

1. *Conditional sentences*

There are three conditional particles **ҁíza, ҁin,** and **law,** of
which **ҁíza** is the most frequent. Let us consider the two types of
sentence illustrated in English by

(*a*) 'If you come tomorrow, I will give you the money.'

and

(*b*) 'If you had come yesterday, I would have given you the
money.'

(i) The possibilities in Arabic under (*a*) are as follows:

⎧ **ҁíza kúntï tíigi búkra, ḩaddíilak ilfilúus.**
⎨ **ҁin**　　　,,　　　,,　　　,,　　　,,
⎩ **law**　　　,,　　　,,　　　,,　　　,,

---

[1] Use *ҁábadan.*
[2] *ṭáyyib.*
[3] Use imperative.

⸨ ˤiza géet búkra, ḥaddíilak ilfilúus.
⸨ ˤin   ,,   ,,   ,,
⸨ law   ,,   ,,   ,,

   law tíigi búkra,   ,,   ,,

Notes

1. **kaan**, inflected for person, gender, and number, may be associated with any of the particles. If **kaan** is included, the following verb is in the imperfect; if **kaan** is omitted, the verb is in the perfect but may be in the imperfect following **law**. The most usual practice is to include **kaan** with ˤiza and ˤin, and to omit it after **law**. Notice that the imperfect form **yikúun** is never used after the conditional particles.

2. If **kaan** is included, either **kaan** or the following verb takes **ma -ʃ** of the negative, i.e. either ˤiza ma kúntiʃ tíigi or ˤiza kúntï ma-tgíiʃ, &c.

(ii) In sentences of type (*b*), **kaan** is best included after the particle and is followed by the perfect, i.e.

   ˤiza kúntï géet imbáariḥ, kúnt iddétlak ilfilúus.
   ˤin   ,,   ,,   ,,   ,,
   law   ,,   ,,   ,,   ,,

Notes

1. You may be told by some speakers with a 'Classical bias' that only **law** is possible in this context. In fact, all three particles are currently used.

2. Notice the need for **kaan** in the second clause. In the example given, since the money was not actually handed over, **ḥaddíilak** is possible for ˤiddétlak, i.e. ˤana kúntï ḥaddíilak ilfilúus *I was going to give you the money*. In most contexts, however, the perfect is essential, e.g. ˤiza kúntï géet imbáariḥ, kúntï ʃúftï ɣáli *If you had come yesterday, you would have seen Ali*.

3. Negative forms are as for those under (*a*) above (see (i), note (2)).

4. **law** is often used for greater emphasis and is then sometimes followed by ˤinn (see Lesson 11, 2), e.g. law ˤínnak kúntï géet imbáariḥ, kúntï ḥadárt ilḥáfla *If* ONLY *you had come yesterday, you would have been at the party* (see (ii), note (2) above for ḥadárt).

2. *Verbal sequences*

Verbal forms may sometimes succeed each other in close relation where in translation a linking 'and' or a punctuation device is necessary. This feature is perhaps particularly common with imperatives, of which the following are examples:

   xúd íʃrab   *Take and drink !*
   xúdu-ʃrábu(h)   *Take it and drink it !*

taɣáalu-qɛúdu   *Come* (pl.) *and sit down !*
rúuḥ ráwwaḥ   *Go on home !*
rúuḥ qáblu dilwáqti   *Go and see him now !*

An example of perfect tenses in sequence may be seen in Lesson 27, Exercise B, 1 (**gum ɛaṭṭalúuna**).

3. qaam

The perfect of the verb **qaam, yiqúum** *to stand up* is frequently used as an auxiliary with a following perfect, e.g. **qáam ḍarábni** *he hit me.* The sentence with **qaam** has the force of the somewhat jocular English 'he upped and hit me'. Other examples are:

qúmtĭ nímt   *I went off to bed* or *I fell asleep.*
miʃíit qam ḥáʃni   *I started off but he stopped me.*

qaam is used in a similar way in narratives when it is little more than a device serving to punctuate or mark off incidents as they are related, and can be translated (if at all) by 'then', 'whereupon', &c. It is particularly common in association with **qaal** *he said*, e.g.

géh wi qálli . . . qúmt ana qultĭlu(h) . . . qam irráagil qálli. . . .   *He came and said to me . . . whereupon I said to him . . . then the man said to me. . . .*

EXERCISES

A

1. mumkin áaxud sigáara, law samáḥt?
2. ʕisʕálu-za kan yíqdar yigi[1] búkra walla láʕ.
3. ʕiza-ʃtayáltĭ-kwáyyis, ḥazawwídlak ilmahíyya.
4. ruḥ iɛmílli fingáal[2] qáhwa.
5. ʕúdxul ʃúufu gúwwa walla láʕ.
6. ʕin xallásṭu bádri, tiqdáru-trawwáḥu.

B

1. If we'd left when I wanted to (*tr.* said to you), we'd have been there by now.
2. If you'd asked him, he would have given it to you.

---

[1] See Introduction, B, (c), (i), and Appendix B.
[2] Or *fingdan.*

3. That's far too dear. If you reduce the price, I might buy.

4. It doesn't matter whether they come or not.

5. Ask him if he's married and whether he has any children.

6. I wish[1] I knew whether they were coming or not.

LESSON 29

Comparison of adjectives; colours and physical defects

1. *Comparison of adjectives*

(*a*) **náadi ʃílli̊-f máṣr ʕákbar min náadi-zzetíyya**   *The Shell Club in Cairo is bigger than the Refinery Club.*

(*b*) **ʕiṭṭáqsi̊-kwáyyis ɣan imbáariḣ**   *The weather is better than yesterday.*

(*c*) **ʕissibáaḣa** (or **ʕilɣúum**)[2] **ɣándi ʕahámmi̊ min ittínis**   *I prefer swimming to tennis* (lit. *swimming for me is more important than tennis*).

(*d*) **ʕissagáayir lingilíizi fingiltíra ʕáɣla min máṣr**   *English cigarettes in England are dearer than* (*in*) *Egypt.*

(*e*) **húwwa mitɣállim ʕáktar mínha**   *He is more educated than she is.*

Notes

1. (exx. (*a*) and (*e*)). The comparative pattern is usually that illustrated by **kibíir** *big*—**ʕákbar** *bigger*, **ṣuɣáyyar** *small*—**ʕáṣɣar** *smaller*, **kitíir** *many, much*—**ʕáktar** *more*, &c:

2. (ex. (*c*)). When the 2nd and 3rd radicals are the same, the pattern is that of **xafíif** *light*—**ʕaxáff** *lighter*, **qalíil** *little, few*—**ʕaqáll** *less, fewer*, **ʃidíid** *strong*—**ʕaʃádd** *stronger*, **muhímm** *important* (with prefix **mu-**)—**ʕahámm** *more important*.

3. (ex. (*d*)). Of adjectives ending in **-w** or **-i**, the comparative form ends in **-a**, e.g. **ḣilw** *sweet*—**ʕáḣla** *sweeter*, **ɣáali** *dear, expensive*—**ʕáɣla** *dearer*, **ɣáali** *high*—**ʕáɣla** *higher*.

4. The comparative form is invariable, e.g. **ʕilwálad/ʕilbínt/ʕilwiláad/ ʕilbanáat ákbar** *The boy/girl/boys/girls/ is/are bigger.*

5. **ʕákbar** is to be translated *bigger* or *biggest* according to context. Thus, **ilwálad ilʕákbar** is either *the bigger boy* or *the biggest boy*. Without the article,

---

[1] *ya réet.*

[2] Or *ɣoom.*

however, a comparative-superlative distinction may be marked by position. **wálad ákbar** is *a bigger boy* but **ʕákbar wálad** can only be *the biggest boy*: **ʕilwálad ilʕákbar filwiláad dóol** and **ʕákbar wálad filwiláad dóol** *the biggest among those boys* are variants. Notice the omission of the article when the comparative precedes the noun; we have already encountered this feature with **ʕánhu** (Lesson 15, 8) and shall meet it again with the ordinal numerals (Lesson 30, 2, note (2)).

6. Notice the use of the comparative with a following numeral, e.g. **ʕiddíinákbar wáḥda/ʕitnéen/taláata milburtuqánda** *Give me the biggest one/two/three of those oranges.*

7. Pronominal suffixes may be added to the comparative form, e.g. **ʕayláahum** *the dearest of them.*

8. The particle **min** precedes a second noun or pronoun with which comparison is made (exx. (*a*), (*c*), (*d*), and (*e*)). It is possible but less customary to use the positive form of the adjective followed by the particle **ɣan** (cf. ex. (*b*)), e.g. **ʕilwálad kibíir ɣan ilbínt** for **ʕilwálad ákbar milbínt**.

9. With words having no comparative form, e.g. the participial form **mitɣállim** (see Lesson 33) in ex. (*e*), **ʕáktar** *more* and **ʕaqáll** *less* are used in the example quoted.

2. Colours and physical defects

(*a*) **ʕalwáan iʃʃírka ʕáṣfar w-áḥmar** *The colours of the Company are yellow and red.*

(*b*) **ɣándak ḥaríir ázraq?** *Have you any blue silk?*

(*c*) **lóon ɣenéeh ʕíswid lakin ɣenéen issittǐ-btáɣtu zárqa** *His eyes are* (lit. *the colour of his eyes is*) *black but his wife's eyes are blue.*

Notes

1. Examples of this category form their masculine and feminine singulars and common plurals as follows. Notice that the masculine singular pattern is also that of the comparative with which we have just been concerned.

Masc. sing.	Fem. sing.	Plural		Masc. sing.	Fem. sing.	Plural	
ʕáḥmar	ḥámra	ḥumr	red	ʕáṭraʃ	ṭárʃa	ṭurʃ	deaf
ʕáxḍar	xáḍra	xuḍr	green	ʕáxraṣ	xárṣa	xurṣ	dumb
ʕázraq	zárqa	zurq	blue	ʕáɣrag	ɣárga	ɣurg	lame
ʕáṣfar	ṣáfra	ṣufr	yellow				

2. **w** and **y**, as elsewhere, bring their own special difficulties. It may help in learning separately the following examples to realize that **oo** and **ee** usually correspond to Classical Arabic **aw** and **ay** respectively, and **ii** and **uu** to the pronunciation of **iy** and **uw**:

Masc. sing.	Fem. sing.	Plural		Masc. sing.	Fem. sing.	Plural	
ʕíswid	sóoda	suud	black	ʕáɣwar	ɣóora	ɣuur	one eyed
ʕábyaḍ	béeḍa	biiḍ	white	ʕáɣma	ɣámya	ɣumy	blind

3. The comparative form—as far as it can be distinguished—is regular and,

therefore, identical with the masculine singular. It should preferably be followed by ʒan rather than min, e.g. ʕilḥaʃiiʃ dá ʕáxḍar ʒan dá *This grass is greener than that* (see 1, note (8), above).

EXERCISES

A

1. ʕilʒámal illi ʒamaltúuh innahárḍa ʕáḥsan kitíir min bitaʒ imbáariḥ.
2. ʕinnahárḍa ḥárrĭ-ktíir ʒan imbáariḥ.
3. ʕissákan fi bursaʒíid binnísba-l máṣr, ʕáhda w-árxaṣ.
4. ʕálṭaf ḥáaga ʒamaltăha-nnahárḍa-nnak géet bádri.
5. ʕilqúuṭa dí lissa xáḍra-ʃwáyya, miʃ mistiwíyya.
6. ʕilʒálam ilmáṣri lóonu ʕáxḍar wi-f wúṣṭu-hláal wi tálat nugúum.

B

1. It's easier said than done (*tr.* talking[1] is easier than doing).
2. Do you think it's quicker by rail (*tr.* the journey by the train is quicker) than by road (*tr.* than the car)?
3. I prefer to go by air because it's quicker than anything else.
4. Don't shout as if I were deaf![2]
5. It isn't as hot today as it was yesterday.
6. Have you a cheaper room than the one I'm in at the moment?

LESSON 30

Numerals (*concluded*)

1. *Numeral-noun concord* (*concluded*)

We have seen (Lesson 18) that **wáaḥid/wáḥda** and **ʕitnéen** may follow the noun. This is not true of other numerals unless the article is present. The following examples exhaust the possibilities with and without the article—notice that when the article is included, if the noun precedes the numeral it is always in the plural:

---

[1] ʕilkaláam.
[2] Translate 'as if I were deaf' by *húww-an-áṭraʃ* lit. 'is it that I am deaf?'

talat riggáala	three men	xamasṭáaʃar ráagil	fifteen men
Ɂittálat riggáala	the	Ɂilxamasṭáaʃar ráagil	the
or	three	or	fif-
Ɂirriggáala-ttaláata	men	Ɂirriggáala-lxamasṭáaʃar	teen
			men

Notes

1. If the noun is defined by the article or a pronominal suffix, then a following numeral takes the article, cf. examples above, to which add **banáatu-ttaláata** *his three daughters*. This feature has already been noted with reference to noun-adjective agreement (Lesson 1, 1 and Lesson 6, 1, note (5)).

2. Notice the regular 'feminine' form of **taláata** following the noun (see Lesson 18, 1, note (4)).

2. Ordinals

láazim tirgáɣu-ʃʃúɣl táalit yóom ilɣíid   *You* (pl.) *must return to work on the third day of the feast.*

Notes

1. There is a special ordinal pattern for the numerals 3–10. The fact that the pattern is also that of the active participle of the simple verb-form (see Lesson 33, 2) may help you to remember it.

Masc.	Fem.		Masc.	Fem.	
táalit	tálta	third	sáabiɣ	sábɣa	seventh
ráabiɣ	rábɣa	fourth	táamin	támna	eighth
xáamis	xámsa	fifth	táasiɣ	tásɣa	ninth
sáatit	sátta	sixth	ɣáaʃir	ɣáʃra	tenth

N.B. **sáadis** occurs as a 'learned' form for **sáatit**.

2. The noun with the ordinal is, of course, always singular, but the ordinal may precede or follow. If it follows, then there is the usual agreement with regard both to the article and to gender, e.g. **ráagil táalit** *a third man,* **Ɂirráagil ittáalit** *the third man,* **Ɂissítt ittálta** *the third woman.* As we have seen for **ɣánhu** (Lesson 15, 8) and the comparative form of the adjective (Lesson 29, 1, note (5)), the ordinal may precede the noun with definite reference but without the article. When the ordinal precedes, it is invariable in the masculine form whatever the gender of the noun, e.g. **táalit ráagil** (or **Ɂirráagil ittáalit**) *the third man,* **táalit sítt** (or **Ɂissítt ittálta**) *the third woman.*

3. Like **wáaḥid** and **Ɂitnéen** among the cardinals, so the words for 'first' and 'second' need special notice.

ɣáwwil *first* may precede or follow the noun, e.g. **ɣáwwil fáṣl** or **ɣilfáṣl ilɣáwwil** *the first chapter.* Following the noun, however, the adjective **ɣawwaláani** (with fem. and pl. forms **ɣawwalaníyya** and **ɣawwalaniyyíin**) is used more frequently than **ɣáwwil**, i.e. **ɣilfáṣl ilɣawwaláani, ɣiṣṣáfḥa-lɣawwalaníyya** *the first page.* For the feminine **ɣawwalaníyya, ɣúula** is sometimes heard from educated speakers, i.e. **ɣiṣṣáfḥa-lɣúula.**[1]

[1] You may also hear from such speakers **ɣáwwal** for **ɣáwwil**.

táani (masc.), tánya (fem.) *second,* cf. xúd ittáani ҳalyimíin *take the second on the right,* are also used, together with the plural tanyíin, in the sense of 'other, another', e.g. ҁiddíini waḥid táani *give me another one,* ҁittanyíin féen? *where are the others?* The 'learned' forms ҁáaxar (masc.) and ҁúxra (fem.) are sometimes heard from educated speakers for the more usual táani and tánya in the sense of *other,* e.g. ҁilkitáab ilҁáaxar *the other book.*

ҁáaxar should not be confused with ҁáaxir *last* which behaves like ҁáwwil above, i.e. ҁáaxir fáṣl or ҁilfáṣl ilҁáaxir *the last chapter.* Like ҁawwaláani above, the adjectival forms ҁaxráani, ҁaxraníyya, ҁaxraniyyíin are commoner than ҁáaxir following the noun, i.e. ҁilfáṣl ilҁaxráani, ҁiṣṣáfḥa-lҁaxraníyya. The 'learned' forms ҁaxíir (masc.) and ҁaxíira (fem.) are sometimes heard from educated speakers for the commoner ҁaxráani and ҁaxraníyya.

4. Ordinals from 'eleventh' on have the same shape as the cardinals but are distinguished as ordinals by the facts that (*a*) the numeral always follows the noun and (*b*) the noun is always in the singular, e.g. ҁirráagil ilxamasṭáaʃar *the fifteenth man,* ҁirráagil ilmíyya *the hundredth man,* ҁirráagil ilwáaḥid¦ wi ҳiʃríin *the twenty-first man.* Contrast, therefore, for example, ҁirráagil ilxamasṭáaʃar with the forms under 1 above, i.e.

xamasṭáaʃar ráagil   *fifteen men*
ҁilxamasṭáaʃar ráagil or ҁirriggáala-lxamasṭáaʃar   *the fifteen men*
ҁirráagil ilxamasṭáaʃar   *the fifteenth man*

EXERCISES

A

1. ҁiʃʃáqqa-btaҳítna fiddóor issáatit. xúd ilҁaṣanṣéer.
2. ҁíbni ṭiliҳ ilxáamis fimtiḥáan issanáadi.
3. xud ҁáwwil taḥwíida (*or* ḥáwwid fi ҁáwwil síkka) ҳalaymíinak wi baҳdéen táalit wáḥda ҳala-ʃmáalak.
4. ҁana báqbaḍ mahiyyíti-f ҁáaxir yóom fiʃʃáhr.
5. síibu-lḥiḍáaʃar fáṣl ilҁawwalaniyyíin w-ibtídu min fáṣl iṭnáaʃar.
6. ҁilḥáfla ḥatkúun yom sabaҳṭáaʃar iʃʃáhr illi gáay.

B

1. This is the last time I shall tell you.
2. Where are the twelve pounds I lent you some time ago?
3. This isn't the first time you've told me (*tr.* you tell me) about it.
4. What ought I to say (*tr.* what do you think I shall say) to him when I see him another time?
5. Translate the first thirty lines into English.
6. Take the third on the left, then go straight on and you'll see it (*tr.* you'll find it) after two or three hundred metres.

LESSON 31

Collectives and units

1. (a) **ʕíktib iggawabáat ɣala wáraq ábyaḍ xafíif** *Write the letters on thin, white paper.*

(b) **dáwwar ɣalwáraqa-lli katábtĭ fíiha miswáddit iggawáab** *Look for the sheet on which I wrote the draft letter.*

(c) **ʕiggawáab illi géh min lándan kan min tálat waraqáat** *The letter from London had* (lit. *was of*) *three sheets.*

(d) **ʕiṣṣufrági qáddim lína béeḍ lilfuṭúur. káltĭ mínhum béeḍa wáḥda, wi ṣáḥbi kal tálat beḍáat, wi fíḍil baɣdĭ kída beḍtéen**[1] *The waiter brought us eggs for breakfast. I ate one of them, my friend ate three, and there still remained two after that.*

Notes

1. Certain nouns are distinguished from others by the fact that the suffix **-a** or **-aaya** is added to them to form what may be called the 'unit-noun', i.e. one or a piece of a larger whole, cf. **wáraq** and **wáraqa** in (a) and (b) above. These collective nouns are further marked off by the fact that, following a numeral from 3 to 10, they have a plural form in **-aat**, cf. **waraqáat** in (c). The collective form is used, for example, after **ʃuwáyya** *a little* and before **kitíir** *a lot* when other nouns require a plural of the types illustrated in Lessons 4 and 32, e.g. **ʃuwáyyit wáraq** *a little paper*, **wáraq kitíir** *a lot of paper*, but **ʃuwáyyit biyúut** *a few houses*, **biyúut kitíir** *a lot of houses*.

2. The dual is formed from the unit-form (cf. (d) above and, e.g. **waraqtéen** *two sheets* (or *pieces*) *of paper*).

3. Notice that the pronoun referring to a collective is usually in the plural, cf. **mínhum** in (d) above, but an accompanying adjective, verb, &c., is in the singular, e.g. **wáraq kuwáyyis** *good paper*.

4. There are also, for certain collectives, related 'broken' plural forms, e.g. **ʃágar** (coll.) *trees*, **ʕaʃgáar** *different kinds of trees* (cf. **ʃágara** *a tree*, **ʃagaráat** *trees (3–10)*); also **ʕawráaq** *papers*. Such plurals are comparatively rare.

5. Other examples of collectives are:

Collective	Unit	Counted (3–10)
xoox *peaches*	**xóoxa** *a peach*	**xoxáat** *peaches*
lamúun *lemons*	**lamúuna** *a lemon*	**lamunáat** *lemons*
burtuqáan *oranges*	**burtuqáana** *an orange*	**burtuqanáat** *oranges*
figl *radishes*	**fígla** *a radish*	**figláat** *radishes*

[1] Pronounced **beṭtéen**.

Collective		Unit		Counted (3–10)	
báṣal	onions	báṣala or baṣaláaya an onion		baṣaláat	onions
gáẓar[1]	carrots	gáẓara or gaẓaráaya a carrot		gaẓaráat	carrots
baṭáaṭiṣ	potatoes	baṭaṭṣáaya a potato		baṭaṭṣáat	potatoes
míʃmiʃ	apricots	miʃmíʃa or miʃmiʃáaya an apricot		miʃmiʃáat	apricots
mooz	bananas	móoza or mozáaya a banana		mozáat	bananas
qúuṭa	tomatoes	quṭáaya a tomato		quṭáat or quṭayáat tomatoes	

6. Many verbal nouns of the simple form of the verb (see Lesson 35) are treated similarly to collectives, i.e. with -a and -aat added to the 'basic' form; e.g. ḍarb *hitting*, ḍárba *a blow*, ḍarbáat *blows (3–10)*.

2. Certain other nouns, also considered collectives, are not treated as under 1 above. This second type requires one of a series of special words for unit-reference, the latter varying with the collective they accompany. For the 'counted' form the plural of the special word is used followed by the collective. Examples are:

Collective		Unit		Counted (3–10)	
ʒínab	grapes	ḥabbáayit ʒínab[2] a grape		ḥabbáat ʒínab	grapes
faṣúlya	beans	ḥabbáayit faṣúlya a bean		ḥabbáat faṣúlya	beans
bisílla	peas	ḥabbáayit bisílla a pea		ḥabbáat bisílla	peas
qamḥ	wheat	ḥabbáayit qámḥ a grain of wheat		ḥabbáat qámḥ	grains of wheat
súkkar	sugar	ḥíttit súkkar a lump of sugar		ḥítat súkkar	lumps of sugar
láḥma	meat	ḥíttit láḥma a piece or slice of meat		ḥítat láḥma	pieces or slices of meat
ʒeeʃ	bread	lúqmit ʒéeʃ a piece or slice of bread		lúqam ʒéeʃ	pieces or slices of bread
toom	garlic	ráas tóom a garlic plant		rúus tóom	garlic plants

Notes

1. In some parts of the country, e.g. Upper Egypt, ḥábba is used for ḥabbáaya. In Cairo, ḥábba is sometimes used in the sense of 'handful, little'.

2. The dual is, of course, formed on the 'special' word, e.g. ḥittitéen súkkar, raséen tóom.

3. In country districts raas is used with báṣal and gáẓar.

4. ṣubáaʒ (pl. ṣawáabiʒ) lit. *finger* is sometimes used with mooz (see 1, note (5)), i.e. ṣubáaʒ móoz *a banana*, xámas ṣawáabiʒ móoz *five bananas*.

5. For things commonly occurring in pairs, fárda (pl. fírad) is used for reference to one, e.g. fárdit ʃaráab *one sock*, fárdit gázma *one shoe*, fárdit guwánti *one glove*. The plural fírad as in síttï fírad ʃarabáat *six socks* is rarely used thus.

¹ See Introduction, B (ii).
² ʒínaba may be heard.

EXERCISES

A

1. yímkin yikun fíh lamúun fissúuq búkra.
2. wíqqit ilburtuqáan innahárḍa-b xámsa sáaɣ.
3. ʕana miḥtáag li ráṭlĭ láḥma kullĭ yóom.
4. ʕiddíini ḥittit súkkar ziyáada min fáḍlak.
5. wíqqit ilmóoz bitíṭlaɣ ɣáʃar ṣawáabiɣ mutawaṣṣiṭíin (or wáṣaṭ).
6. yilzámna-rɣiféen ɣeʃ afrángi kúllĭ yóom.

B

1. How are you going to make soup without meat or vegetables?
2. I'm not going to pay that price for[1] potatoes.
3. How much are these oranges each (*tr.* one of these oranges), and how much an oke?
4. There are roughly five bananas to half an oke (*tr.* five bananas come (to) half, &c.).
5. One of my socks is missing. Find out[2] from the laundry (*tr.* laundryman) if they still have it.
6. If you look under those papers, I think you'll find it.

LESSON 32

Number (broken plural patterns)

1. (*a*) **ʕilburtuqáan ɣand ilfakaháani-b kúll ilʕatmáan** (or **ʕasɣáar) ilmuxtálifa** *The fruiterer has oranges at various prices.*

(*b*) **ʕiṣṣuḥúun muxtálifa filḥágm** *The plates are of different sizes.*

(*c*) **ʕúwaḍ innóom miḥtáaga-l tartíib** *The bedrooms want tidying.*

(*d*) **ɣummáal izzetíyya-byiʃtáɣalu min issáaɣa sítta ṣabáaḥan** *The refinery workmen work from 6 a.m.*

---

[1] *fi.*   [2] *ʕisʕal.*

(e) **fih maráakib kitíir filmíina-nnahárɖa** *There are a lot of ships in the harbour today.*

(f) **ʕilmanadíil iṣṣuɣayyára-btaɤt issítt, líssa ma ɣasalháaʃ ilmakwági** *The laundryman hasn't yet washed the mistress's small handkerchiefs.*

Broken plural patterns are very numerous and we shall list only the most frequent. Moreover, although there is considerable regularity of correspondence between singular and plural patterns, it is not always possible to forecast from singular to plural or vice versa. You should, therefore, learn both the singular and plural of nouns and adjectives as you meet them. In most cases you will find you can arrive at the plural form by taking into account the syllable structure and the vowelling of the singular.

The commonest plural patterns are as follows (C = consonant):

(i) **ʕaCCáaC** and **ʕiCCáaC: qálam, ʕiqláam** *pen/s, pencil/s*, **ḥiml, ʕiḥmáal** *load/s*, **ʃakl, ʕaʃkáal** *shape/s*, **suuq, ʕaswáaq** *market/s*, **biir, ʕabyáar** *well/s*, **loon, ʕalwáan** *colour/s.*

Note

Some plurals, e.g. **ʕayyáam** *days*, **ʕafráan** *ovens*, have **a** in the first syllable when initial or in isolation, but usually **i** when in close grammatical relation with a preceding noun or particle, e.g. **ʕayyáam ilʕusbúuɤ** *the days of the week* but **liyyáam** *the days*. **ʕilʕayyáam** is possible for **liyyáam** and is perhaps commoner among educated speakers; see also Lesson 19, 3, note (ii) and Lesson 20, 2, notes (iv) and (vi).

(ii) **CuCúuC** and **CiCúuC: ṣaḥn, ṣuḥúun** *plate/s, saucer/s*, **xadd, xudúud** *cheek/s*, **beet, biyúut** or **buyúut** *house/s.*

(iii) **CíCaC** and **CúCaC: ɤílba, ɤílab** *(small) box/-es*, **ɤúmda, ɤúmad** *headman/-men*, **ʃánṭa, ʃúnaṭ** *bag/s, briefcase/s*, **kóora, kúwar** *ball/s*, **ríiʃa, ríyaʃ** *quill/s*, **ṣúura, ṣúwar** *picture/s*, **ʕóoɖa, ʕúwaɖ** *room/s.*

(iv) **CuCáaC: kibíir, kubáar** *big*, **ṭawíil, ṭuwáal** *long, tall*, **ɤaríiɖ, ɤuráaɖ** *broad.*

Note

This is the pattern of a number of common adjectives, with the feminine singular formed in the usual way with **-a** and the plural of common gender.

(v) CuCCáaC: ʒáamil, ʒummáal *workman/-men*, táagir,
tuggáar *merchant/s*, ʃáaṭir, ʃuṭṭáar *clever*.

Note

Nouns and adjectives of this pattern refer to human beings. The singular
form is as that of the active participle of the simple verb-form (Lesson 33, 2).

(vi) CúCaCa: ʃaríik, ʃúraka *partner/s*, xaṭíib, xúṭaba
orator/s, ʃaqíiq, ʃúqaqa *blood brother/s*.

Note

This pattern, referring solely to human beings, is of nouns only: contrast (iv).
The plural pattern CuCaCáaʕ, e.g. xuṭabáaʕ, is sometimes used by educated
speakers.

(vii) CaCáaCi: ʃamsíyya, ʃamáasi *parasol/s*, ṣiníyya,
ṣawáani *tray/s*, kúrsi, karáasi *chair/s*, ʃákwa,
ʃakáawi *complaint/s*.

(viii) ʕaCCíCa and ʕiCCíCa: suʕáal, ʕasʕíla *question/s*, gawáab,
ʕagwíba *answer/s* (contrast gawáab, gawabáat
letter/s), sábat, ʕisbíta *basket/s*.

(ix) CaCáaCiC: máktab, makáatib *office/s*, *desk/s*, gárdal,
garáadil *bucket/s*, márkib, maráakib *ship/s*, fulúuka,
faláayik (*small*) *sailing-boat/s*, bihíima, baháayim
animal/s, sitáara, satáayir *curtain/s*, ʕizáaza, ʕazáayiz
bottle/s, ginéena, ganáayin *garden/s*.

Note

See note to (x).

(x) CaCaCííC: fingáal (or fingáan), fanagíil (or fanagíin)
cup/s, xanzíir, xanazíir *pig/s*, mandíil, manadíil
handkerchief/s, ṭarbúuʃ, ṭarabíiʃ *tarboosh/-es*, fanúus,
fawaníis *lamp/s*, niʃáan, nayaʃíin *medal/s, decoration/s*.

Note

Any singular pattern containing 4 consonants corresponds to one of the plural
patterns (ix) or (x), depending on the length of the vowel between the 3rd and
4th consonants of the singular, viz. short vowel—(ix), long vowel—(x). Notice
that singulars of 3 consonants with a long vowel between the 2nd and 3rd, and
with the ending -a, correspond to plurals of pattern (ix).

2. *Addenda*

(i) A few nouns form their plural by the straightforward addition of a suffix **-aan**, e.g. **ḥeeṭ, ḥeṭáan** *wall/s*, **ɣeeṭ, ɣeṭáan** *field/s*. This suffix also appears in certain broken plural patterns, e.g. **faar, firáan** *mouse/mice*, **gaar, giráan** *neighbour/s*, **toor, tiráan** *bull/s*, **ɣazáal, ɣizláan** *gazelle/s*, **xarúuf, xirfáan** *ram/s*, **fáaris, firsáan** *horseman/-men*, **qamíiṣ, qumṣáan** *shirt/s*.

(ii) The following are examples of nouns for which the type of singular-plural relationship is comparatively rare and not included above: **raas, ruus** *head/s*, **sána, siníin** or **sanawáat** *year/s*, **kitáab, kútub** *book/s*, **madíina, múdun** *city/-ies*, **gámal, gimáal** (a fairly common pattern) *camel/s*, **gábal, gibáal** *mountain/s*, **wálad, wiláad** or **ʕawláad** *boy/s*, **saṭḥ, ʕúṣṭuḥ** or **ṣuṭúuḥ** *roof/s*, **saqf, ʕúsquf** *ceiling/s*, **ráagil, riggáala** *man/men*, **duktúur, dakátra** *doctor/s*, **túrki, tarákwa**[1] *Turk/s*.

(iii) Nouns of relationship are often of special shape and should be learned separately. The most important are **ʕabb, ʕabbaháat** *father/s*, **ʕumm, ʕumma-háat** *mother/s*, **ʕaxx, ʕixwáat** *brother/s*, **ʕuxt, ʕixwáat** *sister/s*, **ʕibn, ʕabnáaʕ** *son/s*, **bint, banáat** *daughter/s*, **ɣamm, ɣaɣmáam** (*paternal*) *uncle/s*, **ɣámma, ɣammáat** (*paternal*) *aunt/s*, **xaal, xiláan** (*maternal*) *uncle/s*, **xáala, xaláat** (*maternal*) *aunt/s*, **gidd, gudúud** *grandfather/s*, **gídda, giddáat** *grandmother/s*. Note **ʕíbnǐ ɣámm/xáal** (*male*) *cousin* (lit. *the son of an uncle*) and **bíntǐ ɣámm/ xáal** (*female*) *cousin*.

(iv) Notice that in some cases a given singular form may correspond to more than one plural, e.g. **másal** *proverb, saying*; *example*, **ʕamsáal** *proverbs*, **ʕamsíla** *examples*, **líɣba** *game*; *toy*, **ʕalɣáab** *games*, **líɣab** *toys*.

EXERCISES

A

1. ma baqáaʃ fawáakih fissúuq. xílṣit xáaliṣ.
2. ʕilʕóoda ma fiháaʃ ʃababíik kifáaya ɣaʃan ittahwíya.
3. lazim tizáakir ilʕamsíla-kwáyyis ɣaʃan tífham.
4. ma titʕaxxárʃǐ búkra, ḥaykúun ɣandǐna-dyúuf.
5. ʕisbáqni biʃʃúnaṭ ɣalmaḥáṭṭa. ʕana ḥalḥáqak ḥáalan.
6. baqáali sitt úʃhur (*or* sittǐ-ʃhúur) ma ʃuftúuʃ, raḥ féen?

B

1. I'd like to see[2] some cheap cigarette boxes.
2. I've some very attractive ivory-inlaid ones.
3. You must be careful of sandstorms in the desert (*tr.* which arise in the desert) at this time of year (*tr.* these days).
4. That's only for rich people, not for poor folk like us.[3]
5. Can you give me the names for the parts of a car?

[1] More commonly ʕatráak.   [2] ʕatfárrag.
[3] zayyǐ ḥalátna.

6. Eye diseases are very widespread in Egypt. For this reason many Egyptian doctors are eye-specialists.[1]

LESSON 33

Participles

1. (a) ʕad-ínta ʃáayif illi ḥáṣal   *But you see* (or *have seen*) *what happened.*

(b) huwwa ráayiḥ yiʃúufu dilwáqti   *He is going to see him now.*

(c) ʃúft iʃʃibbáak maftúuḥ   *I saw the window (was) open.*

(d) ʕana-mnaḍḍáfu-nnahárḍa   *I have cleaned it today.*

(e) humma sakníin fi béet mitráttib kuwáyyis   *They live in a well-appointed house.*

(f) ʕana laqéetu-mgáawib ɣaléeh   *I found he had answered it.*

(g) ʕana laqéetu mitgáawib ɣaléeh   *I found it had been answered.*

(h) ʕana mistaɣmílha min zamáan   *I have used* (or *been using*) *it* (fem.) *for a long time.*

(i) ʕilwálad muxxu mitláxbaṭ innahárḍa, muʃ ɣáarif (or qáadir) yiʃtáɣal   *The boy's mind is topsy-turvy today, he can't* (lit. *doesn't know how to*) *do his work.*

2. *Simple form of the verb*

The simple form of the verb has both an active and a passive participle.

(a) In the active participle pattern, **aa** follows the 1st consonant and **i** the 2nd, e.g. ɣáarif (cf. 1 (i)). **y** appears as the 2nd consonant of hollow verb participles (cf. ʃáayif in 1 (a)). ḥáaṭiṭ illustrates the participle of a doubled verb (ḥaṭṭ, yiḥúṭṭ *to put*). Notice the participial form of weak verbs, e.g. máaʃi.

(b) The passive participle is characterized by a prefix **ma-** and

---

[1] *mutaxaṣṣaṣíin f-amrááḍ ilɣiyúun.*

the vowel **uu** infixed between the 2nd and 3rd consonants, e.g. **maftúuḥ** (1 (c)), **maſdúud** *pulled*. The weak verb is again exceptional, ending in **-i**, e.g. **mánsi** *forgotten*, **mármi** *thrown*. There is no passive participle of the hollow verb (simple form), cf. **minbáaɣ** or **mitbáaɣ** *sold* which are the participles of the derived **ſin-** or **ſitbáaɣ, yin-** or **yitbáaɣ** *to be sold* (cf. **baaɣ, yibíiɣ** *to sell*).

(c) Both participles are inflected for gender and number (see Lessons 3 and 4), e.g. **sáakin/sákna/sakníin** (cf. 1 (e)), **ḥáatiṭ/ḥátta/ḥaṭṭíin, máaſi/máſya/maſyíin** (see Lesson 22, 2, note (2)), **maftúuḥ/maftúuḥa/maftuḥíin, mánsi/mansíyya/mansiyyíin** (see Lesson 3, 1, note (4)).

Notes

  (i) Final **a** of the feminine form is, of course, lengthened when a suffix beginning with a consonant is added, e.g. **híyya maskáah** *she is holding it*, **di mafṣuláali-b sítta-gnéeh** *this was sold to me (after bargaining) for £6*.
  (ii) The verbal suffix **-ni** (not **-i**) of the 1st pers. sing. is used with the participle, e.g. **híyya maskáani** *she is holding me*.

(d) The active participle may sometimes require a 'passive' translation, e.g. **ſilbaqqáal qáafil** *the greengrocer('s) is closed*, cf. **ſiddukkáan maqfúul** *the shop is closed*. A more literal translation of **ſilbaqqáal qáafil** is *the greengrocer HAS closed* (see Lesson 34, 1).

3. *Derived forms of the verb*

Derived forms usually have one participial form only (see, however, (d) below).

(a) Generally speaking, the participle may be formed by substituting **m** for **y** of the 3rd pers. sing. masc. imperfect, e.g. **mitrími** (**ſitráma, yitrími** *to be thrown*), **mináḍḍaf** (**náḍḍaf, yináḍḍaf** *to clean*), **mixálli** (**xálla, yixálli** *to let, allow*), **mitnáḍḍaf** (**ſitnáḍḍaf, yitnáḍḍaf** *to be cleaned*), **migáawib** (**gáawib, yigáawib** *to answer*), **mitgáawib** (**ſitgáawib, yitgáawib** *to be answered*), **mixtílif** (**ſixtálaf, yixtílif** *to differ*), **mixtáar** (**ſixtáar, yixtáar** *to choose*), **minkább** or **mitkább** (**ſin-** or **ſitkább, yin-** or **yitkább** *to be poured*), **minbáaɣ** or **mitbáaɣ** (**ſin-** or **ſitbáaɣ, yin-** or **yitbáaɣ** *to be sold*).

Additional observations, however, are necessary for

   (i) some forms of the weak verb, of which the participle—
       unlike the imperfect—ends in **-i**, e.g. **mitxálli** (**ʕitxálla,
       yitxálla** *to leave, withdraw*), **mitráaḍi** (**ʕitráaḍa,
       yitráaḍa** *to be placated, come to an agreement*), **mistákfi**
       (**ʕistákfa, yistákfa** *to be satisfied, have enough*);

  (ii) the 'colour' verbs (see Lesson 23, 3, note (3)), of which the
       participle has the vowel **i** in the second syllable, e.g.
       miḥmírr (**ʕiḥmárr, yiḥmárr** *to turn red, blush*);

 (iii) the derived form with **ʕista-**, of which the participial
       prefix **musta-**, i.e. with the vowel **u**, is often preferred by
       educated speakers to **mista-**, e.g. **musta-** or **mistáɣlim**
       (**ʕistáɣlim, yistáɣlim** *to inquire*), **musta-** or **mistábʃar**
       (**ʕistábʃar, yistábʃar** *to have good news, be optimistic*),
       musta- or **mistaɣídd** (**ʕistaɣádd, yistaɣídd** *to be ready
       (of persons)*).

(*b*) (i) The passive participle of the simple form is generally pre-
       ferred to the participle of the derived forms with **ʕit** or
       ʕin + simple form, e.g. **mármi** *thrown* rather than
       mitrími, makbúub *poured* rather than **mitkább** or
       minkább.

  (ii) In some contexts, there is little difference between the use
       of a passive participle and the perfect tense of the derived
       forms with **ʕit** or **ʕin**, e.g. **ʕana qabílt innaggáar wi
       qálli maktábak maɣmúul** (or **itɣámal**) *I met the car-
       penter and he told me your desk has been made.* Contrast,
       however, **maftúuḥ** in 1 (*c*) above with **ʃúft iʃʃibbáak
       infátaḥ** *I saw the window open* (i.e. *by itself*).

(*c*) Since **ʕit-** is usually a passive prefix, the participles of the
fahhim- and **gaawib-**forms (see Lesson 23, 3) may be considered
'active', the corresponding **ʕit-** forms providing the 'passive' participles, e.g. **mináḍḍaf** (active)—**mitnáḍḍaf** (passive) *cleaned*,
migáawib (active)—**mitgáawib** (passive) *answered* (cf. 1 (*f*) and
(*g*)). Cf. the quadriliteral **miláxbaṭ**—**mitláxbaṭ** *confused* (ex. 1 (i)).

(*d*) In 'Classical' Arabic, derived forms of the verb have both
an active participle (**i** in the final syllable) and a passive participle

(a in the final syllable). In the Egyptian colloquial, this distinction is maintained by educated speakers for certain **musta-** participles. **mustáɣmir** *colonist* and **mustáɣmar** *colonized*, though 'learned', are both in current use. Compare, too, **da-ktáab mistáɣmil** (or **mustáɣmil**) *this is a second-hand book* and **ʕilkitáab dá mustáɣmal kitíir** *this book is used a lot*. Notice that in the case of **mustáɣmal**, **musta-** (not **mista-**) is obligatory, a further sign of the learned nature of the word. Usage, however, is not always fixed, and you will encounter individual variation.

(*e*) The 'Classical' form is used by educated speakers for some participles of other than the **ʕista-** form, e.g. **muxtálif** for **mixtílif**, **munfáɣil** for **minfíɣil**, **mutaʃákkir** for **mitʃákkir** *thank you*, **mutawáʂʂiṭ** for **mitwáʂʂaṭ**. The use of 'learned' participial forms characterizes *educated* colloquial more than any other single factor. Notice, too, in colloquial usage such contrasts as **miɣállim** (participle of **ɣállim, yiɣállim**) and **muɣállim** *teacher*, **mifáttiʃ** (participle of **fáttiʃ, yifáttiʃ** *to inspect*) and **mufáttiʃ** *inspector*.

EXERCISES

A

1. ʕana mistanníik baqáali saɣtéen.
2. huwwa middíini kílma-nnu gáay.
3. ʕana laqéetu náayim, ma-qdírtiʃ aʂaḥḥíih.
4. ma-tsíbʃ ilbáab maftúuḥ lamma túxrug.
5. maḥkúum ɣaléeh bissígni tálat ʃuhúur ɣaʃan issírqa.
6. ʕana badáwwar ɣalmaɣáaliq ilmaṭlíyya bilfáḍḍa. humma féen?

B

1. He's been sitting there for an hour.
2. There are special letter-boxes marked 'Urgent'.
3. I don't know how to explain it (fem.) to you.
4. The teacher is prepared to help you as much as[1] he can.
5. Here, take it! You need it more than I do. But look after it!
6. I wonder (*tr.* I don't know) where it can be! I saw it hanging behind the door this morning.

---

[1] ɣala qáddi ma.

LESSON 34

Use of the (active) participle

1. The participle is nominal in form with no distinction of person. It is possible, therefore, to consider **káatib iggawáab** in the sentence **huwwa káatib iggawáab** as a sequence of two nouns in the construct and translate *he is the writer of the letter*. But the participle of many verbs (e.g. **kátab, yíktib**) may be said to refer to the state of having performed the verbal action. In the appropriate context the translation of **huwwa káatib iggawáab** is *he has written the letter*. Other verbs, for example, verbs of motion, behave differently from **kátab, yíktib** and it is not surprising that translation in English will often take different forms. Notice that the following examples with the participle are of the typical nominal sentence pattern, completed by the initial pronoun.

> **huwwa ɣáarif ʃúɣlu-kwáyyis** *He knows* (i.e. *has learned*) *his job well.* (Both **yíɣraf** and **biyíɣraf** are possible here for **ɣáarif.**)
>
> **hiyya-mnaḍḍáfa-lʕóoḍa** *She has cleaned the room.* (Cf. **bitnáḍḍaf ilʕóoḍa** *She is cleaning the room.*)
>
> **huwwa ráakib ilḥuṣáan** *He is riding* (i.e. *has mounted*) *the horse.* (Cf. **biyírkab ilḥuṣáan** *He is mounting the horse.*)
>
> **ʕana wáakil** *I have eaten, am full.*
>
> **ʕana-mráhnak (= miráahin+ak)**
> **ʕana mitráahin wayyáak** } *I have bet you.*
>
> **ʕana-mráttib ilhudúum** *I have arranged the clothes.*

There is no past-time sense with verbs of motion in the following examples:

> **huwwa ṭáaliɣ baɣdi-ʃwáyya** *He will be coming out soon.* (**ḥa-**, i.e. **ḥayíṭlaɣ**, is possible here and in the following two examples.)
>
> **ʕana-msáafir búkra** *I am travelling (leaving) tomorrow.*
>
> **huwwa náazil dúɣri** *He will be (coming) down right away.*

Past reference may also be absent in negative forms with **muʃ** or **miʃ**, e.g.

ʔana miʃ wáakil   *I am not going to eat* (or *I have not eaten*).

hiyya míʃ minaḍḍáfa-lḥóoḍa   *She is not going to clean the room* (or *she has not cleaned the room*).

Compare the tenses and the participle in the following:

ʃúftu xáarig milbéet   *I saw him coming out of the house.*

ʃúftu xárag milbéet   *I saw him come out of the house.*

ʃúftu biyúxrug milbéet (kullï yóom)   *I have seen him come* (or *coming*) *out of the house* (*every day*).

ʃúftu ḥayúxrug milbéet   *I saw him about to come out of the house.*

and contrast

laqéetu káatib iggawáab   *I found he had written the letter.*

laqéetu kátab iggawáab   *I found he had written the letter.*

laqéetu-byíktib iggawáab   *I found him writing the letter.*

laqéetu ḥayíktib iggawáab   *I found him about to write the letter.*

2. Like the tenses (see Lesson 10, 1), the participle may be preceded by **kaan, yikúun** with corresponding differences in the time-reference of the whole.

kaan, yikúun may precede either perfect or participle of **kátab**-type verbs with little difference of meaning, e.g.

ʔissíttï kanit naḍḍáfit (or **minaḍḍáfa**) **ilbéet**   *The woman had cleaned the house.*

There is little difference between the inclusion or omission of **kaan** in, e.g.

laqéetu kan ɣáamil (or **ɣámal**) **ʃúɣlu(h)**   *I found he had done his work.*

but if **kaan** is included, it is certain to refer to a perfect tense elsewhere in the context, e.g.

A. **ʔilwálad miʃi bádri léeh?**   *Why has the boy gone early?*

B. **laqéetu kan ɣáamil** (or **ɣámal**) **ʃúɣlu-w qultílu ráwwaḥ**   *I found he had done his work and told him to go home.*

where **káan ɣáamil** refers back to **míʃi.**

Once again verbs of motion behave differently, e.g.

kuntĭ máaʃi fiʃʃáariɣ *I was walking in the street.*
kan náazil dúɣri lakin ma-nzílʃ *He was going to come down right away but has not done so.*

In contrast with the last example, you cannot say **kan kaatib iggawaab lakin ma katabuuʃ**; cf. **kan ḥayíktib iggawáab lakin ma katabúuʃ** *He was going to write the letter but has not done so.*

The following additional examples include some with the imperfect **yikúun** which usually requires *will* in the English translation:

lamma daxált kan káatib iggawáab *He had written the letter when I went in.*

kan biyíktib iggawáab lamma daxált *He was writing the letter when I went in.*

qabílna ṣáaliḥ fissíkka w-iḥna-mrawwaḥíin[1] *We met Ṣāliḥ in the street as (= **wi**) we were going home.*

qabílna ṣáaliḥ fissíkka w-iḥna-bnitkállim wayya báɣḍ[1] *Ṣāliḥ met us in the street as we were talking together.*

filwáqtĭ dá-ykunu xargíin *They will be leaving at that time.*

filwáqtĭ dá-ykunu xáragu *They will have left by then.*

filwáqtĭ dá-tkun minaḍḍáfa- (or **naḍḍáfit**) **lɁóoḍa** *She will have cleaned the room by then.*

filwáqtĭ dá-tkun bitnáḍḍaf ilɁóoḍa *She will be cleaning the room at that time.*

EXERCISES

A

1. ma-txafíiʃ! Ɂana-mɣállim ʃunáṭna, míʃ ḥaydíɣ.
2. mantaʃ ɣáamil zayyĭ ma baqúllak!
3. ɣándak ḥáqq. Ɂana kuntĭ náasi-nnĭ kan ɣándi maɣáad wayyáak.
4. kuntĭ fáakir axállaṣ innahárḍa lakin ma-qdírtĭʃ.

---

[1] Notice the use of the particle *wi.*

5. káttar xéerak, m-aqdárʃ akul táani. ʕana mityáddi líyya (*or* min) sáaʒa.

6. ʕana-msallimúulu quddam ʒáaṭif afandi.

B

1. I didn't know that was the arrangement.
2. Who was that I saw passing by just now?
3. I've been sitting here for the past half hour.
4. Where are you going? Who has given you permission to leave?
5. As we were going along, I happened to see him[1] standing on the other side of the road.
6. I saw him wearing European clothes the other day. He doesn't usually, does he?

LESSON 35

The verbal noun; nouns of place and instrument

A. *The verbal noun*

1. (*a*) **ḍárbu lilʒiyáal biʃʃaklída muʃ kuwáyyis** *It's not right for him to beat the children like that* (lit. *His beating the children in that way is not right*).

   (*b*) **taʒlíim ilbanáat biyitqáddim[2] fi máṣrï dilwáqti** *The education of girls is progressing in Egypt nowadays.*

   (*c*) **bi-ʃwáyyit tafáahum tíqdar tiḥílli masʕáltak maʒáah** *With a little understanding you can overcome your difficulty with him.*

2. The verbal noun, sometimes called the infinitive, behaves differently from other nouns in a number of ways. One of these is illustrated in 1 (*a*) where, since **ḍarb** is defined by the suffix **-u,** the noun **ʕilʒiyáal** governed by **ḍarb** must be preceded by the particle **li. li** is also necessary when the verbal noun governs two

---

[1] ʃúftu biṣṣúdfa.
[2] Or, more familiarly, *máaʃi-kwáyyis.*

nouns of which the first is in construct with it, e.g. **kitábt** (or
kitáabit) **ilwálad liggawáab ɣámḍa gíddan** *The boy's writing
of the letter is completely illegible* (**kitáaba** = *writing*).

Certain verbal nouns of the simple form, e.g. **ḍarb,** may be
suffixed with **-a** and **-aat** when reference is to the number of times
the action is performed, e.g. **ḍarábtu ḍárba gámda qáwi** *I struck
him a really hard blow,* **ḍarábtu tálat ḍarbáat ɣala wíʃʃu(h)** *I hit
him three times on the* (lit. *his*) *face* (see Lesson 31, 1, note (6)). In
this use the verbal noun usually follows a given tense-form of the
same verb and is often used for emphasis; thus the first of the two
examples is better translated *I hit him really hard.*

3. Verbal nouns of the simple form are of more than one pattern;
ḍarb *striking,* **ʃurb** *drinking,* **duxúul** *entering* are examples, among
which **ḍarb** illustrates the commonest pattern.

Patterns of derived forms are fixed and are exemplified below.
Where plural forms occur these are regularly in **-aat,** e.g. **taɣlimáat**
instructions, **miɣaksáat** *quarrels.*

Verb (Perfect)	Verbal noun
(a) ɣállim (*to teach*)	taɣlíim (pl. taɣlimáat)
(b) ɣáakis (*to quarrel*)	miɣáksa (pl. miɣaksáat)
(c) ʔiɣtáraf (*to confess*)	ʔiɣtiráaf (pl. ʔiɣtirafáat)
(d) ʔiḥmárr (*to turn red*)	ʔiḥmiráar
(e) ʔitkábbar (*to be self-satisfied*)	takábbur
(f) ʔitfáahim (*to come to an understanding*)	tafáahum
(g) ʔinfágar (*to explode*)	ʔinfigáar (pl. ʔinfigaráat)
(h) ʔistáɣlim (*to inquire*)	ʔistiɣláam (pl. ʔistiɣlamáat)

Notes

(i) There is no ʔit- form corresponding to ʔinfigáar with ʔin- (see (g)).

(ii) The verbal nouns of weak verbs corresponding to (a), (b), and (c) end in
-iya, -ya, and **-a** respectively, e.g. **tasníya** (sánna, yisánni *to second*
(*motion*), *support*), **minádya** (náada, yináadi *to call*), **ʔibtída** (ʔibtáda,
yibtídi *to begin*). The verbal noun of weak verbs is common only in these
forms.

(iii) The consonant **y** appears in the verbal noun of hollow verbs corresponding to (c), e.g. **ʔixtiyáar** (ʔixtáar, yixtáar *to choose, elect*).

(iv) Educated speakers generally use **mu-** for **mi-** in verbal nouns with this
prefix; cf., too, **muʃáwra** *consultation,* **munáwra** *manœuvre.*

4. The verbal noun of quadriliteral verbs is regularly of the pattern illustrated by **laxbáṭa** (**láxbaṭ, yiláxbaṭ** *to confuse, muddle*). This is perhaps the main difference between quadriliteral verbs and those of the derived form in which the 2nd radical is doubled, i.e. **náḍḍaf, yináḍḍaf, ɤállim, yiɤállim,** &c.

B. *Nouns of place and instrument*

These two classes of noun are characterized as follows: nouns of place by initial **ma-** and the vowel **i** or **a** in the second syllable, e.g. **máglis** (pl. **magáalis**) *council, council-room* (cf. **gálas, yíglis** *to sit*), **máktab** (pl. **makáatib**) *office, desk* (cf. **kátab, yíktib** *to write*); nouns of instrument by initial **mu-** (sometimes **mi-**) or **ma-** and the vowel **aa** or **a** in the second syllable, e.g. **muftáaḥ** (pl. **mafatíiḥ**) *key* (cf. **fátaḥ, yíftaḥ** *to open*), **maqáṣṣ** (pl. **maqaṣṣáat**) *scissors* (cf. **qaṣṣ, yiqúṣṣ** *to cut with scissors or shears*). Final **-a** is also a feature of certain nouns of instrument, e.g. **maknása** (pl. **makáanis**) *broom* (cf. **kánas, yíknis** *to sweep*).

EXERCISES

A

1. xad wáqtĭ ṭawíil fi ɤamálha laṭíifa biʃʃaklída.
2. baláaʃ taʃdíid ɤalɤummáal, ʕáḥsan yizháqu.
3. fih máaniɤ min quɤáadi hína?
4. warríini-mráaya-ṣɤayyára ɤaʃan ilḥiláaqa.
5. ʕana-smíɤtĭ ɤan muqablítku maɤa báɤḍĭ-l ʕáwwil márra.
6. ma baḥíbbĭʃ migíyyu hína-ktíir. qúllu ma-ygíiʃ táani.

B

1. There is a lot of rivalry between them at work.
2. There's no point (*tr.* meaning) in waiting. They must have gone.
3. Keep to the pavement! It's dangerous[1] to walk in the middle of the road.
4. He's counting on their helping him.
5. By doing it this way, you'll save a lot of time (*tr.* doing it this way saves, &c.).
6. It's no use arguing! The room badly[2] wants painting.

---

[1] *xáṭar ɤaléek.*   [2] Use *ḍarúuri.*

APPENDIX A

Prominence or accentuation

The place of the prominent syllable in Cairene words is subject to certain definite rules which can be stated simply if we first know something of the syllable in the language.

Assuming that every syllable must begin with a consonant and contain a vowel, there are the following five syllable types: CV, CVV, CVC, CVVC, CVCC (C = consonant, V = vowel, VV = long vowel). Here are a few examples expressed in terms of C and V:

maf-húum *understood*	**ḍa-rábt** *I/you hit*	**fa-na-gíin** *cups*
CVC-CVVC	CV-CVCC	CV-CV-CVVC
qáa-bil *he met*	**ḍá-rab** *he hit*	**ḍá-ra-bit** *she hit*
CVV-CVC	CV-CVC	CV-CV-CVC

The five syllable types may be reduced to three quantities:
- (i) CV —Short (quantity)
- (ii) CVV —Medium (quantity)
  - CVC
- (iii) CVVC—Long (quantity)
  - CVCC

Prominence depends on the quantitative pattern of the whole word in accordance with the following three rules:

1. If the ultimate syllable is long, that syllable is always prominent, e.g. **manadíil** *handkerchiefs*, **fihímt** *I/you understood*, **ḍarabúuh** *they hit him*.

2. Words of which the ultimate syllable is not long have for the most part the penultimate syllable prominent (exceptions are catered for by rule (3)), e.g. **muɣállim** *teacher*, **maknása** *broom*, **dáawa** *he treated, cured*, **ʕitwágad** *it was found*, **mahiyyíti** *my pay*, **fihmúuha** *they understood her*, **ḍarabítu(h)** *she hit him*.

3. When both the penultimate and antepenultimate syllables

are short, e.g. **kátabit** *she wrote*, and, in the case of words of four or five syllables, the pre-antepenultimate is not a further short syllable, e.g. **ʕinkásarit** *it* (fem.) *was broken*, then the antepenultimate syllable is prominent as shown in the examples. Contrast, therefore, the pairs

$$\begin{cases} \textbf{ʕitwágad} & (CVC\text{-}C\acute{V}\text{-}CVC) \\ \textbf{ḍárabit} & (C\acute{V}\text{-}CV\text{-}CVC) \end{cases}$$

$$\begin{cases} \textbf{ʕinkásarit} & (CVC\text{-}C\acute{V}\text{-}CV\text{-}CVC) \\ \textbf{ḍarabítu(h)} & (CV\text{-}CV\text{-}C\acute{V}\text{-}CV) \end{cases}$$

Notes

(a) The above rules apply to 'simple' and suffixed forms alike with the following two exceptions:

   (i) If a suffix beginning with a vowel is added to the 3rd pers. sing. fem. perfect of weak verbs (type **ráma**), then the penultimate syllable is prominent, e.g. **rámit+u(h)=ramítu(h)** *she threw it*: contrast **kátab +u = kátabu** *they wrote* or *he wrote it* (see rule (3) above). Notice that in some parts of Egypt **rámit+u(h) = ramáatu(h)**.

   (ii) The plurals **ḍubúɡa** *hyenas*, **subúɡa** *lions*, **libísa**[1] *underpants*, and **yiríba**[2] (or **yirbáan**) *crows*. Notice the rare vowel-sequences **u-u** and **i-i** in the first two syllables of these words, and contrast other sequences —and other prominence—in **kátaba** *clerks*, **búxala** *misers*, **ɡínaba** *grape*. Contrast also **kútubu(h)** *his books*, the grammatical structure of which differs from that of **ḍubúɡa** and **subúɡa**.

(b) Notice that the *initial* syllable of the numeral is prominent in the numeral-noun construction of Lesson 19, 3, note (ii), e.g. **xámast** (not **xamást**) **iyyáam** *5 days*. t could, however, be regarded as a feature of the whole complex, and is only arbitrarily allotted to the numeral.

(c) The rules given in this Appendix apply, of course, to Cairo. The facts may differ slightly elsewhere—this is so, for example, in Upper Egypt— but similar analysis on the basis of syllable pattern may be applied to any form of Egyptian Arabic.

APPENDIX B

Long vowels

The student will have noticed throughout that a long vowel in a given word is not necessarily pronounced long in related forms, cf. **qáabil** *he met* but **qabílt** *I/you met*, **máasik** *holding* but **masíkhum**

[1] Or **ʕilbísa**.   [2] Or **ʕiyríba**.

holding them, **manadíil** *handkerchiefs* but **manadílha** *her handkerchiefs.*

The two rules governing the occurrence of long vowels are as follows:

    1. A vowel pronounced long can only occur in a prominent syllable.

    2. A long vowel does not occur in a closed syllable, i.e. type CVVC, unless the syllable is final, cf. **manadíil** but **manadílha** above.

Notes

(*a*) The long vowel **ii**, pronounced short in accordance with the rules, nevertheless retains the quality associated with **ii**, not **i** (see Introduction, p. 10). The qualities of **ii** and **i** in ʃ**íili** *take away* (fem.)!, ʃ**ilíih** *take* (fem.) *it* (masc.) *away!*, **siib** *leave!* and **síbha** *leave it* (fem.)! are substantially the same, and the **i** of, e.g. **síbha** is not pronounced as **i** in, e.g. **bint** *girl*.

For many speakers similar remarks would apply to **uu** and **u** as in ʃ**uuf** *see!* and ʃ**úfha**, but in this case pronunciation of (single) **u** as laid down in the Introduction (p. 11) is acceptable.

(*b*) A short vowel (corresponding to a long one in related forms) sometimes occurs very long contrary to rule (2) above when the word containing it is singled out for emphasis, e.g. ɣ**áalya gíddan!** *very dear!*, cf. the commoner ɣ**álya** (masc. ɣ**áali**).

(*c*) In 'Classical' Arabic as pronounced in Egypt, long vowels occur in non-prominent syllables. Contrary to rule (1) above, this feature can be noticed in a few 'learned' words such as ʕ**adátan** *usually*, ʕ**ilqahíra** *Cairo* which, in slow colloquial style, educated speakers often pronounce with a long or half-long vowel in the pre-tonic syllable, i.e. ʕ**aadátan, ʕilqaahíra.**

Similarly, in accordance with rule (2), a long vowel does not normally occur in a non-final closed syllable, but most educated speakers make a difference of vowel-length between ʕ**ámmi** *my uncle* and the 'learned' ʕ**áammi** *ignorant*, as well as between ʕ**amm** *uncle* and ʕ**aamm** *public, general*; in neither ʕ**áammi** nor ʕ**aamm** is the vowel pronounced as long as in, say, ʕ**áamil**, where it is, of course, in an open syllable.

(*d*) The style of utterance on which this book is based may be termed *slow colloquial*. In *rapid* style, vowels are commonly pronounced long only before a pause. It may be noted in passing that difference of style also correlates with differences of vowel-quality: for example, in rapid style, the difference between short **i** and **e**, and short **u** and **o**, is greatly reduced.

APPENDIX C

Elision

Elision concerns the omission under certain conditions of the short vowels **i** and **u** and of the consonant **ʕ**.

1. Elision of i and u.

Contexts involving elision of **i** and **u** are subdivided under (*a*) and (*b*).

(*a*) If a suffix beginning with a vowel is added to a word of which (i) the ultimate syllable is of the type CiC or CuC and (ii) the penultimate syllable is open (i.e. type CV or CVV), then **i** or **u** of the ultimate syllable is almost invariably elided, e.g.:

ɣáawiz *wanting* (masc. sing.) + **a** = **ɣáwza** *wanting* (fem. sing.).

qáabil *he met* + **u** = **qáblu** *they met* or *he met him.*

yáaxud *he takes* + **u** = **yáxdu** *they take* or *he takes it.*

yistáahil *it is worthy* + **ak** = **yistáhlak** *it is worthy of you.*

wíḥiʃ *unpleasant* (masc. sing.) + **a** = **wíḥʃa** *unpleasant* (fem. sing.).

fíhim *he understood* + **it** = **fíhmit** *she understood.*

yitwígid *it is found* + **u** = **yitwígdu** *they are found.*

Notes

(i) Contrast the facts when the suffix begins with a consonant, e.g. **qáabil + hum** = **qabílhum** *he met them*, or when the penultimate syllable is closed, e.g. **fáhhim+u(h)** = **fahhímu(h)** *he explained to him* (cf. **qáabil + u(h)** = **qáblu(h)**).

(ii) **u** occurs very rarely in context (*a*) and in words of the pattern CúCuC is not elided, e.g. **kútub + u(h)** = **kútubu(h)** *his books.*

(iii) **i** of the suffix -**it** (3rd pers. sing. fem. perfect) is never elided, e.g. **kátabit + u(h)** = **katabítu(h)** *she wrote it*, **rámit + u(h)** = **ramítu(h)** *she threw it.* Contrast, **qáalit + u(h)** = **qalítu(h)** *she said it* with **qáabil + u(h)** = **qáblu(h)** above. Contrast, too, -**it** of the feminine noun in construct, of which **i** is regularly elided, e.g. **tigáara + u(h)** = **tigártu(h)** *his business* (not **tigarítu(h)**; cf. **tigaríthum** *their business*).

(iv) Unlike **i** and **u**, the vowel **a** is not elided in comparable contexts. With **fíhim + it** = **fíhmit** and **yitwígid + u** = **yitwígdu** above, contrast **ḍárab + it** = **ḍárabit** *she hit* and **ʕitwágad+u** = **ʕitwágadu** *they were found.*

(v) Elision is not a feature of the 'Classical' language, and is absent also from 'learned' forms in educated colloquial. This is particularly applicable to participles; for example, the educated forms **munfáʒil, munfáʒila, munfaʒilíin** *angry, upset* correspond to the less-educated but more 'characteristically colloquial' **minfíʒil, minfíʒla, minfiʒlíin.**

(*b*) **i** and **u** occurring in an initial syllable which is short and not prominent, are elided when the preceding word ends in a vowel, e.g.:

ʕinta + tiʒibt = ʕinta-tʒíbt   *you are tired.*
ʕana + fihimt = ʕana-fhímt   *I understood.*
ʕiddiini + huduumak = ʕiddíini-hdúumak   *give me your clothes!*
ʕabu + ḥuséen = ʕabu-ḥséen   *Husein's father.*

Notes

(i) Contrast the facts when the initial syllable is prominent, e.g. **fáḍḍa ʒílabu(h)** *he emptied his boxes,* **ʕabu ʒúmar** *Omar's father.*
(ii) Once again **a** in comparable contexts is not elided. With the above examples of elided **i** and **u**, contrast **ʕinta katábt** *you wrote,* **ʕana ḍarábt** *I hit,* **ʕiddíini ʃaráabak** *give me your socks,* **ʕabu faríid** *Fareed's father.*
(iii) Although the vowel **u** is elided according to rule in, say, **ʒándi + ḥumáar = ʒándi-ḥmáar** *I have a donkey,* nevertheless **ḥ** is pronounced with the lips rounded as for **u**. The markedly different pronunciation which results from keeping the lips spread throughout the -diḥ- syllable, is quite unacceptable.
(iv) In emphatic utterances, elision may not occur: cf. **yáa xuṣáara** (emphatic) and **ya-xṣáara** (non-emphatic) *What a pity!*

2. Elision of initial **ʕ.**

The contexts in which **ʕ** is elided when no longer initial in the word or sentence are subdivided under (*a*) and (*b*). Notice that if a pause is made before the word in which **ʕ** is initial, then the consonant is not, of course, elided.

(*a*) **ʕ** preceded by a consonant.

When the preceding word ends in a consonant, **ʕ** is frequently elided unless the word containing it is singled out for emphasis or contrast, e.g. **ʃuɣl íbnak** *your son's work,* **ʒamalt éeh** *what have you done?.* **ʃúɣli ʕíbnak** might be used for example in contrast with **ʃúɣlak ínta** *your work,* while a more emphatic rendering of **ʒamalt éeh?,** showing surprise, indignation, sarcasm, &c., would be ɣamáltï ʕéeh? Initial ʕ of, for example, ʕábadan *ever*, *never*, a word which is frequently used emphatically, is rarely elided.

Elision of ʕ is more frequent among less educated speakers. In educated speech, the most important grammatical forms in which ʕ is regularly elided are as follows:

1st pers. sing. imperfect (e.g. ʕáktib *I write*); imperative forms (e.g. ʕíktib *write!*); derived forms (perfect tense) of the verb (e.g. ʕitbáɣat *it was sent*); the article ʕil; the pronouns ʕána, ʕínta, ʕínti, ʕíntu, and ʕíḥna; verbal nouns of the derived forms (e.g. listiɣláam *the inquiry*, lintixabáat *the elections*); the nouns of relationship ʕabb, ʕumm, ʕibn, ʕaxx, ʕuxt; the demonstrative series ʕaho, ʕahe, ʕahum, ʕáadi; the interrogatives ʕeeh *what*, ʕímta *when*, ʕánhu *which*; the connective particle ʕinn; the relative ʕílli; a few nouns such as ʕism *name*.

In addition, ʕ is commonly elided in nouns and adjectives of certain patterns, e.g. liyyáam (notice the i vowel) or ʕilʕayyáam *the days*, ʕiqfáal libwáab (or ilʕabwáab) *the locks of the doors*, lákbar or ʕilʕákbar *the bigger one*. In other patterns, however—especially those in which there are only two other consonants—ʕ is NOT elided: examples are ʕizn *permission*, ʕakl *food*, *eating*, ʕúgra *rate*, *hire*, ʕamíin *trustworthy*, ʕasáami *names*, ʕagáaza *leave*, ʕasáasi *basic*, ʕiḥáala *retirement*, *resignation*, ʕiṣáaba *injury*, ʕizáaza *bottle*.

ʕ in its rare occurrence as the 1st radical of a quadriliteral noun or of a verbal form is never elided: e.g. ʕárnab/ʕaráanib *rabbit/s*, ʕámar *he ordered*, ʕáxxar *he delayed*.

Notes

(i) ʕ of ʕeeh is not elided following h in fíih ʕéeh? *what is there?*, *what's the matter?*, and following the doubled consonants in zayyï ʕéeh? *such as?*, qaddi ʕéeh? *how much, how far?*

(ii) For further illustration of elision and non-elision of ʕ, with particular reference to a preceding numeral, see Lesson 19, 3, note (ii) and Lesson 20, 2, note (iv).

(*b*) ʕ preceded by a vowel.

When the same vowel both precedes and follows ʕ, then one of the vowels is usually elided together with ʕ, e.g. ʕinta + ʕaḥmar = ʕint-áḥmar *you are red*, fi + ʕiidu(h) = fíidu(h) *in his hand*. In

emphatic·speech, however, the vowel and ʕ both remain, i.e. ʕínta
ʕáḥmar, fi ʕíidu(h); cf. also ʕáɣla ʕálfï márra *a hundred times
dearer*. Notice, then, that as a result of elision it is impossible to
tell from the single sentence ʕana ɣawz-áakul *I want to eat*
whether a man or a woman is speaking, since ɣaawiz + ʕaakul and
ɣawza + ʕaakul may both give the same result. Notice, too, how
fi + ʕafraan = fifráan *in ovens* is 'more colloquial' than fi ʕafráan
(cf. liyyáam and ʕilʕayyáam under (*a*) above).

When the vowels preceding and following ʕ differ, then, with
the exceptions noted in the following paragraph, both vowels and ʕ
remain, e.g. ʕismǎha ʕéeh *What is her name ?*, biyiɣmílu ʕéeh
What are they doing?

The exceptions concern the vowel **i. i,** as well as ʕ, is elided
before **a,** e.g. bi+ʕaktib = báktib *I write, am writing*, naawi +
ʕaruuḥ = náaw-arúuḥ *I intend to go*, xalliini + ʕarawwaḥ =
xallíin-aráwwaḥ *let me go home*, ɣali + ʕafandi =ɣál-afandi
Ali Efendi. Initial ʕi is regularly elided, whatever the vowel
that precedes, e.g. da+ʕilli + ʕana+ɣawzu(h) = dá-ll-ana
ɣáwzu(h) *that's what I want*, ʕissána-lli fáatit *last year*, ʕana-
ddetháalu(h) *I gave it* (fem.) *to him*, ʃúufu-lli quddámku *look*
(pl.) *who is in front of you!*

Notes

(i) With the relatively few words in which ʕ of an initial open syllable ʕi- is
not elided, elision of i occurs in accordance with the rules under 1 above,
e.g. ʕabu+ʕimaam (proper name) = ʕábu-ʕmáam *Imam's father*.

(ii) ʕalláah is treated exceptionally, ʕa being elided whatever vowel precedes,
e.g. li+ʕallaah = lilláah *to God*, yarḥámkumu-lláah *may God have
mercy on you* (see also Introduction, pp. 6 and 10).

PART II

TEXTS

The contents of Part II are listed again below.

Texts 1–6 and 25–27 are comparatively short and, together with Appendixes A and B, are studied separately by candidates at the 1st examination of the Shell Company of Egypt, Ltd., and the Anglo-Egyptian Oilfields, Ltd nationalized in 1964 and 1956 respectively.

The remaining texts are divided according to type and subject-matter: 7–16 are dialogues on a variety of topics; 17–19 popular stories; 20–24 dialogue and narrative on Egypt and Islam; 25–33 dialogues and narrative specifically concerning the oil industry in Egypt. The oil texts are not, however, unduly technical and contain much of general interest and use; similar material might be collected by others who are concerned to meet their particular needs.

A few of the texts are very well known and have appeared in similar form elsewhere, for example in the works of Gairdner and Elder.

Notes. In the English translations of the texts, noteworthy additions to and omissions from the Arabic are included in round and square brackets respectively. Other necessary remarks, e.g. indication of literal translation, are given also in round brackets.

Text and translation cannot always be exactly accommodated on facing pages. Where there is overlapping an oblique stroke is inserted to indicate the point reached by the text or translation on the opposite page.

Text No.   *Page*

1. tawbíix bi ʕádab   120
    (A polite rebuke)

2. ʕittáʓlab ilmakkáar   120
    (The cunning fox)

3. ʕiṭṭámaʓ yiqíllǐ ma gámaʓ   120
    (The best-laid schemes of mice and men . . .)

4. ʕinnaggáar ilkasláan   122
    (The lazy carpenter)

5. ʕilyaʃíim w-innaṣṣáab   122
    (The simpleton and the cheat)

6. muḥáwra ben ṣáaḥib béet wi xaddáamu(h).   .   . 124
    (Conversation between a man and his servant)

7. muḥáwra ben ʓáamil w-ilmúʃrif ʓaléeh   .   .   . 126
    (Exchange between a workman and his supervisor)

8. muḥáwra ben síttǐ-w xaddámha   128
    (Dialogue between a woman and her servant)

9. listiʓdáad lissáfar min máṣrǐ li-ʃbíin ilqanáaṭir   .   . 130
    (Setting-out from Cairo for Shibin el Qanatir)

10. máktab ilbúṣṭa   132
    (The Post Office)

11. muḥáwra ben síttǐ-w gózha   134
    (Dialogue between a woman and her husband)

12. muḥáwra ben ʕagnábi-w máṣri 138
    (Conversation between a foreigner and an Egyptian)

13. xáan ilxalíili 140
    (The Muski)

14. muḥáwra ben wáḥda síttǐ maṣríyya w-iṭṭabbáax bitáʓha 142
    (Dialogue between an Egyptian woman and her cook)

15. takmílit ilmuḥáwra-ssábqa   146
    (Conclusion of the preceding text)

16. fiṣáal ben táagir wi-zbúun   148
    (Bargaining between a merchant and a customer)

17. ʕilḥaʃʃáaʃ wi-ḥmíiru(h)   150
    (The hashish smoker and his donkeys)

18. gúḥa filmáṭʓam   152
    (Guha in the restaurant)

Text No.   *Page*

19. ʕilfalláaḥ w-ilɣarḍiḥálgi 154
    (The peasant and the scribe)

20. ʕidáarit ilḥukúuma-f máṣr 156
    (Government administration in Egypt)

21. ʕiṭṭáqsï-f máṣr 158
    (The weather in Egypt)

22. ʕaháali-lqúṭr ilmáṣri 160
    (The people of Egypt)

23. ʕiddíin ilʕisláami 160
    (The Muslim religion)

24. ʕilmuwaṣaláat fi máṣr 162
    (Communications in Egypt)

25. ʕistixráag izzéet ilxáam 164
    (The production of crude oil)

26. takríir izzéet ilxáam 166
    (Refining crude oil)

27. tawzíiɣ wi béeɣ ilmuntagáat ilbitrolíyya . . . 168
    (The distribution and marketing of petroleum products)

28. ḥuqúul ʕabáar izziyúut 170
    (The Oilfields)

29. ʕizzetíyya 172
    (The Refinery)

30. furúuɣ ʃírkit ʃíllï-l máṣr 174
    (The branches of the Shell Company of Egypt)

31. ʕidáarit iʃʃarikáat fi máṣr 176
    (The administration of the companies in Egypt)

32. ʕistiɣmáal ilmuntagáat ilbitrolíyya 178
    (The use of petroleum products)

33. máktab ilmustaxdimíin 180
    (The Personnel Department)

App. A. Greetings (taḥiyyáat) 184

App. B. Exclamations and 'Oaths' 190

1. *tawbíix bi ʕádab*

fi yóom milʕayyáam kan ráagil ɣagúuz ráakib ḥumáaru fissíkka-w qáblu walad ʃáqi. fa qáal ilwálad 'naháarak saɣíid,[1] y-ábu-lḥumáar'; qam qállu-lɣagúuz 'naháarak saɣíid yá-bni'.

2. *ʕittáɣlab ilmakkáar*

yóom milʕayyáam xárag ʕásad ɣalaʃáan yiṣṭáad wi kan maɣáah díib wi táɣlab.

ʕilʕásad iṣṭáad ḥumáar wi ṭálab middíib innu yíqsim ilḥumáar bénhum húmma taláata, fa-ddíib qáal 'ʕittáɣlab yáaxud rígl, w-an-áaxud rígl, w-ilbáaqi ɣalaʃáanak'. fa qáam ilʕásad ḍárab iddíib ṭáyyar[2] ráasu-w ṭálab mittáɣlab innu yíqsim. fa-ttáɣlab qállu(h) 'xúd kúllǐ ḥáaga! ʕilli yífḍal mínnak yikfíini'.

ʕilʕásad istáɣrab qáwi mittáɣlab wi qállu(h) 'gíbt iʃʃaṭáara di-mnéen?' fa-ttáɣlab qáal 'min ráas[3] iddíib illi ṭáarit'.

3. *ʕiṭṭámaɣ yiqíllǐ ma gámaɣ*

káan fih márra falláaḥa ṭammáaɣa maʃya fissíkka-w ʃáyla ɣala rásha ḥállit lában rayḥa-tbíiɣu fissúuq.

wi hiyya máʃya qáalit li nafsǎha 'ʕana dilwáqt-abíiɣ illában w-aʃtíri-b támanu béeḍ, ʕilbéeḍ yiṭalláɣli katakíit, ʕabíiɣ ilkatakíit w-aʃtíri-b tamánha náɣga w-innáɣga tíwlid xirfáan kitíir. ʕabíɣhum w-aʃtíri ḥíttit ʕárḍǐ w-ilʕárḍǐ-ṭṭalláɣli[4] qúṭn. ʕabíiɣu w-aḥáwwiʃ w-aʃtíri ʕárḍǐ-lɣáayit ma yíbqa ɣandi ɣízba.'

wi hiyya máʃya dáasit fi ḥúfra fissíkka-w wíqɣit w-inqálabit ilḥálla fa raḥ mínha-llában w-aḥlámha sáwa.

[1] See Appendix A to this Part.
[2] Notice the sequence ʋf verbs without any linking particle (see Lesson 28).
[3] *n* before *r* or *l* is frequently pronounced as the following consonant: *min raas* may be pronounced *mir raas*.
[4] Pronounced *ṭṭ-*.

1. *A polite rebuke*

One day [from the days] an old man was riding his donkey along (*lit.* in) the road when (*lit.* and) he was met by a rude boy (*lit.* a rude boy met him). Said the boy, 'Good-day, you (*lit.* O) father of a (*lit.* the) donkey'. 'Good-day, my son,' replied the old man.

2. *The cunning fox*

Once upon a time a lion went out hunting accompanied by (*lit.* and with him were) a wolf (*or* jackal) and a fox.

The lion caught a donkey and asked the wolf to divide it between the three of them. The wolf said, 'The fox shall have (*lit.* take) a leg, I'll take a leg, and the rest is for you.' Whereupon the lion struck off the wolf's head (*lit.* hit the wolf and made his head fly) and asked the fox to do the dividing. And the fox said, 'Take the lot (*lit.* everything), and what's left [from you] will do for me.'

The lion was greatly surprised at the fox and said to him, 'Where did you get (*lit.* bring) such (*lit.* this) cleverness from?' And the fox said, 'From the wolf's head that flew off.'

3. *The best-laid schemes of mice and men . . .* (lit. *Greed lessens what is gathered*)

A greedy peasant woman was once walking along the road, carrying on her head a pot of milk she was going to sell [it] in the market.

As she was going along she said to herself, 'I'll sell the milk now and with what I get for it (*lit.* with its price) buy some eggs: the eggs will give me (*lit.* bring out for me) chickens. I'll sell the chickens and buy [with their price] a ewe: the ewe will bear many sheep. I'll sell them and buy a piece of land: the land will yield me cotton. I'll sell it, save and buy land till I finish up with a farm (*lit.* until there remains with me a farm).'

But as she went she stepped into a hole in the road, tripped, and (there) was the pot up-ended: away went (*lit.* went from her *or* she lost) the milk and with it (*lit.* at the same time) her dreams.

4. ˤinnaggáar ilkasláan

kan márra ráagil ɣandu wálad ṣuɣáyyar sínnu tálat siníin wi ḥábbï yiɣmíllu-sríir fa ráaḥ li naggáar w-ittáfaq maɣáah w-innaggáar qállu-nn issiríir ḥaykun gáahiz baɣd usbúuɣ.

wi fáat usbúuɣ w-itnéen wi taláata w-innaggáar ma kánʃï líssa xállaṣ issiríir. wi kúllï ma (kan) yirúuḥ linnaggáar yiqúllu(h) 'taɣáala baɣd usbúuɣ' liɣáayit irráagil ma[1] tíɣib xáaliṣ wi ma ráḥʃï táani linnaggáar.

ˤilwálad kíbir w-iggáwwiz[2] wi xállif wálad fa ṭálab min abúuh siríir lí-bnu(h) f-abúuh qállu(h) 'rúuḥ linnaggáar w-úṭlub mínnu-ssiríir'. fa lámma ráaḥ linnaggáar yuṭlub mínnu-ssiríir illi ṭalabúuh min xámsa-w ɣiʃríin sána, ˤinnaggáar qállu(h) 'xud filúusak ahéh! ˤana m-aḥíbbïʃ astáɣgil fi ʃúɣli.'

5. ˤilɣaʃíim w-innaṣṣáab

márra falláaḥ ɣaʃíim géh min ilˤaryáaf li máṣrï ˤáwwil márra-f ḥayáatu(h) w-istánna wáaḥid qaríibu-f midáan báab ilḥadíid ɣalaʃáan yáxdu-yfarrágu ɣala máṣr.

ˤilfalláaḥ ʃáaf innï kúllï wáaḥid kan yibúṣṣï fissáaɣa-w baɣdéen yímʃi-b súrɣa-w yirúuḥ yídfaɣ filúus filkúʃk illi táḥt issáaɣa.

ˤistáɣrab ilfalláaḥ qáwi lilmanɣárda. wi kan fih ráagil wáaqif quráyyib mínnu fa qáal lilfalláaḥ 'tigáara-kwayyísa qáwi. ˤan-áksab mínha xáaliṣ ilḥámdu lilláah.'

ˤilfalláaḥ qáal lirráagil 'tigáara ˤéeh?' fa-rráagil qállu(h) 'ˤáṣlï ˤana ṣáaḥib issaɣáadi wi záyyï ma ʃúft, kúllï wáaḥid yibúṣṣï fíiha-yruḥ yídfaɣ filúus lilkáatib bitáaɣi filkúʃk. náas kitíir ḥabbu yiʃtirúuha mínni w-ana ma-rḍítʃ.'

ˤilfalláaḥ ṭálab mirráagil innu yiʃtiríiha-w ɣáraḍ ɣaléeh ɣáʃara-gnéeh fa-rráagil qáal lilfalláaḥ 'náas kitíir ḥabbu yiʃtirúuha mínni-b

[1] See p. 84, footnote.
[2] See Lesson 24, 2, Note (5).

4. *The lazy carpenter*

There was once a man who had a small three-year old son. He wanted [to have] a bed made for him, so he went to a carpenter and came to an arrangement (*lit.* agreed) with him, the carpenter telling (*lit.* told) him that the bed would be ready in a week.

One, two, three weeks passed and still the carpenter had not finished the bed. Every time he went to him (*lit.* to the carpenter), he would say [to him], 'Come in a week's time (*lit.* after a week),' till (finally) the man grew very tired (of it) and gave up going (*lit.* did not go again) to the carpenter.

The boy grew up, married and a son was born to him (*lit.* he begat a son). He asked [from] his father for a bed for his son, and his father told him, 'Go to the carpenter and ask him [for the bed].' But when he went to the carpenter to ask him for the bed which had been ordered (*lit.* they ordered it) twenty-five years before, the carpenter said to him, 'Here, take your money (back)! I don't like hurrying [in] my work.'

5. *The simpleton and the cheat*

A simple peasant once came from the country to Cairo for the first time in his life, and was waiting (*lit.* waited) in Bab el Hadiid Square for a relative of his to take him and show him round Cairo.

The peasant noticed that everyone would look at the clock, then quickly walk on and go to pay [money] at the kiosk under the clock. He (*lit.* the peasant) was very surprised at this [sight], and [there was] a man standing beside him [who] said to him, '(This is) An excellent business! I make a lot out of it, praise God.' 'What business?', said the peasant [to the man], and the man said to him, 'The fact is that I'm the owner of that clock and, as you've seen, everyone who looks at it goes and pays [money to] my clerk in the kiosk. A lot of people have wanted to buy it from me but I haven't wanted to sell (*lit.* haven't agreed).'

So the peasant asked the man if he could buy it (*lit.* that he will buy it) and suggested to him ten pounds. Then the man said to him, 'Many have wanted to pay (*lit.* buy it from) me/ twenty

ʕiʃríin ginéeh w-ana ma-rḍítʃ. ʕinnáma ɣalaʃáanak ma ɣandííʃ
máaniɣ liʕánnak ragil ṭáyyib.'

dáfaɣ ilfalláaḥ ilɣáʃara-gnéeh wi ráaḥ lilkúʃk ɣalaʃan yíqbaḍ
ilfilúus. qáamu qalúulu(h) 'da ʃibbáak ittazáakir w-innáas biyidfáɣu-
flúus ɣalaʃáan yirkábu-lqáṭr'. wi lámma símiɣ kída kan ilfalláaḥ
zaɣláan wi maksúuf fi wáqtĭ wáaḥid.

6. muḥáwra ben ṣáaḥib béet wi xaddáamu(h)

A. y-áḥmad! *B.* ʕafándim. *A.* ʕana-msáafir búkra-w ɣáwzak
tiṣaḥḥíini-ssaɣa sítta-w núṣṣĭ wi-tgíbli ʃáay. *B.* ḥáaḍir y-afándim.
(ʕissaɣa sítta-w núṣṣĭ-f táani yóom ʕáḥmad yixábbaṭ ɣala báab
ʕóḍt¹ innóom)

B. ṣabáaḥ ilxéer ya xawáaga. ʕissáaɣa sítta-w núṣṣ. ʕitfáḍḍal iʃʃáay.
A. ṣabáaḥ ilxéer ɣaléek. ḥaḍḍárli-lfuṭúur baɣdĭ tíltĭ sáaɣa min
faḍlak. *B.* ḥáaḍir. ɣawiz táakul éeh filfuṭúur ya xawáaga? *A.* béeḍ
maḍrúub wi túst, w-ana ɣáwzak tiḥaḍḍárli-lhudúum wi-tḥuṭṭắha-f
ʃánṭa-ṣɣayyára. *B.* ḥáaḍir. ḥaḍrítak ráagiɣ ímta? *A.* baɣdĭ yoméen,
yaɣni búkra filmísa, wi ḥatɣáʃʃa hína. *B.* wi ḥaḍrítak ḥatílbis bádla
dilwáqti? *A.* náɣam. *B.* wi ḥatílɣab gúlf. *A.* ʕáywa.
(ʕáḥmad baɣdĭ tíltĭ sáaɣa-yxábbaṭ táani ɣalbáab)

B. ʕilfuṭúur ḥáaḍir. *A.* ʕana gáay ḥáalan. *B.* (lamma ṣáaḥib ilbéet
biyíʃṭar) ʕilɣarabíyya mawgúuda ya xawáaga. *A.* káttar xéerak.
qúul lissawwáaq inni gáay ḥáalan. háat ittúst y-áḥmad. *B.* ḥáaḍir,
y-afándim. ʕissawwáaq mistánni, ʕanazzíllu-ʃʃánṭa? *A.* ʕáywa,
baɣdĭ daqíiqa. ʕana ɣáwzak tigíib láḥma wi-xḍáar lilɣáʃa búkra, wi
ɣawzíin ḥáaga lilfuṭúur báɣdĭ báɣdĭ búkra? *B.* láa ya xawáaga,
ɣandína kúllĭ ḥáaga, bássĭ ɣawzíin láḥma. *A.* kuwáyyis. ʕadi-gnéeh
li maṣrúuf ilyoméen. níɣmil² ilḥisáab bitaɣ imbáariḥ baɣdĭ m-árgaɣ.
B. ṭáyyib. fih ḥáaga tánya ya xawáaga? *A.* ʕáywa. yímkin waḥid
ṣáḥbi yírgaɣ wayyáaya. ʕana ɣáwzak tiḥáḍḍar ʕoḍt¹ iḍḍuyúuf.

---

¹ Pronounced ʕoṭṭ.
² Notice the use with future time-reference of the imperfect without ḥa-.
See also Lesson 8, Exercise B, 3 and Lesson 9, Exercise B, 3. Notice that in these
examples the verb is in the 1st person: ḥa- can be used with the second person, for
example in Lesson 9, Exercise B, 3, i.e. *ḥatíḍrab líhum tilifóon?* 'Are you going
to phone them?'

pounds and I haven't agreed, but you're a good fellow, so in your case (*lit.* for you) I don't mind.'

The peasant paid the ten pounds and went to the kiosk to collect the money, whereupon he was told (*lit.* they said to him), 'This is the ticket-window where (*lit.* and) people pay [money] to go by (*lit.* ride the) train.' And when he heard this the peasant was at once both confused and angry (*lit.* angry and ashamed).

6. *Conversation between a man* (lit. *the master of a house) and his servant*

A. Ahmad! *B.* Sir! *A.* I'm going away tomorrow. I want you to wake me at half-past six and bring me tea. *B.* Yes, sir.

(At half-past six the next day Ahmad knocks on the bedroom door)

B. Good-morning, sir. It's half-past six. Here is the tea! *A.* Good-morning. Have breakfast ready for me in twenty minutes please. *B.* Yes. What do you want [to eat] for breakfast, sir? *A.* Scrambled eggs and toast. And I want you to look out my clothes for me and pack (*lit.* put) them in a small bag. *B.* Yes. When are you coming back? *A.* In two days' time (*lit.* after two days), that's to say tomorrow evening, and I shall have dinner here. *B.* Certainly, and are you putting a suit on now? *A.* Yes. *B.* Will you be playing golf? *A.* Yes.

(After twenty minutes Ahmad knocks on the door again)

B. Breakfast is ready. *A.* I'm coming right away. *B* (When the master of the house is having breakfast). The car's here, sir. *A.* Thank you. Tell the driver I'm coming at once. Bring the toast, Ahmad. *B.* Yes, sir. The driver's waiting, shall I take the bag down to him? *A.* Yes, in a minute. I want you to get some meat and vegetables for dinner tomorrow. Do we want anything for breakfast the day after [tomorrow]? *B.* No, sir, we've everything (we need). We just want meat. *A.* Good. Here's a pound for the two days' expenses. We'll settle up (*lit.* do the account) for yesterday after I get back. *B.* Yes. Is there anything else, sir? *A.* Yes. A friend of mine may come back with me. I want you to get the spare (*lit.* guests') room ready./ *B.* All right, sir. Your

B. ħáaḍir. ʕiʃʃánṭa-btáɣtak filɣarabíyya. *A.* káttar xéerak, y-áħmad.
B. maɣa-ssaláama. *A.* ʕalláah yisallímak.

7. muħáwra ben ɣáamil w-ilmúʃrif ɣaléeh

A. ya ɣál-afándi! *B.* ɣawiz éeh, ya síidi? *A.* ʕana ɣándi muʃkíla
filbéet ʃayláani gíddan wi miʃ ɣáarif áɣmil éeh. *B.* qúlli ʕéeh
ilmuʃkíla di kamáan. ħakim ínta kullï yóom fi maʃáakil. *A.* láʕ,
ʕana ráagil míʃ bitaɣ maʃáakil. ʕidduséeh bitáaɣi-ndíif. di muʃkíla
ɣaʕilíyya ṣírfa. *B.* ʕéeh ilħikáaya? *A.* ʕíbni ɣayyáan filbéet wi
ɣáawiz awaddíih lilħakíim wi bíddi yom ʕagáaza. *B.* ya ʕáxi,
ʕinta wáaxid yoméen ʕagáaza-b ʕízn ilʕusbúuɣ illi fáat. *A.* y-afándi,
ʕilyoméen illi bitqúul ɣaléehum, dóol ʕagáaza maraḍíyya-b ʕiznï
midduktúur liʕánni kuntï maríiḍ. *B.* ṭáyyib, w-ilyóom illi ħatáxdu
dilwáqti-ykun izzáay? *A.* yinħísib min agázti-ssanawíyya. *B.* ʕinta
bitqúul innak ragil míʃ bitaɣ maʃáakil w-idduséeh bitáaɣak niḍíif
wiláakin inta wáaxid síttiyyáam bi ʕízn w-inta líssa ma xadtïʃ[1]
ilʕagáaza-ssanawíyya. *A.* wi máalu(h)? yígra ʕéeh? ʕissítt iyyáam
dóol maxṣumíin. *B.* ʕinta ħatúqɣud tigadílni? *A.* ma fíiʃ luzúum
lizzáɣal, y-afándi. xálli-lmáktab yíxṣim ilyóom dá, záyyï báɣḍu(h).
B. wi ɣalaʃan éeh? ʕinta ráagil ṣáaħib ɣiyáal wi miħtáag li ʕúgrit
ilyóom. *A.* ʕáɣmil éeh baqa? yaɣni baláaʃ awáddi-lwálad lilħakíim
w-asíibu filbéet yimúut. *A.* ʕana ma baqullákʃï síibu xallíih
yimúut. ʕana ɣáawiz aqúllak lamma-tráwwaħ baɣd iḍḍúhr,
waddíih lilħakíim. *A.* ʕana baráwwaħ wáxri, wi-ɣyadt[2] ilħakíim
bitkúun malyáana náas. *B.* huwwa-lwálad ɣayyáan qáwi? ɣándu
ʕéeh? *A.* ʕáywa, ɣayyáan qáwi, ɣándu ħáṣba w-ana xáayif innu
yíɣd-axúuh[3] iṣṣuɣáyyar. *B.* ṭáyyib, madam ilwálad ɣayyáan
bilħáṣba-w da máraḍ múɣdi-w ḍarúuri-twaddíih lilħakíim, ʕan-
axúdlak ʕíznï milmáktab. *A.* ʕáqdar arúuħ wayyáak ilmáktab?
B. ʕísmaɣ, wi lámma-yqulúulak filmáktab 'gara ʕéeh? ʕinta kúllï
yóom w-ittáani ʕagáaza,' tiqúul ʕéeh? / *A.* madáam inta ɣáarif

---

[1] Pronounced *xáttïʃ.*
[2] Pronounced *ɣyatt.* In isolation, *ɣiyáada.*
[3] See Part I, App. C, 2 (*b*).

bag's in the car. *A.* Thank you, Ahmad. *B.* Goodbye (sir).
A. Goodbye.

7. *Exchange between a workman and his supervisor*

A. Ali Efendi! *B.* What do you want? *A.* I've a problem at home
which is worrying me a lot, and I don't know what to do (about it).
B. Tell me what it is this time (*lit.* what this problem is, too). Just
like you,[1] in trouble every day. *A.* No, I'm not (*lit.* I am not a man
of troubles), my record's clean. This is entirely a family matter.
B. What's it about (*lit.* what's the story)? *A.* My son is ill at home.
I want to take him to the doctor and would like a day's leave.
B. My dear chap, you had two days leave granted (*lit.* with permission) last week. *A.* Sir, the two days you're talking of were sick-
leave on the doctor's recommendation, since I was ill. *B.* All right,
and the day you're going to take now, what (*lit.* how) will that be?
A. It can be taken off my annual leave. *B.* You say you aren't a
troublesome man and that your record's clean, and (yet) you've
had six days off and still not taken your annual leave. *A.* What of it!
What does that matter? Those six days have been deducted.
B. Are you still going to argue with me? *A.* There's no need to be
angry (*lit.* for anger), sir. Let the office deduct the day! It's all the
same (to me). *B.* Why? You're a family man and need the day's
pay. *A.* Well, what am I to do? Do you mean (*lit.* that is to say)
I shouldn't take the boy to the doctor but leave him at home to die.
B. I'm saying no such thing (*lit.* not telling you to leave him, &c.).
I want to suggest that you take him to the doctor when you go
home this afternoon. *A.* I go home late, and the doctor's surgery
will be full of people. *B.* Is the boy very ill? What has he got?
A. Yes, very. He has measles and I'm afraid he'll give it to (*lit.*
infect) his small brother. *B.* All right, since the boy has measles,
which (*lit.* and it) is an infectious disease, and it's essential for you
to take him to the doctor, I'll get (*lit.* take) you permission from the
office. *A.* Can I go with you to the office? *B.* Listen, when they
say to you [in the office], 'What's the matter, you're always looking
for leave (*lit.* every day and the next day)!', what will you say?

[1] This is the force of *ḥdakim.*

innŭhum ḥayqúulu kída-w yiᵹmílu wayyáaya dáwʃa, ma fíiʃ
luzúum arúuḥ. qullŭhum ínta-w xallíin-aráwwaḥ aʃúuf ilwálad.
B. ṭáyyib, ráwwaḥ inta! lakin ʃúuf, di ʕáaxir márra! ʕana miʃ
ᵹáawiz ilmáktab yiftíkir innak bitíkzib walla-btíᵹmil ḥíyal. maᵹa-
ssaláama. rabbína yiʃfíilak íbnak. A. ʕalláah yisallímak. káttar
xéerak.

8. muḥáwra ben síttĭ-w xaddámha

A. yá-ṣṭa![1] ḥáḍḍar ilfuṭúur ᵹalaʃáan ilxawáaga ᵹawiz yífṭar bádri-
nnaharḍa. B. ḥáaḍir. ʕilʕáklĭ gáahiz fi ʕóḍt[2] iṣṣúfra, bássĭ ma fíiʃ
zíbda-w béeḍ. A. léeh baqa![3] wi gáahiz izzáay iza kan ma fíiʃ
zíbda-w béeḍ! B. nisíit aʃtiríihum imbáariḥ. A. ʕahó-nta tamálli
kida! lamm-asʕálak ᵹan ḥáaga, tiqul 'nisíit, nisíit', wi baᵹdéen
wayyáak baqa! B. ya sítt ana bánsa min kútr iʃʃúyl. A. ʕéeh
huwwa-ʃʃúyl ikkitíir! baqa kúllĭ wáaḥid yiʃtáᵹal yínsa? baláaʃ
ḥíyal, ʕana ᵹarfáak innak ḥíyali. B. láa walláahi ya sítt, ʕana ráagil
ʕamíin fi ʃúyli. A. ʕúskut, ma-trúddĭʃ ᵹaláyya! baláaʃ kaláam!
yálla, rúuḥ ʃúuf ʃúylak! w-inta tamálli kasláan. B. ya sítt iddíini-
flúus ᵹalaʃáan baᵹd ilfuṭúur arúuḥ issúuq aʃtíri-lláazim ᵹaʃan ilᵹáda
w-ilᵹáʃa. A. láʕ, ma-trúḥʃ, ʕaná-lli[4] ḥarúuḥ. ʕínta náḍḍaf ʕúwaḍ
innóom wi rattíbha-w kamáan ʕóḍt[2] iggulúus, w-íᵹsil ilbaláaṭ
w-ímsaḥ ilʕizáaz w-íftaḥ iʃʃababíik. B. ṭáyyib, ʕaṭállaᵹ issagagíid
bárra kamáan? A. ʕáywa-w naffáḍhum wi ma tinsáaʃ tiwáddi-
lbayaḍáat lilᵹasíil. B. ḥáaḍir. fíih hudúum lilmákwa, ya sítt?
A. ʕáywa, di ḥáaga-mhímma. ʕínta fakkartíni. fih hína ʕárbaᵹ
fasatíin wi badlitéen lilxawáaga wi tálat qumṣáan wi núṣṣĭ dástit
manadíil wi núṣṣĭ dástit fúwaṭ ṣúfra-w fustanéen lilbínt.
B. w-awáddi máfraʃ iṣṣúfra kamáan? A. maᵹlúum, da láazim qáwi
liʕannĭ ᵹandína-dyúuf innahárḍa filᵹáʃa, wi láazim/ tiqúul lilmak-

---

[1] = ya + ʕúṣṭa, a form of address used chiefly to craftsmen and artisans.
[2] Pronounced ʕoṭṭ.
[3] See Appendix B to this Part.
[4] = ʕána + ʕílli.

A. Since you know they will say that and make it difficult (*lit.* make trouble) for me, there's no need for me to go. *You* tell them and let me go home to see (to) the boy. *B.* All right, off you go! But look, this is the last time. I don't want the office to think that you tell lies or are up to tricks. Goodbye. I hope your son gets better (*lit.* may our Lord cure your son for you). *A.* Goodbye (and) thank you.

8. *Dialogue between a woman and her servant*

A. Cook, get breakfast ready for the master, he wants it (*lit.* to breakfast) early today. *B.* Certainly, it (*lit.* the food) is ready in the dining-room, only there isn't any butter or eggs. *A.* What next! How can the meal be ready then (*lit.* if there isn't any butter, &c.)! *B.* I forgot to buy any (*lit.* them) yesterday. *A.* You're always the same! Whenever I ask you about anything, you say, 'I forgot'. What's wrong with you? *B.* Madam, I forget because I've so much work to do (*lit.* from the great amount of work). *A.* What's this about a lot of work? So anyone who works has to be (*lit.* is) forgetful, has he? Enough of these exaggerations (*lit.* tricks)! I know you too well (*lit.* I know you that you are a trickster)! *B.* Oh, no, really, madam, I'm an honest man in my work. *A.* Be quiet and don't answer me back! That's enough talk, off you go and see to your work! You're always idle. *B.* Madam, will you give me some money to go to the market after breakfast and buy what's necessary for lunch and dinner? *A.* No, I'm going, not you (*lit.* don't go, I'm the one who's going). You dust and tidy up the bedrooms, and the lounge too, then wash the floor, and clean and open the windows (*lit.* wipe the glass and open the windows). *B.* All right. Shall I put the carpets out, too? *A.* Yes, and beat them. And don't forget to take the (bed and table) linen to the wash. *B.* Yes. Are there any clothes for the laundry, madam? *A.* Oh, yes, that's important, you've reminded me. There are four dresses, two of the master's suits, three shirts, half a dozen handkerchiefs, half a dozen napkins, and two of the young mistress's (*lit.* of the girl's) dresses. *B.* Shall I take the table-cloth, too? *A.* Yes, of course, that's very necessary since we have guests for dinner today. And you must

wági yistáʒgil wi yikwíihum kuwáyyis. Ꜥíwʒa yitꜤáxxar zayy
ilmárra-lli fáatit. *B.* ya sítt, Ꜥiza kuntï ḥáʒmil kúllï dá, míin
ḫayíƴsil iṣṣuḫúun w-issakakíin w-iʃʃúwak w-ilmaʒáaliq wi Ꜥabríiq
illában wi Ꜥabríiq iʃʃáay? *A.* Ꜥínta, liꜤánnï da ʃúƴlak w-inta malzúum
tiʒmílu(h). *B.* muʃ áḥsan, ya sítt, ḥaḍrítik tigíibi ṣufrági-ysaʒídni?
Ꜥana ʒaláyya-lmáṭbax, liꜤánni ṭabbáax wi húwwa-ykun ʒaléeh
iṣṣúfra-w tanḍíif ilbéet. *A.* míin yídfaʒ Ꜥugrítu(h)? Ꜥiḥna fúqara
míʃ ayníya. *B.* Ꜥismaḥíili ya sítt, Ꜥiggáras biydúqq. Ꜥazúnn
ilmakwági géh. *A* (lilmakwági). ʃúuf yá-ṣta, ʒandína-hdúum
lilmákwa-w ʒawzáak tikwíihum kuwáyyis wi-traggáʒhum innahárḍa
baʒd iḍḍúhr. múmkin? *C* (Ꜥilmakwági). humma káam ḥítta ya
sítt? *A.* Ꜥahúm! ʒiddúhum! *C.* ya sítt, dóol arbáʒa-w ʒiʃríin
ḥítta. muʃ múmkin axalláʃhum kullúhum innahárḍa. *A.* láakin
iḥna mustaʒgilíin wi ʒawzínhum innahárḍa. *C.* ʃúufi ya sítt!
Ꜥilḥáaga-lmustaʒgíla, Ꜥakwíiha-nnahárḍa ʒalaʃan xáṭrik w-ilbáaqi
búkra. *A.* ṭáyyib, ma fíiʃ máaniʒ. Ꜥíkwi bádla lilxawáaga-w fustanéen líyya-w máfraʃ iṣṣúfra w-ilfúwaṭ wi raggáʒhum issáaʒ-arbáʒa
filmaʒáad tamáam. *C.* ḥáaḍir, ya sítt.

9. *listiʒdáad lissáfar min máṣrï li-ʃbíin ilqanáaṭir*

A. saʒíida ya sídna. *B.* saʒíida-mbárka. *A.* Ꜥállah! gara Ꜥéeh!
ʒala féen? *B.* walláahi ʒandi Ꜥagáaza múddit ʃáhr, wi-msáafir
aƴáyyar háwa-w manáazir w-astaráyyaḥ ʃuwayya. *A.* misáafir
féen? li Ꜥáyyï gíha? *B.* lilꜤaryáaf ʒalaʃáan ilꜤinsáan yitmáttaʒ bi
manáazir ilƴeṭáan w-ilxúḍra. *A.* saddáqni Ꜥáḥsan, liꜤánn ilmúdun
ma fiháaʃ ráaḥa, Ꜥílla-ddáwʃa w-ilxáwta-w qáraf iʃʃúƴl. yáll-amm-
áxrug[1] wayyáak.

(fiʃʃáariʒ)

B. táksee![2] yá-ṣta, ḫúṭṭ iʃʃúnaṭ wára-f ʃánṭit ilʒarabíyya w-íṭlaʒ
ʒalmaḥáṭṭa! *C* (Ꜥissawwáaq). Ꜥilmaḥáṭṭa-kkibíira walla maḥáṭṭit

---

[1] = yálla + Ꜥámma + Ꜥáxrug.
[2] In the form used when hailing a taxi, the final vowel is protracted and closer
in quality to *e* than to *i*.

tell the laundryman to hurry but to make a good job of them. See that he's not late like last time! *B*. If I'm going to do all that, madam, who's going to do the washing-up (*lit.* to wash the plates, knives, forks, spoons, milk jug, and teapot)? *A*. You (are), because it's your job and you have to do it. *B*. Wouldn't it be better, madam, if you brought a waiter to help me? I'd have the kitchen to look after for (after all) I *am* a cook, and he would be responsible for the dining-room (*lit.* dining-table) and for cleaning the house. *A*. Who would pay his wages? We're poor, not rich. *B*. Excuse me, madam, the bell's ringing. I think the laundryman has come. *A* (To the laundryman). Look, laundryman, we've some clothes for you (*lit.* for the laundry). I want you to do them well and return them this afternoon. Is that possible? *C* (The laundryman). How many items are there, madam? *A*. There they are! Count them! *C*. There are twenty-four, madam. I can't finish them all today. *A*. But we're in a hurry and want them today. *C*. Look, madam, since it's you (*lit.* for your sake), I'll do the urgent thing(s) today and the rest tomorrow. *A*. All right, then, that will do (*lit.* there is no objection). Press a suit for the master, two dresses for me, (iron) a table-cloth and the napkins and return them at 4 o'clock sharp. *C*. Very well, madam.

9. *Setting-out* (lit. *the preparing for the journey*) *from Cairo for Shibin el Qanatir*

A. Hullo, old man (*lit.* our master). *B*. Hullo. *A*. Well now, what's on? Where are you going? *B*. I've a month's holiday and I'm off for a change of air and scenery (*lit.* travelling to change, &c.), and a rest (*lit.* to rest a little). *A*. Which part are you going to? *B*. The country, to enjoy (*lit.* because a man enjoys the sight of) the fields and greenery. *A*. I agree, there's nothing better (*lit.* believe me, it is best), [since] there's no rest (to be had) in cities, nothing but noise and bustle and the strain of work. Come on, I'll go so far (*lit.* go out) with you.

(In the street)

B. Taxi! . . . Driver, put the luggage in the boot and drive (*lit.* go out) to the station. *C* (The driver). The main station or / Pont

kúbri-llamúun? *B.* Ṣilmaḥáṭṭa-kkibíira, ʒalaʃáan ana-msáafir li-
ʃbíin ilqanáaṭir. bassĭ súuq bi súrʒa ʒalaʃan nílḥaq ilqáṭr. *C.* ḥáaḍir.

(filmaḥáṭṭa)

B. ya ʃayyáal! ʃíil iʃʃúnaṭ wi ḥuṭṭúhum filqáṭr illi qáayim ʒala
xáṭṭĭ-ʃbíin ilqanáaṭir. nimrítak káam? *D* (Ṣiʃʃayyáal). míyya
xámsa-w talatíin. ḥaḍrítak ḥatírkab dáraga Ṣéeh? *B.* dáraga tánya.
bassĭ ʃúuf diwáan yikun niḍíif w-ana gáyyĭ waráak, bássĭ ḥáqtaʒ
ittazkára.

(baʒdĭ dáfʒĭ Ṣúgrit ittáksi ḥasab ilʒaddáad wi huwwa wáaqif
    quddáam ʃibbáak ittazáakir)

B. ya ḥáḍrit, Ṣiddíini tazkára-skúndu li-ʃbíin ilqanáaṭir. *E* (Ṣit-
tazkárgi). Ṣistánna-ʃwáyya lamm-amáʃʃi-lli quddáamak. *B.* y-afán-
di-ddíini-ttazkára, Ṣilqáṭrĭ qárrab yiqúum w-ilʒáfʃĭ maʒa-ʃʃayyáal.
E. y-afánd-ana ʒáarif maʒáad qiyáam ilqáṭr w-ana fáahim ʃúɣli.
míʃ mistánni lamma ganáabak¹ tifahhímni. ḥaḍrítak ʒawiz tazkára
ráayiḥ gáay? *B.* láṢ, ráayiḥ báss. *E.* Ṣitfáḍḍal, Ṣittazkára-héh!

(filqáṭrĭ liʃʃayyáal)

B. kúll iʃʃúnaṭ mawgúuda? Ṣitfáḍḍal ilṢúgra. *D* (Ṣiʃʃayyáal).
Ṣéhda! ṢilṢúgra di míʃ kifáaya. *B.* Ṣana-ddétlak ilṢúgra-w baqʃíiʃ
ziyáada. yálla baqa!

10. *máktab ilbúṣṭa*

A. Ṣáhlan, Ṣizzáyyĭ ḥaḍrítak w-izzáyy ilṢawláad? *B.* walláahi-
lwálad iṣṣuɣáyyar súxnĭ-ʃwayya, w-izzáyyĭ ma ʒándak? *A.* Ṣilḥáal
min báʒdu bárḍu-lbintĭ rígʒit milmadrása-w ʒandáha ḥaráara
ʒálya. *B.* salamítha, wi ḥaḍrítak rayiḥ féen dilwaqti? *A.* Ṣana
ráayiḥ ilbúṣṭa ʒalaʃan astílim ṭárdĭ w-aṣóogar gawáab. *B.* Ṣana
kamáan rayiḥ² ilbúṣṭa ʒalaʃan ábʒat gawáab ʒáadi. *A.* ma fíiʃ
luzúum tirúuḥ ilbúṣṭa, Ṣirmíih fi Ṣáyyĭ sandúuq. / *B.* sanadíiq

¹ Notice the retention of honorific terms of address despite the ill humour on
both sides.
² May be pronounced *kamaar rayiḥ*.

Limun? *B*. The main station. I'm going to Shibin el Qanatir. Hurry though (*lit.* just drive quickly), so that we catch the train. *C*. Right.

(At the station)

B. Porter! . . . Take the bags and put them in the train [standing on the line] for Shibin el Qanatir. What's your number? *D* (The porter). A hundred and thirty-five. What class are you going (*lit.* riding)? *B*. Second. Just see that the compartment is clean (*lit.* look out a compartment which is clean) and I'll come on after you. I'm just going to get (*lit.* cut) the ticket.

(After paying the taxi fare according to the meter, he is standing at the window of the booking-office (*lit.* of the tickets))

B. Excuse me (*lit.* your honour), can I have (*lit.* give me) a second-class ticket for Shibin el Qanatir? *E* (The ticket-clerk). Wait a minute while I deal with those in front of you. *B*. My dear sir, do give me the ticket, the train's about to go and my luggage is with the porter. *E*. [Sir] I know what time the train's due out (*lit.* the departure-time of the train), and I know my job. I don't expect (*lit.* haven't been waiting for) you to tell me (it). (Anyway) do you want a return (*lit.* a going-coming) ticket? *B*. No, just single. *E*. Here you are, here's the ticket.

(In the train to the porter)

B. Are all the bags here? There you are (*lit.* take the fee)! *D*. What's this! This isn't enough. *B*. I've paid you and given you a bit extra. Off with you now!

10. *The Post Office*

A. Hullo! How are you and how are the children? *B*. I'm afraid the young one (*lit.* small boy) has a slight temperature, but how are yours? *A*. It's the same story (*lit.* the condition alike, i.e. like yours), the girl's just come home from school with a high temperature. *B*. I hope she'll soon be better. Where are you going now? *A*. I'm off to the Post Office to collect a parcel and register a letter. *B*. I'm going there, too, to post a letter (*lit.* ordinary letter). *A*. You don't need to go to the Post Office. Slip it in any box. / *B*. Street letter

ilbúʂʈa fiʃʃawáariʒ láha mawaʒíid w-iggawábda mistáʒgil. *A.* Ɂiza
kúntĭ mistáʒgil fih sanadíiq lónhum áxdar Ɂirmíih fíihum, maktúub
ʒaléehum 'Ɂilbaríid ilmustáʒgil'. *B.* ɁilmasɁála wáhda, bárdu
yilzámn-arúuh ilbúʂʈa ʒalaʃan awzínu(h). *A.* Ɂiza kan láazim[1]
tirúuh ilbúʂʈa, yálla-nrúuh sáwa. *B.* Ɂitfáddal, Ɂintá-bnĭ haláal,
fakkartín-ana ʒáawiz abʒat filúus lilwálad filbálad. *A.* Ɂaftíkir inta
hatʒaʈʈálna-ʃwayya ʒalaʃan yilzámak tigíib filɁáwwil hiwáala-w
timláaha. *B.* láɁ, miʃ láazim hiwáala, Ɂan-agib Ɂíznĭ baríid ʒalaʃan
ma yinʂiríʃʃ illa-l ʂáhbu(h). *A.* Ɂíhna dilwaqti-wʂílna-lmáktab
w-ismáhl-arúuh liʃʃibbáak iʈʈurúud. *B.* ʈáyyib, Ɂan-astáɁzin.
A (li-mʒáawin ilbúʂʈa). ya hádrit ilmiʒáawin, naháarak saʒíid.
C (Ɂilmiʒáawin). naháarak saʒíid mubáarak.   tílzam xídma?
A. min fádlak, Ɂana líyya ʈárdĭ hína-w ʒáawiz astílmu(h). *C.* féen
ilháfʒa min fadlak? *A.* Ɂilháfʒa-héh. *C.* ʒándak biʈáaqit tahqíiq
iʃʃaxʂíyya? *A.* mutaɁássif, ma ʒandíiʃ. *C.* míin yiʒráfak filmáktab
hina? *A.* walláah-ana m-aʒráfʃĭ háddĭ hína-w ma háddĭʃ yiʒráfni
kamáan. *C.* ʈáyyib, rúuh hat wáahid yiʒráfak wi-ykúun maʒrúuf
lilmáktab. *A.* ʈáyyib. Ɂana ʒáawiz asággil iggawábda. *C.* Ɂiʃʃibbáak
ittáani ʒala-ymíinak. hína ʃibbáak ittawzíiʒ. *A.* y-afándi, tísmah
tisaggílli-ggawábda. *D* (Ɂilmiʒáawin ittáani). háadir. *A.* Ɂana
ʒáawiz kamáan ʈawáabiʒ búʂʈa-w wáraqit dámya. *D.* Ɂilwáraqa
min fíyyit káam? *A.* xámas ʈawáabiʒ min fíyyit qírʃĭ sáaɣ wi
wáraqit dámya-b xámsa sáaɣ. *D.* Ɂitfáddal ahúm. hat ʒáʃara sáaɣ
min fadlak. *A.* mutaʃákkir, Ɂissaláamu ʒaléekum. *D.* ʒaléekumu-
ssaláam.

11. *muháwra ben síttĭ-w gózha*

A. yáa saláam, gara Ɂéeh fiddínya? Ɂéhda! *B.* máalik? háʂal éeh?
zaʒláana léeh kida? *A.* m-azʒálʃ izzáay! kúllĭ ma-nqúul iddínya
hatkúun kuwayyísa w-ilhagáat tírxaʂ, tíyla-zyáada w-iddínya báqit
zayy izzíft. *B.* Ɂinti ɣalʈáana-za kúnti tiftíkri-nn-ilɣála / yintíhi

[1] May be pronounced *kal laazim.*

boxes have collection times and this letter is urgent. *A.* If you're in a hurry, there are green boxes you can post in [them] marked 'Express [Post]'. *B.* That doesn't help (*lit.* the problem is the same), I still have to go to the post to weigh it. *A.* (Well,) if you must go, let's go together. *B.* Certainly. I'm glad I met you (*lit.* you are the child of righteousness), you've reminded me I want to send some money to the boy in the village. *A.* That means (*lit.* I think) you're going to hold us up since first of all you'll have to get a money-order and fill it in. *B.* No, a money-order isn't necessary. I'll get a postal-order and make it payable only to bearer (*lit.* so that it can only be paid to its owner). *A.* Here we are. Excuse me, I must go (*lit.* forgive my going) to the parcels window. *B.* Of course. Goodbye. *A.* (To the postal assistant). Good-morning. *C* (The assistant). Good-morning. Can I help you (*lit.* do you need service)? *A.* I've a parcel here which I want to collect please. *C.* Where is the slip please? *A.* Here it is. *C.* Have you an identity card? *A.* I'm sorry, I haven't. *C.* Who knows you here in the office? *A.* Heavens, I don't know anyone here and nobody knows me either. *C.* All right, fetch someone who knows you and who is known to the office. *A.* All right. I want to register this letter. *C.* The other window on your right. This is the distribution window. . . . *A.* Would you mind registering this letter for me? *D* (The second assistant). Certainly. *A.* I also want some stamps and a fiscal stamp. *D.* [A stamp] for how much? *A.* Five one-piastre stamps and a five-piastre fiscal stamp. *D.* Here you are. That will be (*lit.* bring) ten piastres please. *A.* Thank you. Good day. *D.* Good day to you.

11. *Dialogue between a woman and her husband*

A. I really don't know what's the matter with everything nowadays (*lit.* Good heavens, what has happened in the world? What is it?). *B.* What's the trouble [with you]? What's happened? Why are you so cross? *A.* Why shouldn't I be cross! Whenever we say things are going to be all right and prices go down, up they go still further and things are worse than ever (*lit.* the world has become like pitch). *B.* You're wrong if you think that high prices / are at an

w-ilḥáala titḫássin. *A.* Ṣísmaɤ ya síidi. Ṣana rúḫt issúuq ɤalaʃan aʃtíri-ʃwáyyit xuḍáar. *B.* ṭáyyib, wi ḥáṣal éeh? *A.* Ṣana saṢált ilxúḍari ɤan táman kúllï ṣánf min Ṣaṣnáaf ilxuḍáar wi qálli ɤan táman ilbisílla w-ilbaṭáaṭiṣ w-ilfaṣúlya-w hakáza. *B.* w-iʃtaréeti walla láṢ? *A.* láṢ, ma-ʃtarétʃ. laqéet kúllï ḥáaga ɤálya, Ṣinʃálla ma ḥáddï kál! *B.* wi baɤdï kída ɤamálti Ṣéeh? *A.* síbtu-w rúḫtï-l dukkáan gazᴢáar wi saṢált iggazᴢáar 'ɤándak ɤáḍmï ɤaʃan iʃʃúrba?'. *B.* ṭáyyib, w-iʃtaréeti ɤáḍmï-w láḥma? *A.* Ṣáywa-w ḥaníɤmil bilɤáḍmï-ʃwayyit ʃúrba. *B.* baɤdï kída ruḥti féen? *A.* lafféet ʃuwáyya-w biṣṣúdfa laqéet ráagil sammáak biybíiɤ sámak w-iʃtaréet mínnu-ʃwáyya, zayyï wíqqa. *B.* kuwáyyis, w-iʃtaréeti fákha walla láṢ? *A.* Ṣamm-aqúllak ilfákha-ṭṭáaᴢa ɤálya gíddan wi muʃ ḍarúuri náakul fákha kullï yóom. *B.* ɤandína Ṣéeh filbéet hína ya sítti? *A.* ɤandína ɤéeʃ wi gíbna-w zíbda-w béeḍ wi-mrábba-w ʃuwáyyit makaróona-w ɤandína sámak. *B.* ɤáal. Ṣiɤmilílna-ʃwáyyit makaróona-b ʃúrbit ilɤáḍm, wi ɤandína sámak. *A.* Ṣaho kída. wi báɤdï búkr-aʃtíri fárxa-w núṭbux ɤaléeha Ṣáyyï ṣánfï-xḍáar rixíiṣ. *B.* ya sítt, garáalik éeh? Ṣinti-tgannínti?[1] di-lfiráax ɤálya xáaliṣ ilyoméen dóol. *A.* ḥaníɤmil éeh baqa? kúllï yóom láḥma, láḥma? láazim niɤáyyar ilṢáklï-ʃwayya. *B.* Ṣismáɤi baqa, lazim tifattáḥi ɤéenik. ma-tgibíiʃ firáax ɤayyaníin wi ma-txallíiʃ ilfarárgi-yɤíʃʃik. *A.* ma-txáfʃ! ma yiqdárʃi yíḍḥak ɤaláyya. *B.* ṭáyyib, lamm-aʃúuf ʃaṭártik baqa.

(fi dukkáan ittáagir bayyáaɤ ilfiráax)

A. ṣabáaḥ ilxéer. *C* (Ṣittáagir). Ṣáhlan wi sáhlan, ṣabáaḥ innúur. Ṣáyyï xídma ya háanim?[2] *A.* Ṣana ɤáwza fárxa fayyúumi-smíina. *C.* bi kúllï mamnuníyya. Ṣitfaḍḍáli, Ṣáadi fárxa zayyï ṭálabik ɤalaʃan xáṭrik. *A.* tamánha káam? *C.* ya sítt an-awzinháalik liṢann ilfiráax dilwáqti-btitbáaɤ bilmizáan. *A.* ɤáawiz káam?

---

[1] Pronounced Ṣinti-ggannínti.
[2] A term of address generally used to a young woman.

end and that things are improving. *A.* Listen, I've been to the market to buy a few vegetables. *B.* Yes, and what happened? *A.* I asked the greengrocer the price of every kind of vegetable, [and he told me the price of] peas, potatoes, beans, and so on. *B.* And did you buy (anything) or not? *A.* No, I didn't. I found everything a sight too dear (*lit.* I found everything dear, may nobody eat!). *B.* What did you do then? *A.* I left [him] and went to the butcher's and asked him whether he had any soup bones. *B.* Did you get (*lit.* buy) bones and meat? *A.* Yes, and we'll make some soup from the bones. *B.* Where did you go after that? *A.* I looked round a bit and came across a man selling fish, so I bought some from him, an oke, I should say. *B.* Good, and did you buy any fruit? *A.* [Let me tell you] Fresh fruit is very dear and we don't have to eat fruit every day. *B.* What have we got [here] in the house [my wife]? *A.* We've bread, cheese, butter, eggs, jam, and a little macaroni. Oh, and fish, too. *B.* Fine. Make us some macaroni (to go) with the soup [from the bones], and we've (already) got some fish. *A.* That's it. And the day after tomorrow I'll get a chicken and we'll have (*lit.* cook on it) some (*lit.* any kind of) cheap vegetables with it. *B.* What's come over you? Have you gone crazy? Chicken is terribly expensive these [two] days. *A.* Well, what are we going to do then? Are we going to have nothing but meat day after day? We must have a change (*lit.* change the food a little). *B.* Listen then, you must use your brains (*lit.* open your eye). Don't get diseased chicken and don't let the poulterer swindle you. *A.* Don't worry (*lit.* be afraid), he can't get the better of me (*lit.* laugh at me). *B.* All right, we (*lit.* I) shall see how clever you are, then.

(At the poulterer's (*lit.* in the shop of the merchant seller of chickens)

A. Good morning. *C* (The poulterer (*lit.* merchant)). Good morning, what can I do for you, madam? *A.* I want a fat Fayoumi chicken. *C.* With pleasure. Here you are, just the chicken you want [for your sake]. *A.* How much is it? *C.* I'll weigh it for you, madam, as chickens are sold by weight (*lit.* scales) nowadays. *A.* What does it come to (*lit.* how much do you want)? / *C.* Sixty

C. sittíin qirʃĭ sáaɣ. *A.* yáa saláam! hiyya káam rátl? *C.* xámsa-w
núṣṣ w-irrátlĭ-b ḥidáaʃər ḥasab ittasɣíira. *A.* káttar xéerak. xúd
ginéeh w-iddíini-lbáaqi. *C.* ʕitfaḍḍáli, maɣa-ʃʃúkr. ʕin ʃáaʕ
alláah tiʃarráfi marra tánya.

12. *muḥáwra ben ʕagnábi-w máṣri*

A (ʕilʕagnábi). naháarak saɣíid. *B* (ʕilmáṣri). naháarak saɣíid
mubáarak. *A.* ʕizzáyy ilḥáal? ʕinʃálla-tkúun mabṣúuṭ. *B.* ʕilḥámdu lilláah, ʕahe máʃya. wi ḥadrítak ínta mabṣúuṭ hína?
A. ʕana gáay ziyáara hína-l muddit ʃáhr. *B.* ʕáhlan wi sáhlan, wi
ḥadrítak ʃarráftĭ máṣrĭ ɣalaʃan ʃúɣlĭ walla fúsḥa? *A.* ɣalaʃan fúsḥa-l
múdda-qṣayyára. *B.* ḥadrítak ʕáwwil márra géet máṣrĭ wi-btitkál-
lim ɣárabi zayy íbn ilbálad. *A.* láʕ, ʕana batkállim ɣarabi-ʃwáyya
báss, ɣalaʃan ana kúntĭ hína-f máṣrĭ márra min zamáan, w-ilmásal
biyqúul, 'ʕilli yíʃrab min máyyit inníil yirgáɣlu táani.' *B.* déhda!
ʕinta latíif qáwi. ɣala kída ҳúrtĭ[1] maṭá ariḥ ʕasaríyya-f máṣr?
A. ʕáywa, ҳúrtĭ baɣḍ ilmaṭáariḥ. *B.* záyyĭ ʕéeh baqa? *A.* ҳúrtĭ
lúqṣur w-itfarrágtĭ ɣalʕasáar ilqadíima-lfarɣuníyya w-irrumaníyya,
w-ilmaɣáabid, wi ṭúrab ilmulúuk. *B.* ɣáal, ɣáal. w-itfarrágtĭ ɣala
ʕéeh hína-f máṣr? *A.* ʃúft iggáamiɣ ilʕázhar, wi gáamiɣ maḥámmad
ɣáli w-ilqálɣa, wi gáamiɣ íbnĭ ṭulúun[2] wi gáamiɣ irrifáaɣi-w
gáamiɣ iṣṣulṭáan ḥásan, wi gáamiɣ ɣámr ibn ilɣáaṣ fi máṣr ilqadíima.
B. yáa saláam, ʕinta ҳúrtĭ ʕamáakin ʕasaríyya-mhímma, wi ḥadrítak
ҳúrt ilkanáayis ilqadíima-f máṣr ilqadíima? *A.* láʕ, lakin ҳúrtĭ
madíinit ɣámr ittarixíyya-lli-ktaʃafítha maṣláḥit ilʕasáar. *B.* wi ҳúrtĭ
ʕéeh kamáan maṭáariḥ tarixíyya-lli-ssawwaḥíin ʕáwwil ma-byíigu
máṣrĭ-byitfarrágu ɣaléeha? *A.* ʃuft ilháram ilkibíir w-ilʕahramáat
illi ḥawaléeh, w-ábu-lhóol wi saqqáara. *B.* báaqi ɣaléek baqa-tʃúuf
ilʕantikxáana w-ilkutubxáana. *A.* ʕin ʃáaʕ alláah ʕiza káan ɣandi
wáqt, ʕana náaw-arúuḥ lilqanáaṭir ilxayríyya-w ginént ilḥayawanáat.
B. bássĭ ḥadrítak nisíit ḥáaga-mhímma. *A.* ʕéeh híyya? / *B.* xáan

---

[1] See Introduction, B (ii).
[2] Often *ṭalúun* is less educated speech.

piastres. *A.* Good heavens, how many pounds is it? *C.* Five and a half, at eleven piastres a pound according to the (official) price-list. *A.* Thank you. Here is a pound. Give me the change. *C.* There you are, thank you. I hope you will come (*lit.* honour) again.

12. *Conversation between a foreigner and an Egyptian*

A (The foreigner). Good-day. *B* (The Egyptian). Good-day to you. *A.* How are you? Well, I hope (*lit.* I hope you are happy). *B.* Yes, pretty well, thank you (*lit.* praise God, it (*fem.*) is going). Are you enjoying yourself here (*lit.* are you happy here)? *A.* (Yes.) I've come here on a month's visit. *B.* How nice (*lit.* welcome)! Have you come to (*lit.* honoured) Egypt on (*lit.* for) business or pleasure? *A.* For a short holiday. *B.* This is the first time you've been to Egypt and (yet) you speak Arabic like a native (*lit.* a son of the country). *A.* No, I only speak a little Arabic, but (*lit.* because) I was here in Egypt once a long time ago, and the proverb says, 'Whoever drinks from the water of the Nile will return to it again.' *B.* Ah, you are very kind. You've been to historical places in Egypt, I suppose (*lit.* therefore). *A.* Yes, I've visited some. *B.* Such as? *A.* I've been to Luxor and done the rounds of the old Pharaonic and Roman remains, the temples, and tombs of the kings. *B.* Fine, and what have you seen here in Cairo? *A.* [I've seen] The Azhar Mosque, the Muhammad Ali Mosque, and the Citadel, [the mosques of] Ibn Talun, the Rifa'i, Sultan Hasan, and 'Amr Ibn el-'As in Old Cairo. *B.* Really! You (certainly) have visited some interesting historical places. And have you been to the old churches in Old Cairo? *A.* No, but I've been to the ancient city of 'Amr which was discovered by the Department of Antiquities. *B.* And what about (*lit.* what have you also visited of) the places of interest that tourists make for as soon as they come to Egypt? *A.* I've seen the Great Pyramid and those around it, as well as the Sphinx and Sakkaara. *B.* Then you've only the Antiquities Museum and the Literary Museum left to see. *A.* I hope I shall (also) have time to go to the Barrages and the Zoo. *B.* But there's one important thing you've forgotten. *A.* What's that? / *B.* The Muski and the

ilxalíili w-ilʕaḥyáaʕ ilwaṭaníyya-w miqyáas¹ inníil. *A.* káttar
xéerak. ʕana-smíƹtï-w qaréet kitíir ƹan miqyáas inníil wi di ḥáaga
tarixíyya-mhímma. *B.* ƹala kída yilzámak tiẕúur kúll ilmaṭáariḥ
illi qultílak ƹaléeha ƹalaʃáan izziyáara-tkúun fi maḥallǎha. *A.* lák
ḥáqq. ʕana ḥatʕáxxar kamáan muddit usbúuƹ ƹalaʃan aʃúuf kúll
ilḥagáat ilmuhímma díyyat. *B.* ʃúuf ya xawáaga, ʕana-f ʕatámmï
listiƹdáad awarríilak kúllï máṭraḥ bidúun muqáabil.² *A.* ʕaʃkúrak
gíddan ƹalaʃan lúṭfak wi-msaƹdítak líyya. *B.* qúlli baqa, ʕéeh
ilmanáaẕir illi ƹagabítak fi máṣr? *A.* ʕaqúllak bi kúllï ṣaráaḥa báƹḍ
ilmanáaẕir kuwayyísa gíddan wi baƹḍǎha míʃ qaddï kída. *B.* gamíil,
wi ʕéeh ʕáḥsan ḥáaga-nbaṣáṭtï mínha milmaṣriyyíin? *A.* ʕáḥsan
ḥáaga ƹagabítni filmaṣriyyíin ikrámhum liḍḍéef. *B.* kuwáyyis.
ganáabak rúḥtï lúqṣur fiṣṣaƹíid, ʕéeh fíkrak ƹan innáas hináak?
A. ʕilḥaqíiqa-ṣṣaƹáyda kúrama gíddan. *B.* ʕin ʃáaʕ alláah nitqáabil
yóom litnéen w-ána-f xidmítak. maƹa-ssaláama. *A.* ʃúkran,
ʕalláah yisallímak.

13. *xáan ilxalíili*

A. ʕásƹad alláah misáak. *B.* ʕalláah yimassíik bilxéer. *A.* ʕana
saʕáltï ƹaléek fiṣṣúbḥ, wi ma kúntïʃ mawgúud w-iftakárt innak
tikúun mawgúud billéel. *B.* ʕáywa, qábl iḍḍúhr ana rúḥtï xáan
ilxalíili ƹalaʃáan aʃtíri báƹḍ ilḥagáat. *A.* muʃ ƹéeb innï-f xáan
ilxalíili ḥagáat kitíir muhímma w-ilmaṣriyyíin ma-yʃufuháaʃ wala
yiʃtiruháaʃ. *B.* saddáqni tíqdar tiqúul huwwa súuq lilʕagáanib
w-issawwaḥíin. *A.* ṣáḥḥ, liʕánn ilʕagáanib ilmawgudíin fi máṣr
w-issawwaḥíin illi-byíigu fiʃʃíta min biláad bárra, biyiʃtíru ʕáktar
ḥagáthum iṣṣuƹayyára-l zíinit biyúthum min xáan ilxalíili liʕannu
súuq ʃárqi. *B.* walláah-ana ʃúftï-hnáak baḍáayiƹ kitíira baƹḍǎha
hindíyya-w ƹagamíyya-w ṣiníyya, ʕinnam-aktárha-ṣnáaƹa maṣríyya
daqíiqa-w mutqána. *A.* ʕána liḥaddï dilwáqti ma rúḥtïʃ xáan
ilxalíili, la ʃúft ilḥagáat wal-áƹraf ismǔhum ḥátta. *B.* ʕan-aqúllak
ƹalá-smï³ báƹḍ ilḥagáat ilmuhímma w-illi láazim kullï / máṣri

¹ *maqáas* (*inníil*) is more 'characteristically colloquial'.
² Pronounce *q* as in 'Classical' (see Part I, Introduction). *bidúun miqáabil* is
used by less educated speakers.
³ = *ƹala* + *ʕism*.

native quarters, and (also) the Nilometer. *A*. Thank you, I've heard and read a good deal about the Nilometer which is very interesting historically. *B*. [Then] You must visit all the places I've told you about so that your stay shall be really profitable (*lit.* in its place). *A*. You're right. I'll stay on another week to take them all in (*lit.* see all those interesting things). *B*. Look, sir. I'm quite ready to show you everywhere without any obligation. *A*. Thank you very much for your kindness and help [to me]. *B*. Tell me, what are the sights that have impressed (*lit.* pleased) you most in Egypt? *A*. I'll tell you quite frankly, some things are very nice and others not so nice. *B*. Fair enough. And what has pleased you most about (*lit.* the nicest thing you have been pleased from it from) Egyptians? *A*. Chiefly their generosity (*lit.* the thing I've been most pleased with is the Egyptians' generosity) to a guest. *B*. Good. You've been to Luxor in Upper Egypt, what do you think of the people there? *A*. Sa'idis are certainly very generous. *B*. I hope we shall meet on Monday, when I shall be (*lit.* and I am) at your service. Good-bye. *A*. Good-bye and thank you.

13. *The Muski*

A. Good evening. *B*. Good evening. *A*. I called on (*lit.* asked after) you this morning and you weren't here, but I thought you'd be in in the evening. *B*. Yes, I went to the Muski this morning (*lit.* before noon) to buy a few things. *A*. Isn't it a shame that there are so many delightful (*lit.* important) things in the Muski which Egyptians neither see nor buy. *B*. The truth of the matter is (*lit.* believe me you can say) it's a bazaar for foreigners and tourists. *A*. True, [since] foreigners domiciled in Egypt and tourists coming from abroad in winter buy most of their small household ornaments (*lit.* small things for the adornment of their houses) from the Muski because it's an Eastern bazaar. *B*. I've certainly seen a lot of things (*lit.* goods) there, including (*lit.* some of them) Indian, Persian and Chinese (articles), although it's mostly fine Egyptian inlaid work. *A*. [Up to now] I've never been to the Muski. I haven't seen these (*lit.* the) things nor do I even know what they're called. *B*. I'll tell you the names of a few of the outstanding things which every

yiʃtirííha. bássï ɣálya. *A.* záyyï Ɛéeh? *B.* fíih zuhriyyáat gamíila maṣnúuӡa min nihჳáas áhჳmar w-áṣfar, wi ӡaléeha-ktáaba-w náqʃ, wi kamáan ӡílab xáʃab ṣuɣayyára lissagáayir muṭaӡӡáma-b sínn ilfíil. *A.* Ɛísmaӡ, Ɛana ʃúftï-f béet wáahჳid ṣáhჳbi ṣáhჳnï-nhჳáas wi ṭaqṭúuqit sagáayir, gumáal¹ gíddan muṭaӡӡamíin¹ bi fáḍḍa. *B.* míʃ bassï kída. fíih kamáan kiyáas mixaddáat li Ɛóḍt iggulúus min hჳaríir bi Ɛalwáan muxtálifa-w ӡaléehum kitáaba milqurƐáan². *A.* báqa yaӡni-hnáak hჳagáat Ɛantikáat listiӡmálha lizzíina-f fárʃ ilbéet. *B.* maӡlúum, fíih sagagíid ӡágami wi-klimáat báladi-w síbahჳ kahramáan ɣálya gíddan. *A.* Ɛilɣaráaba-nni rúhჳt iṣṣáaɣa-w hiyya gámbï xáan ilxalíili-w m-aftakártïʃ arúuhჳ hináak. *B.* Ɛiṣṣáaɣa di ӡalaʃáan innáas ilƐaɣníya-lli-byiʃtíru dáhab wi fáḍḍa. *A.* láa ya hჳabíibi, Ɛihჳna fúqara. báss ana rúhჳtï wayya-ssítt iʃtaréena lilbínt hჳálaq ṣuɣáyyar wi-rxíiṣ. *B.* wi ṭábӡan fúttï ӡalmúski w-ilham-záawi-w baḍḍáӡtï-w ḍayyáӡt ilqirʃéen. *A.* láa Ɛábadan, Ɛíhჳna dilwáqti Ɛáaxir iʃʃáhr w-iggéeb fáaḍi. *B.* Ɛaftíkir géeb issábӡï ma yixláaʃ. *A.* láa y-axúuya, ṣáahჳib ilӡiyáal láahu³ sábӡï wala ḍábӡ. *B.* ӡala kúllï hჳáal int-anistína-w nawwartína. *A.* Ɛalláah yiƐánsak wi-ynáwwar ӡaléek. Ɛismáhჳli baqa, ӡándi maӡáad. *B.* Ɛitfáḍḍal, m-aӡaṭṭaláakʃ.

14. *muhჳáwra ben wáhჳda síttï maṣríyya w-iṭṭabbáax bitáӡha*

A (Ɛissítt). y-áhჳmad. *B* (Ɛiṭṭabbáax). náӡam ya sítt. *A.* búkra hჳatkúun ӡandína-ӡzúuma-kbíira, yaӡni hჳáfla ӡalaʃan / ӡíid miláad

---

¹ See Lesson 5, 1, note (2).
² q pronounced as in 'Classical' Arabic (see Part I, Introduction).
³ = *la + hu.* For *hu,* cf. *mahúuʃ* as a variant of *mahuwwáaʃ* (Lesson 12, 4).

Egyptian should buy. They're dear, though. *A.* Such as? *B.* [There are] Beautiful engraved (*lit.* and on them writing and ornamentation) flower-vases of brass and copper, and small wooden cigarette-boxes, ivory-inlaid. *A.* [Listen] I've seen at a friend's house a brass platter and ash-tray, (both) very lovely and inlaid with silver. *B.* Not only that. There are also silk cushion covers in different colours for the lounge, with quotations (*lit.* writing) from the Koran on them. *A.* You mean they've *objets d'art* there for use as household ornaments (*lit.* for their use for adornment in furnishing the house). *B.* (Yes,) Of course, and there are (also) Persian carpets and local rugs, and very expensive rosaries of ambergris. *A.* The extraordinary thing is that I've been to the Sagha which is just beside the Muski but I haven't thought of going to the Muski itself (*lit.* there). *B.* The Sagha's only for rich people who buy gold and silver. *A.* No, my dear fellow, we're poor. I only went with the wife to buy (*lit.* and we bought) some cheap little ear-rings for the daughter. *B.* Then you must (*lit.* of course) have passed through the Muski and Hamzaawi, and spent the odd piastre on things (*lit.* bought things and wasted the two piastres). *A.* Not at all (*lit.* No, never). This is the end of the month and we're hard up (*lit.* the pocket is empty). *B.* I don't think a king's (*lit.* lion's)[1] pocket is ever empty. *A.* My dear fellow, a father (*lit.* owner of the children) is neither king nor courtier (*lit.* neither lion nor hyena).[1] *B.* Never mind (*lit.* it's all the same), it's been a pleasure seeing you (*lit.* you have cheered us and given us light). *A.* It's been a pleasure for me, too. Would you excuse me [now], I have an appointment. *B.* Of course, I won't keep you.

14. *Dialogue between an Egyptian woman and her cook*

A (The woman). Ahmad! *B* (The cook). Yes, madam. *A.* We're having a big party tomorrow [that is to say a party] for / the boy's

[1] *sabɛ* 'lion' is used to refer to a person who is outstandingly gifted in one way or another. *ɖabɛ* 'hyena' in the following sentence refers to one who is also, but somewhat less, well endowed. Reference is presumably to the strength of both animals which enables them to overcome difficulties. In the present context, B's implication, denied by A, is that A is a man of some means.

ilwálad. B. wi máalu(h), ˁana mistaɣídd. ˁilmaɣzumíin ḥaykúunuktíir ya sítt? A. ḍarúuri, liˁánnĭ lafándi ɣáazim kúll aṣḥáabu w-ana ɣázma kúll aṣḥáabi kamáan. B. yikúun ɣáʃa walla ʃáay? A. ḥaykúun ɣáʃa zayy issána-lli fáatit, ˁinta-nsíit? B. láˁ, ma-nsítʃ, ˁana básˁal ɣalaʃáan agíib ṭabbáax wayyáaya w-itnéen ṣufragíyya-ysaɣdúuni. A. ˁinta láazim tisˁálni filˁáwwil ˁéeh ilḥagáat illi ɣawzíin niɣmílha lilˁákl ɣalaʃáan tiḥaḍḍárha. B. maɣlúum, líki ḥáqq. qulíili ḥaḍrítik ɣawza tiɣmíli ˁéeh, ɣalaʃáan aʃtíri-lḥagáat illi tilzámna-nnahárḍa. A. ʃúuf baqa, ˁana ɣáwza kúllĭ ʃéeˁ yikúun mawgúud wi ḥáaḍir, ma-tkúnʃĭ fih ḥáaga náqṣa ˁábadan. B. maɣbúuṭ, ɣalaʃan búkra fiṣṣúbḥ ḥakúun maʃɣúul fi tanḍíif ilbéet wi tartíib ˁóḍt iṣṣúfra-w ˁóḍt iggulúus. A. ˁísmaɣ y-áḥmad, ˁinnáas ilmadɣiyyíin¹ múʃ ḥayáklu-w yiʃrábu-w humma qaɣdíin². dóol kitíir w-ilquɣáad móoḍa qadíima. B. ˁummáal³ aɣmil éeh? A. ʃúuf, rúṣṣ iṭṭarabeɣáat gambĭ báɣḍĭ-b ṭúul ṣafféen wi ma-tḥúṭṭíʃ karáasi ˁábadan. B. ˁana fáahim dilwáqti-nnĭ ḥaḍrítik ɣawzáan-aḥáḍḍar ṭarabeɣáat buféeh. A. ˁáywa kída, dá-ll-ana ɣawzáah, liˁannĭ kúll innáas dilwáqti-byiɣmílu bufeháat filḥafaláat. B. dilwáqti qulíili ɣala kúllĭ ṭalabáatik illi ɣawzáaha min iṣnáaf⁴ ilxuḍáar w-ilfawáakih w-ilḥalawiyyáat w-iṭṭuyúur w-illáḥma. A. ˁiʃtíri díik rúumi-w tálat farxáat, wi fáxdit xarúuf wi ɣáʃart irṭáal láḥma-btíllu min ɣéer ɣáḍm, w-illáḥma tiɣmílha kulláha sandawitʃáat. B. w-agíib xuḍáar éeh? A. háat bisílla xáḍra-w faṣúlya xáḍra wi-ʃwáyyit gázar wi baṭáaṭiṣ báss. ˁana muʃ ɣáwza ṭabíix kitíir, ˁana ɣáwz-áktar ilˁáklĭ nawáaʃif. B. ḥaníɣmil ṣálaṭit ˁéeh? A. ˁíɣmil ṣanféen, wi ma tinsáaʃ tiḥáḍḍar gíbna túrki-w gíbna báladi⁵-w sardíin ɣalaʃáan ilḥagáat di-tkun mázza liˁánnĭ ḥaykúun fih ʃúrb. B. ḥáaḍir ya sítt. w-agíib iṣnáaf fákha ˁéeh? A. háat tiffáaḥ wi móoz wi mánga-w kommítra w-iza káan fih míʃmiʃ fissúuq háat ʃuwáyya. B. bássĭ ḥaḍrítik ma qultíiʃ ɣalḥalawiyyáat. niɣmílha filbéet walla niʃtiríiha? A. xud báalak inta ḥatkúun maʃɣúul li ˁáaxir dáraga filmáṭbax, múʃ ḥatíqdar tíɣmil ḥalawiyyáat, / ya dóobak tigáhhiz

---

¹ madɣuwwíin (sing. mádɣu) is also used by educated speakers.
² Notice the construction with wi. See also Lesson 34, 2.
³ Pronounced with 'back' a.
⁴ Or min ˁaṣnáaf, although this is less likely from the cook than from his employer.
⁵ See Lesson 3, 1, note (7).

birthday. *B*. That's quite all right (*lit*. what of it, I am ready). Will
there be many guests (*lit*. invitees)? *A*. Of course. [Since] The
master and I have both invited all our friends. *B*. Will it be dinner
or tea? *A*. Dinner, the same as last year. Have you forgotten?
B. No, I haven't forgotten, I'm (only) asking so that I (can) get
a cook and two waiters to help me. *A*. You'd better ask me first
what food we want (*lit*. what things we want to make them for
eating), so that you can get it ready. *B*. Yes, of course, you're
right. Tell me what you want [to do] so that I can buy the things
we need today. *A*. Listen (*lit*. see), then. I want everything here
ready, there mustn't be anything missing. *B*. I agree, for tomorrow
morning I shall be busy cleaning the house and putting the lounge
and dining-room in order. *A*. Look, Ahmad, the guests (*lit*. people
asked) aren't going to sit down to eat and drink. There are too
many of them, and sit-down parties (*lit*. sitting) are old-fashioned.
B. What shall I do, then? *A*. [Look] Draw the tables together
lengthways (in) two rows, and don't put out any chairs at all.
B. I understand now, [that] you want me to prepare buffet tables.
A. Yes, that's it, that's what I want. [Because] Everybody has a
buffet for parties nowadays. *B*. Would you tell me now what you
want by way of (*lit*. all the orders you want of kinds of) vegetables,
fruit, sweets, poultry, and meat. *A*. Get (*lit*. buy) a turkey, three
chickens, a leg of lamb, and ten *rotls* of boned veal. We'll have
(*lit*. you'll make) all the meat (in) sandwiches. *B*. And what
vegetables shall I get? *A*. Just some peas, green beans, a few carrots
and potatoes. I don't want too much hot food but would rather
have most of it cold. *B*. What sort of salad shall we have? *A*. Make
two kinds, and don't forget to get Turkish cheese, local cheese, and
sardines to use as (*lit*. so that those things may be) 'mezzy',[1] since
there'll be drinks (beforehand). *B*. Yes, madam, and what sort of
fruit shall I get? *A*. Apples, bananas, mangoes, and pears, and if
there are any apricots in the market, bring some. *B*. There's just
the sweets you haven't said anything about. Shall we make them
here or buy them? *A*. Be careful, you're going to be extremely
busy in the kitchen. You won't be able to make sweets / or (do)

[1] The name given by Europeans in Egypt to the titbits of food at a cocktail
party.

iṭṭabíix w-ilˤákl. *B.* ṭáyyib, ˤaʃtiríiha min ˤáyyï maḥáll? *A.* láˤ, ma tiʃtiríiʃ inta, ˤána ḥakállim ilḥalawáani fittilifóon w-awaṣṣíih yíˠmil lína-lḥalawiyyáat ill-ana ˠawzáaha ṭáaẓa, wi yibˠathálna.[1]

15. (*takmílit ilmuḥáwra-ssábqa*)

(báˠd intiháaˤ[2] ilḥáfla)

B. ya sítt, ḥaḍrítik mabṣúuṭa milḥáfla? *A.* ˤáywa-nbaṣáṭtï[3] gíddan w-ilḥáfla kanit ˠaˠíima-l ˤáaxir dáraga. *B.* ˤilḥámdu lilláah, rabbína sátar. w-ilˤáklï kan kifáaya-w kan fíih ziyáada min kúllï ṣánf. *A.* múʃ bassï kída, ˤilˤáklï kan lazíiz lilyáaya, w-ilḥaqíiqannak ma ṭabáxtïʃ ṭabíix zayyï kída ˤábadan. *B.* ˤinʃálla-ykunuḍḍiyúuf inbáṣaṭu min kúllï ḥáaga-w xáragu mabṣuṭíin. *A.* ˤinta láazim tikun muṭmaˤínnï[4] milgíha di, liˤann ilmaˠazíim qalúuli-nn inniẓáam w-ittartíib kan gamíil wi múdhiʃ. *B.* kúllï dá-b náfasik w-ilfáḍlï líki. *A.* láa y-áḥmad. ˤilfáḍlï lilláah w-inta kamáan tiˠíbtï-ktíir. *B.* láˤ, ma fíiʃ táˠab iza káanit innatíiga-kwayyísa-w mufríḥa, wi táˠabik ráaḥa ya sítt. *A.* y-áḥmad, taˠáala hína-w háat wáraqa-w qálam ˠalaʃan tíˠmil ḥisáab ilmaṣaríif illi ṣaraftǎha. *B.* ḥáaḍir. bássï lamm-áyli-llában w-áysil báaqi-lḥagáat . . . *B.* náˠam ya sítt. ˤana xallǎṣtï kúll ilḥagáat illi filmáṭbax. *A.* qúlli ˠala táman kúllï ḥáaga-ʃtarétha. *B.* ˤiʃtaréet díik rúumi bitnéen ginéeh wi núṣṣ, wi-fráax bi míyya-w ˠiʃríin qírʃ, wi fáxda ḍáani-b míyya-w xamsíin qírʃ, wi láḥma-btíllu min ˠéer ˠáḍmï-b míyya-w sabˠíin qírʃï-w sábˠa mallíim. *A.* ˠala kída-ykun ilḥisáab suttumíyya-w tisˠíin qírʃ. *B.* láa ya sítt, líss-ana ma qúltïʃ ˠala táman iṣṣálaṭa w-ilxáll w-illamúun w-ilmuṣṭárḍa, w-issardíin w-iggíbna w-ilbéeḍ, w-ilxiyáar w-ilxáṣṣ w-ilxuḍáar w-ilfákha. *A.* ṭáyyib, qúul, mistánni ˤéeh? ˤistáˠgil! ˤana ˠándi maˠáad wi ˠawz-áxrug

---

[1] Pronounced *yibˠathánna*.
[2] A 'classicism'. The 'more colloquial' form ˤintíha is not used by educated speakers. See Lesson 35, 3, note (ii).
[3] Pronounced (*i*)*mbaṣáṭt*(*i*).
[4] A word of very rare pattern.

anything other than (*lit.* you just) prepare the food.[1] *B.* All right, where (*lit.* from which place) shall I buy them? *A.* No, you're not to buy (anything). I'll phone the pastry shop (*lit.* confectioner) and ask them (*lit.* charge him) to make us some fresh sweets (*lit.* sweets that I want fresh) and to send them [to us].

15. (*Conclusion of the preceding dialogue*)

(After the [end of the] party)

B. Were you satisfied with the party, madam? *A.* Yes, I was very pleased, the party was a great success (*lit.* wonderful to the last degree). *B.* Good (*lit.* praise God. God has protected (us))! And there was more than enough food of every kind. *A.* Not only that, the food was extremely tasty, in fact you've never cooked so well. *B.* I hope the guests were pleased and went away satisfied. *A.* You can rest assured of that, for they (*lit.* the invitees) told me that the arrangements were first-rate. *B.* It was your idea and the merit is yours. *A.* No, Ahmad. Things went well (*lit.* the merit is God's) and you yourself went to great trouble (*lit.* tired yourself a lot). *B.* No, it's no trouble (*lit.* there is no tiredness) if the result is worthwhile (*lit.* good and happy). I am happy to do my best for you, madam (*lit.* tiredness for your sake is rest). *A.* Come here, Ahmad, and bring a pencil and paper to reckon up (*lit.* make the account of) what you spent. *B.* Certainly, but let me just boil the milk and finish the washing-up (*lit.* wash the rest of the things. .).
B. Now, madam. I've finished everything in the kitchen. *A.* Tell me the price of everything you bought. *B.* I bought a turkey for two and a half pounds, chickens for a hundred and twenty piastres, a leg of lamb for a hundred and fifty piastres, and the boned veal for a hundred and seventy piastres and seven millemes. *A.* That comes to six hundred and ninety piastres, then. *B.* No, madam, I still haven't told (you) the cost of the salad, vinegar, lemons, mustard, sardines, cheese, eggs, cucumbers, lettuce, vegetables, and fruit. *A.* All right, speak up! What are you waiting for? Come on! I've an appointment and want to go out. / I'm late (already).

---

[1] There is little or no difference of meaning between *ṭabīx* and *ʕakl* in this set expression.

w-itˁaxxárt. *B.* táman kúll ilḫagáat díyyat wayya báᵹd mitéen
tísᵹa-w sabᵹíin qírʃĭ-w núṣṣ. *A.* ˁana-ddétlak ᵹáʃara-gnéeh w-ilḫi-
sáab dilwáqti tusᵹumíyya tísᵹa-w sittíin wi núṣṣ, báaqi talatíin
qírʃĭ-w núṣṣ, dóol ᵹalaʃáanak. *B.* káttar xéerik. ˁalláah yiṭáwwil
ᵹúmrik wi-yxallíilik íbnik.

16. *fiṣáal ben táagir wi-zbúun*

A. ṣabáaḫ ilxéer. *B.* ˁalláah yiṣabbáḫak bilxéer. ˁitfáḍḍal. náᵹam,
láazim xídma? *A.* ˁáywa, lazímni ḫagáat baṣíiṭa. *B.* ˁitfáḍḍal, da
maḫállak. ˁúṭlub w-ana táḫtĭ ˁámrak. báss itfáḍḍal istaráyyaḫ
ᵹalkúrsi. *A.* mutaʃákkir. *B.* tiḫíbbĭ tíʃrab qáhwa sukkar ziyáada
walla mazᵹbúuṭa walla sáada? *A.* láˁ, káttar xéerak, qahwítak
maʃrúuba, ᵹíʃt. *B.* ṣabáaḫ illában wi nahárna zayy ilqíʃṭa. ˁéeh
ṭalabáatak? *A.* walláahi waḫid ṣáḫbi kallífn-aʃtiríilu ṣaníyyit
niḫáas áṣfar mifaḍḍáḍa. *B.* ṣaníyyit qáhwa walla ṣaníyyit ˁéeh?
A. láa, láa, ṣaníyya-b kúrsi xáʃab maxrúuṭ, ᵹalaʃáan yiḫuṭṭáha
zíina-f ˁóḍt iggulúus. *B.* ˁitfáḍḍal, záyyĭ dí wall-ákbar wall-áṣyar?
A. láˁ, mutawaṣṣíṭa. *B.* ʃúuf iṣṣawáani-ktíir quddáamak ahéh, wi
náqqi-lli tiᵹgíbak. *A.* ˁana ᵹáawiz dí. bi káam tibíᵹha? *B.* ḫaḍrítak
ᵹawiz tifáaṣil walla ᵹáawiz kalam wáaḫid? *A.* ˁiza kúntĭ-tqúlli
ᵹattáman bilḫáqqĭ-w titsáahil filbéeᵹ, ma fíʃ luzúum lilfiṣáal.
B. walláahi maḫallína maᵹrúuf wi zabayínna ᵹarfínna láa binzáw-
wid wala binnáqqaṣ wi kalámna wáaḫid. *A.* ṭáyyib, da-kwáyyis
kida. ˁittáman káam baqa? *B.* ˁittáman biṣṣála ᵹannábi, ˁarbáᵹa-
gnéeh. *A.* ya ʃéex inta xaḍḍétni. ˁéeh ittáman dá? *B.* láa ma
titxáḍḍĭʃ, yixalláʃak tídfaᵹ káam. *A.* ˁan-ádfaᵹ itnéen ginéeh
liˁanni-ʃtaréet uxtắha tamáam bittamánda. / *B.* y-afándi, ˁikkaláam

B. The cost of all those things together is two hundred and seventy-nine piastres and a half. *A.* I gave you ten pounds and the total now is nine hundred and sixty-nine and a half. That leaves thirty and a half. That's for you. *B.* Thank you very much, madam (*lit.* may God lengthen your life and leave you your son).

16. *Bargaining between a shopkeeper* (lit. *merchant*) *and a customer*

A. Good morning. *B.* Good morning. Do come in. Well, is there anything I can do for you? *A.* Yes, I want a few small things. *B.* Certainly [this is your place]. I'm at your service (*lit.* ask and I am under your order). But do sit down (*lit.* please rest on the chair). *A.* Thank you. *B.* Do you like (your) coffee very sweet (*lit.* much sugar), half and half, or without sugar? *A.* No, no coffee, thank you all the same. *B.* Not at all.[1] What are you looking for, then (*lit.* what are your requests then)? *A.* Well now, a friend of mine has asked me to buy him a brass silver-inlaid tray. *B.* A coffee tray or what? *A.* No, a tray with a turned wooden stand (*lit.* chair) to use (*lit.* so that he put it) as an ornament in the lounge. *B.* Take your pick. Like this one, bigger, or smaller? *A.* No, average size. *B.* Look over this lot of trays in front of you and pick the one you like (*lit.* which pleases you). *A.* I'd like this one. How much do you want for it (*lit.* sell it at)? *B.* Do you want to bargain or (me to give you) a fixed price (*lit.* one word)? *A.* If you give me a fair price (*lit.* tell with truth) and are reasonable (*lit.* easy in selling), then there's no need for bargaining. *B.* My dear sir,[2] our shop (*lit.* place) is well-known and our customers know that we don't put our prices either up or down, they're fixed. *A.* Good, that's fine. How much then? B. Well, let's arrive at a fair price.[3] Four pounds! *A.* You've frightened me off, my friend. What kind of a price is that? *B.* Don't be put off, say how much you're prepared to pay. *A.* I'll give two pounds, since that was what I gave for one exactly like it (*lit.* exactly its sister). / *B.* Not these days, sir (*lit.* that

---

[1] A rough approximation in the context to *ṣabáaḥ ,. . . qíſṭa.* See App. A.

[2] Roughly the force of *walláahi.*

[3] This is perhaps as near as one can get in translation to *biṣṣála ɣannáabi* (lit. 'by praying on the Prophet').

dá w-ittáman dá míʃ dilwáqti.   da kan zamáan lamma-lḥagáat kanit
rixíiṣa.   A. Ṣana ɣáarif innĭ dilwáqti ɣála w-ilḥagáat ɣálya, wi
ɣalaʃáan kíd-adfáꜧlak itnéen ginéeh wi núṣṣ.   B. láa, láa, líssa bádri,
yíꜧhar innak gáay titfárrag báss walla gáay tifáaṣil, míʃ gay tiʃtíri.
Ṣana qultĭlak milṢáwwil, Ṣíḥna ma ꜧandĭnáaʃ fiṣáal.   A. déhda!
Ṣinta raḥḥábtĭ bíyya filṢáwwil w-ana ꜧáawiz akun zibúun ilmaḥáll.
B. Ṣáhlan wi sáhlan, Ṣilmaḥállĭ maḥállak.   xúd ill-inta ꜧáwzu-w
baláaʃ ilfilúus.   A. láa ma-yꜧáḥḥĭʃ, wi madáam qúltĭ min ɣéer filúus
w-ana-ʃríbtĭ qáhwa-f dukkáanak¹, níqsim ilbálad nuṣṣéen adfáꜧlak
taláata-gnéeh.   B. y-afándi, ḥaráam tixaṣṣárni núṣṣ ittáman.   A. láa
ma fíiʃ xuṣáara. Ṣan-aꜧawwaḍháalak fi béeꜧa tánya. ̣B. tiꜧawwádli-
lxuṣáara-f béeꜧa tánya-zzáay?   A. filṢusbúuꜧ illi gáay ḥági hína
w-aʃtíri-ʃwayyit ḥagáat abꜧátha hadáaya-l Ṣaṣḥáabi², wi kamáan
ḥagíblak maꜧáaya zabáayin gudáad.   B. Ṣiza kan kída ma fiʃ
máaniꜧ.   Ṣitfáḍḍal iṣṣaníyya-héh!   mabrúuk!   A. Ṣalláah yibarik
fíik.   Ṣitfáḍḍal ilfilúus.   B. maꜧa-ssaláama.   Ṣana muntáz̦irak
tiʃárraf filṢusbúuꜧ illi gáay.   A. bi Ṣíznĭ-lláah.

17. Ṣilḥaʃʃáaʃ wi-ḥmíiru(h)

káan fih ráagil ḥaʃʃáaʃ ꜧandu ꜧáʃar ḥimíir filbéet, wi-f yóom min
dóol ilḥaʃʃáaʃ ḥáʃʃiʃ wi xád ḥimíiru-w xárag milbéet, wi ríkib
ḥumáar mínhum wi ꜧádd ittanyíin.   fa laqáahum tísꜧa-w qáal fi
náfsu(h) 'gára Ṣéeh!   Ṣana ꜧándi ꜧáʃar ḥimíir wi dilwáqti húmma
tísꜧa!   Ṣana ɣalṭáan walla-mḥáʃʃiʃ walla sakráan walla Ṣéeh?'
    qam nízil min fóoq ilḥumáar illi kan³ rákbu wi ꜧaddŭhum wi
laqáahum ꜧáʃara.   fa qáal fi náfsu(h) 'Ṣéeh ḥáṣal li múxxi, láazim
ana magnúun.'
    fa rígiꜧ li béetu-w qáal li-mráatu⁴ ꜧalli⁵ ḥáṣal wi ṭálab mínha-
nnǎha-twaddíih lilxánka.   fíhmit maráatu-nnu-mḥáʃʃiʃ wi qalítlu(h)
'ṢilṢáḥsan innak tímʃi wi-txálli-ḥmáar mínhum yirkábak.'   fa-

¹ Coffee had been brought despite the customer's earlier protestations.
² Or (hadáaya) laṣḥáabi.
³ May be pronounced kar, since r follows.
⁴ Notice the elision of a. mára is a word of rare pattern.   Notice the long
vowel in the suffixed form maráatu(h).   ⁵ = ꜧan + Ṣilli.

speech and price are not (of) now). That was a long time ago when things were cheap. *A.* I know that things are dear nowadays and therefore I'll go to two and a half pounds. *B.* Oh, no. You're still a long way away (*lit.* it's (i.e. the price) still early). It looks as if you've just come to look round or to bargain, not to buy. I've told you from the beginning that we don't bargain (*lit.* we haven't bargaining). *A.* Indeed! What about the welcome you gave me at first and (the fact that) I want to be a customer [of the shop]. *B.* Certainly (*lit.* welcome), the shop is yours. Take what you want and never mind about paying. *A.* No, that's impossible, but since you say never mind the money and since I've drunk coffee in your shop, let's split the difference (*lit.* divide the town in two) and I'll pay you three pounds. *B.* It's wrong to make me lose half the price. *A.* But you lose nothing (*lit.* there isn't any loss), (since) I'll make it up to you another time (*lit.* in another sale). *B.* How will you do that? *A.* I'll come here next week and buy a few things to send as presents to my friends, and I'll also bring some new customers with me. *B.* If that's the case, I've no objection. Here, take the tray. Congratulations! *A.* Thank you. Here's the money. *B.* Goodbye, and I'm expecting you [to honour (me)] next week. *A.* Yes, I trust so (*lit.* with God's permission).

17. *The hashish smoker and his donkeys*

There was (once) a hashish smoker who had ten donkeys in his (*lit.* the) house. One day, after smoking some hashish, he took his donkeys and left the house. He mounted one of them, counted the remaining nine (*lit.* counted the others and found them nine), and said to himself, 'What's happened? I have ten donkeys but now they are (only) nine. Am I wrong, drugged, drunk, or what?'

So he got off the donkey he was riding, and counting (*lit.* he counted) them again and finding them ten, said to himself, 'What's happened to my brain? I must be crazy.'

So he returned home, told his wife [about] what had happened and asked her to take him to the asylum. His wife realized (*lit.* understood) that he was drugged so she said to him, 'The best thing is for you to walk and let one of the donkeys ride *you.*' The

nbáṣaṭ ilḥaʃʃáaʃ wi qáal li-mráatu(h) 'kuwáyyis gíddan, ɀalaʃáan yikun ɀándik filbéet ḥiḋáaʃar ḥumáar, tirkábi-lli yiɀgíbik mínhum.'

qáamit maráatu qalítlu(h) 'ʕan-arkábak ínta' w-itṣáwwar[1] ilḥaʃʃáaʃ innu húwwa ʕáḥsan ilḥimíir kulláha w-ibtáda-ynáḥhaq bi ṣóot ɀáali gíddan, fa ḋíḥkit ɀaléeh maráatu w-itlámmu-lgiráan wi fíḋlu yiḋḥáku.

wi lamma fáaq ilḥaʃʃáaʃ wi fíhim innúkta, ṭállaq maráatu bittaláata.[2]

18. *gúḥa*[3] *filmáṭɀam*

fi yóom min záat ilʕayyáam gúḥa-txáaniq wayya-mráatu fa ṭaraḋítu milbéet, fa xárag zaɀláan wi kan gaɀáan gíddan wi-mfállis.

fa ɀámal ʃaḥḥáat wi fíḋil yilíffĭ min ʃáariɀ li ʃáariɀ wi min ḥáara-l ḥáara-w min béet li béet, yíʃḥat wi-yqúul 'ḥásana lilláah, míin yiʃaḥḥátni qírʃĭ walla lúqmit ɀéeʃ ʕarúddĭ bíiha gúɀti? min yoméen ma káltĭʃ wi-mráati ṭarḋáani milbéet.'

báɀḋ innáas istaɣrábu-w qáalu 'da ráagil magnúun', wi báɀḋ innáas kanu-byiʃtimúuh wi baɀḋúhum kanu biyqulúulu(h) 'ɀal-álla, ʕalláah yiɀṭíik.'[4]

wi biṣṣúdfa ʃaf wáaḥid yahúudi fissíkka masik lúqmit ɀéeʃ biyáakul fíiha, qáam qárrab mínnu-w máddĭ ʕíidu-w qállu(h) 'ʕiddíini ḥítta milli-btáakul mínnu(h)' fa ʃáxaṭ fíih ilyahúudi-w qállu(h) 'ʕana ʃaḥḥáat záyyak, ḥatímʃi wall-andáhlak waḥid ʃawíiʃ yiwaddíik ilkarakóon.'

qam sáabu-w míʃi, wi huwwa máaʃi ʃammĭ ríiḥit ʕákl, fa báṣṣĭ ɀala-ymíinu wi ʃáaf máṭɀam wi ɀala ṭúul dáxal ilmáṭɀam wi ṭálab ʕákl, wi kál liḥáddĭ ma ʃíbiɀ wi lámm ilbáaqi-w ḥáṭṭu-f géebu-w qáam. wi báɀḋĭ kída ráaḥ ɀandĭ ṣáaḥib ilmáṭɀam wi sáʕalu(h) 'ʕiza káan wáaḥid ṭarḋáah maráatu milbéet wi géh hína-w kál / wi ma-

---

[1] Pronounced iṣṣáwwar (see Lesson 24, 2, note (5)).

[2] The husband utters the appropriate formula three times if he wishes the divorce to be irrevocable.

[3] Guha, the picaresque character of the simpleton who is rarely outwitted and never at a loss for words, is the hero of innumerable anecdotes told throughout the Arabic-speaking countries. The student could profitably make his own collection of Guha stories, which provide excellent colloquial material.

[4] Standard refusal of a beggar's request for alms.

hashish smoker was delighted (with this) and said to his wife, 'Excellent (idea)! You'll have eleven donkeys in the house and (be able to) ride whichever one you please (*lit.* pleases you of them).'

Then his wife said to him, 'I'll ride *you*', and the man imagined he was the best of all the donkeys and began to bray very loudly (*lit.* in a very loud voice). His wife laughed at him and the neighbours, gathering round, laughed until they couldn't stop.[1]

When the man sobered up and realized the joke, he (at once) divorced his wife.

18. *Guha in the restaurant*

One day Guha quarrelled with his wife and she turned him out of the house. So he took himself off (*lit.* went out) angry, very hungry, and penniless.

He took to begging (*lit.* made a beggar), doing the rounds of the streets, side-streets, and houses, saying, 'Alms for the sake of God! Who'll give me a piastre or a crust (*lit.* piece of bread) to take the edge off my appetite (*lit.* that I may answer my hunger with it)? I haven't eaten for two days, and my wife has turned me out of the house.'

And some [of the people] said in astonishment (*lit.* were astonished and said), 'That's a madman!', while others abused him and some again said to him, 'May God give you (alms)!'

Then suddenly he saw in the street a Jew holding a piece of bread and eating it. So he went up to him, held out his hand and said, 'Give me a little of what you're eating.' Thereupon the Jew shouted at him [saying], 'I'm a beggar like you. Are you going or shall I call a policeman to take you to the station?'

So Guha left him and went off, and as he was walking along, he smelt food (*lit.* the odour of food). Looking to his right and seeing a restaurant, he went straight in and ordered a meal. He ate his fill (*lit.* until he was satisfied), collected what was over, put it in his pocket and got up. Then (*lit.* after that) he went to the proprietor of the restaurant and asked him: 'If someone whose wife had turned him out of the house came here and ate / without having (the)

[1] The force of *fiḍlu* is that they began to laugh and went on and on.

mᵹáhʃĭ-flúus yídfaᵹ táman ilꜤákl, tiᵹmil fíih Ꜥéeh?' fa qállu ṣáaḥib
ilmáṭᵹam 'Ꜥaḍrábu w-axarʃímlu wíʃʃu w-akassárlu-dmáayu(h)'. fa
qállu gúḥa 'ṭáyyib, ʃáhhil! yálla laxbáṭli wíʃʃi-w kássar ráasi
ᵹalaʃan ana mistáᵹgil wi bádal m-anáam ᵹarraṣíif, Ꜥanáam ᵹala-sríir
filmustáʃfa, wi bádal m-alíffĭ fiʃʃawáariᵹ w-áʃḥat, Ꜥáakul filmustáʃfa
maggáanan, wi miʃ ᵹáawiz aʃuf xílqit maráati táani márra.'

19. Ꜥilfalláaḥ w-ilᵹarḍiḥálgi

fi yóom milꜤayyáam wáaḥid falláaḥ gáahil géh milꜤaryáaf li máṣr,
wi di káanit Ꜥáwwil márra lú(h), wi ma kánʃĭ yíᵹraf yíqra wala
yíktib.

wi lámma kan máaʃi fiʃʃáariᵹ ʃáaf ilbúʃṭa-w náas kitíir maskíin
gawabáat wi baᵹḍúhum biyírmu gawabáat fi sandúuq ilbúʃṭa, wi
ráagil qáaᵹid biyíktib wi náas qaᵹdíin ḥawaléeh.[1]

fa sáꜤal ilfalláaḥ wáaḥid wáaqif wi qállu(h) 'Ꜥirragílda-byíktib
éeh?' fa qállu(h) 'biyíktib ᵹaráayiḍ wi gawabáat'.

fa ráaḥ ilfalláaḥ ᵹándu-w qállu(h) 'ya síid-ana ᵹáwzak tiktíbli
gawáab w-addíilak Ꜥugrítak qírʃĭ sáay bádal qírʃĭ taᵹríifa, liꜤinnĭ[2]
kúllĭ ḥáaga yálya dilwaqti'.

fa qállu-rráagil 'ḥatíbᵹat iggawábda féen, wi ᵹáawiz tiqúul fih
Ꜥéeh?' fa qállu-lfalláaḥ 'ḥabᵹátu baládna w-ásꜤal ᵹan gamústi
liꜤínni sibtǎha ᵹayyáana-w muʃ ᵹáarif ḥaṣal láha Ꜥéeh'. fa qállu-
rráagil 'muʃ múmkin aktíblak gawáab liꜤannĭ rígli-btiwgáᵹni-w
m-aqdárʃ amʃi ᵹaléeha'. fa ráddĭ ᵹaléeh ilfalláaḥ wi qállu(h) 'Ꜥana
muʃ ᵹáwzak tiktíbli-ggawáab bi ríglak wi kamáan muʃ ᵹáwzak
tirúuḥ baládna ᵹala rigléek'. fa qállu-rráagil 'ya síidi, Ꜥiza kúnt
aktíblak gawáab li báladak lazímn-arúuḥ lilbálad bitáᵹtak ᵹalaʃan
aqráah quddáam gamústak liꜤánnĭ ma ḥáddĭʃ yíᵹraf yíqra xáṭṭi
ᵹéeri Ꜥána'.

---

[1] Notice the suffixed form of *ḥawaléen*.   [2] For *liꜤann*.

money to pay the price of the meal, what would you do to him?'
The proprietor said to him, 'I'd knock his head off (*lit.* hit him and
scratch his face and smash his brains).' So Guha said to him,
'All right, get on with it (*lit.* hurry)! Give me a drubbing (*lit.*
mangle[1] my face for me and break my pate) for I'm in a hurry.
Instead of sleeping on the pavement, I shall sleep in (*lit.* on) a
hospital bed, and rather than go round the streets begging, I shall
eat for nothing [in hospital], and I never want to see my wife's face
again!'

19. *The peasant and the scribe*

One day an ignorant peasant came from the country to Cairo. It
was his first visit (*lit.* the first time for him) and he could neither
read nor write.

As he was walking along the street, he saw the post-office and a
lot of people with (*lit.* holding) letters in their hands, among them
some posting (*lit.* throwing) letters in the box. And (he also saw)
a man sitting writing with people [sitting] around him.

The peasant said to a bystander (*lit.* asked one standing and said
to him), 'What's that man writing?' to which the man replied (*lit.*
and he said to him), '[He is writing] Petitions and letters.'

So the peasant went up to him and said, 'Sir, I want you to write
a letter for me. I'll give you [(as) your fee] a piastre instead of
half a piastre since everything is so expensive nowadays.'

The man said to him, 'Where are you going to send this letter
and what do you want to say in it?' 'I shall send it to our village
and ask after my water buffalo since she was ill when I left (*lit.* I
left her ill), and I wonder (*lit.* don't know) what's become of (*lit.*
happened to) her.' 'I can't write a letter for you because my foot
hurts me and I can't walk on it.' [And the peasant answered],
'I don't want you to write me the letter with your foot nor do I want
you to walk to our village.' '[Sir] If I write a letter for you to your
village, I'm bound to go [to your village] in order to read it to (*lit.*
before) your buffalo, because nobody can read my writing except
me.'

---

[1] The language of Guha stories is often picturesque.

20. Ɛiddáarit ilḥukúuma-f máṣr

A. Ɛissaláamu ḏaléekum. *B* (Ɛilḏúmda). ḏaléekumu-ssaláam wi raḥmátu-lláah wi barakáatu(h). *A.* tismáḥli min fáḍlak ásɛal ḥaḍrítak suɛáal. *B.* Ɛitfáḍḍal bi kúll ilmamnuníyya, Ɛáyyï xídma? *A.* ya ḥáḍrit ilḏúmda, Ɛana ḥasáafir máṣr, líyya ʃúɣla filmiḥáfẓa-w muʃ ḏarífha féen. *B.* Ɛinta ḥatsáafir máṣrï-w muʃ ḏáarif ḥáaga-zzáay? *A.* láɛ, Ɛana muʃ ḏáarif ḥáaga ḏan dawawíin ilḥukúuma-w maṣalíḥha. *B* ṭáyyib, Ɛan-afahhímak kúllï ḥáaga. *A.* káttar xéerak. walláah-ana ḏándi ḥáẓẓï-w ḥaḍrítak ráagil ṭáyyib. *B.* Ɛéeh illi ḏáawiz tiḏráfu(h)? *A.* wiẓáarit Ɛéeh ilmasɛúula ḏalɛidáara-lḏámma-f máṣr? *B.* wiẓáarit iddaxlíyya híyya-lmasɛúula w-ilmuʃrífa ḏalmuḥafẓáat w-ilmudiriyyáat w-ilmaráakiz. *A.* mitʃákkir gíddan, bássï ḏandi suɛáal wáaḥid. Ɛísmï raɛíis ilbulíiṣ éeh? *B.* fi kúllï-mḥáfẓa wi-mdiríyya-w márkaz raɛíis ilbulíiṣ ismu-lḥikimḍáar. *A.* Ɛísmï raɛíis ilmiḥáfẓa Ɛéeh? *B.* Ɛísmu-lmuḥáafiẓ. *A.* Ɛéeh ilfárqï ben ilmudiriyyáat w-ilmiḥafẓáat? *B.* Ɛilmuḥafẓáat filmúdun ikkibíira zayyï máṣrï w-iskindiríyya w-issuwées w-ilmudiriyyáat filɛaryáaf zayyï-mdiríyyit ilɣarbíyya w-iʃʃarqíyya-w qína. *A.* maf-húum innï raɛíis ilmudiríyya-smu-lmudíir. *B.* Ɛáynaḏam,[1] w-ilmudiríyya mitqassíma-l maráakiz kitíira wi raɛíis ilmárkaz ismu maɛmúur. *A.* Ɛiza kan fíih maráakiz kitíira láazim ilmaɛmúur yikun masɛúul ḏan biláad kitíira-ṣɣayyára. *B.* ṣaḥíiḥ wiláakin rúɛasa-lbiláad iṣṣuɣayyára húmma-lḏúmad. *A.* ṭáyyib ana fáahim dilwáqti-za káan ḏándi ḥáaga filbálad walla ʃákwa, Ɛaqaddímha lilḏúmda. *B.* tamáam w-iza ma kúntïʃ áqdar arúddï ḏaléek, Ɛaqáddim ilmawḍúuḏ lilmaɛmúur w-iza kan fíih luzúum ilmaɛ-múur yiqaddímu lilmudíir w-ilmudíir yiqaddímu lilwazíir. *A.* ʃéeɛ ɣaríib, wiláakin éeh ilḥagáat ill-ana-smiḏṭáha-b xuṣúuṣ ilmagáalis ilbaladíyya? *B.* Ɛilmagáalis ilbaladíyya muntáxaba[2]-b Ɛaṣwáat Ɛáhl ilbálad záyyï ma-ntaxábna Ɛaḏdáaɛ[3] máglis ilmudiríyya-f mudiriyyítna. *A.* yaḏni ma fíiʃ máglis báladi-f baládna? *B.* láɛ, wiláakin ilmúdun ikkibíira-lli fíiha-mḥafẓáat fíiha máglis

---

[1] Pronounced with 'back' *a* in the first syllable.
[2] The pattern is that of the Classical passive participle. The word is used here by the 'Umda: one would expect the form *mintíxba* from the *fellah* talking to him.
[3] 'More colloquially' *Ɛáḏḍa*.

20. *Government administration in Egypt*

A. Good day. *B* (The Umda). Good day to you. *A.* Forgive me
(*lit.* excuse me please) if I ask you a question. *B.* Certainly, please
do [what can I do for you?] *A.* I'm going to Cairo, I've some business at the Governorate but don't know where it is. *B.* How is it
you're going to Cairo and don't know anything about it? *A.* I
know nothing about the Government offices and [its] departments.
B. All right, I'll explain everything to you. *A.* Thank you. I'm
certainly very fortunate and you're being very kind (*lit.* you are a
good man). *B.* What is it you want to know? *A.* Which ministry
is responsible for the general administration of the country?
B. The Ministry of the Interior is responsible for and supervises
the governorates, provinces, and districts. *A.* Thank you, but I've
one question. What is the title of the chief of police? *B.* In every
governorate, province, and district the chief of police is called the
Hakimdar. *A.* What is the head of the governorate called?
B. [He's called] the Governor. *A.* What is the difference between
provinces and governorates? *B.* Governorates are in the large
towns like Cairo, Alexandria, and Suez, while provinces, such as
the Gharbiya and Sharqiya provinces and Qena, are in the
country. *A.* The head of a province is called a Mudir, of course.
B. That's so, and the province is divided into many districts.
A district head is called a Mamur. *A.* If there are many districts
the Mamur must be responsible for a lot of small towns. *B.* True,
but the leaders in the small towns are the Umdas. *A.* Good, I see
now. If I have any village matter (to discuss) or complaint (to
make), I take it to the Umda. *B.* Quite right, and if I can't answer
you, I refer the matter to the Mamur, and if necessary, he forwards
it to the Mudir and the Mudir to the Minister. *A.* Well I never!
But what [is it I've heard] about [the] town councils? *B.* Town
councils are elected by the votes of the townspeople, just as we
voted for the members of the provincial council in our province. *A.* You mean there isn't any town council in our town?
B. No, there isn't, but there is in the big towns where there are

báladi. *A.* mitʃákkir wi dilwáqti ma fíiʃ luzúum asáafir ɣalaʃan
ana ʃáayif innǐ yilzámn-aqaddímlak mawḍúuɣi. ʕaʃúuf wíʃʃak bi
xéer.

21. ʕiṭṭáqsǐ-f máṣr

A. ʕáhlan, ṣúdfa ɣaríiba, ma ʃuftákʃǐ min zamáan. *B.* ʕana saʕáltǐ
ɣaléek marráat kitíira w-iftakárt innak misáafir walla ɣayyáan.
A. ʕaʃkúrak. ʕahó-nta ʃáayif iṭṭáqsǐ tamálli mityáyyar? *B.* ṣaḥíiḥ,
yom ḥárrǐ-w yom bárd, wi yóom háwa wi-tráab. *A.* ʕana miʃ
ɣáarif iḥna dilwáqti-f fáṣlǐ ʕéeh. *B.* ɣándak ḥáqq liʕann iṭṭáqsǐ
muxtálif. *A.* ʕáṣɣab fáṣl huwwa fáṣl iṣṣéef. *B.* min ɣéer ʃákk, fáṣl
iṣṣéef ḥárr. *A.* lák ḥáqq, wiláakin báɣdu ṭaráawit ilxaríif. *B.* ḥatít-
ɣab min bárd iʃʃíta-ʃʃidíid. *A.* qúlli, ʕana ɣáayiz asáafir iskindiríyya
walla ráas ilbárr, ʕánhu-lʕáḥsan wi ʕéeh fíkrak? *B.* ʕana-smíɣt inn
iṭṭáqsǐ fiskindiríyya-rṭúuba, wiláakin bárḍu ʕáḥsan min máṣr.
A. tamáam, lakin irruṭúuba fiskindiríyya-txálli-lhudúum mablúula
tamálli. *B.* ḥatistaḥámma filbáḥr? *A.* ʕummáal, liʕann ilɣúum
filbáḥrǐ-ryáaḍa liggísm. *B.* ṭáyyib, tiftíkir inn issáma ṣáfya fiskindiríyya zayyǐ máṣr? *A.* láʕ, ʕissáma fiskindiríyya fíiha saḥáab wi
ʃabbúura. *B.* qúlli baqa, ʕinta kúntǐ filʕaryáaf, ʕizzáyy iṭṭáqsǐ-
hnáak? *A.* ʕiṭṭáqsǐ filʕaryáaf kuwáyyis gíddan. *B.* ʃéeʕ ɣaríib.
baqá-nta kuntǐ mabṣúuṭ hináak? *A.* maɣlúum, liʕann ittíraɣ fíiha
máyya ḥawaléen ilbiláad w-ilɣízab. *B.* ʕilfallaḥíin biyírwu-
zraɣíthum izzáay? *A.* baɣḍǔhum mittíraɣ wi baɣḍǔhum bil-
maṣáarif. *B.* ʕilfallaḥíin biyḥíbbu-lmáṭar? *A.* gíddan. *B.* léeh?
wi ʕéeh issábab? *A.* liʕánnu-byírwi-zraɣíthum xuṣúuṣan fi ɣádam
wugúud ilmáyya. *B.* mafhúum y-axi-nn ilqúṭnǐ w-ilqámḥǐ
w-ilfúul biyiḥṭáagu lilmáṭar fiʃʃíta báss. *A.* ḥaḍrítak nisíit ilxuḍáar
wi da-mhímm, wiláakin inta máṣri! *B.* ṣaḥíiḥ, wiláakin ɣala kúllǐ
ḥáal iṭṭáqsǐ filʕaryáaf ʕáḥsan miṭṭáqsǐ filmúdun fi wáqt iṣṣéef.
A. ma fíiʃ ʃákk innak bitqúul ilḥáqq, wilakin ilmúdun kuwayyísa fi

governorates. *A*. Thank you. There's no need for me to go now since I see I must bring my business to you. Goodbye.

21. *The weather in Egypt*

A. Hullo there (*lit.* hullo, a strange chance), I haven't seen you for a long time. *B*. I've often been asking about you, too, and I thought you'd gone away or were ill. *A*. Thank you. Isn't the weather changeable (*lit.* you have seen the weather is always changed)! *B*. True, one day hot and the next cold, and another (nothing but) wind and dust. *A*. It makes you wonder what time of year it is (*lit.* I don't know which season we are in now). *B*. Exactly, it's so variable. *A*. Summer's the most difficult time of year. *B*. Yes indeed (*lit.* without doubt), it's (so) hot. *A*. True, but (there's) the cool of the autumn (to come) after it. *B*. (And then) you'll be worn out with the bitter(ly) cold [of] winter. *A*. Tell me, I want to go away to Alexandria or Ras el Barr, which is best, do you think? *B*. I hear (*lit.* heard) it's humid in Alexandria, but even so it's better than Cairo. *A*. Exactly, but the humidity in Alexandria always makes your (*lit.* the) clothes damp. *B*. Are you going bathing? A. Rather! A swim in the sea does you good (*lit.* is exercise for the body). *B*. Yes. Do you think it (*lit.* the sky) is as clear in Alexandria as it is in Cairo? *A*. No, it's cloudy and hazy. *B*. Tell me, you've been in the country, what's the weather like there? *A*. Very nice. *B*. Really! You liked it (*lit.* were happy) there then. *A*. Certainly. The canals around the villages and farms were full of water. *B*. How do the peasants irrigate their crops? *A*. Some of them from the canals and some from irrigation ditches. *B*. Do they like rain? *A*. Very much. *B*. Why is that? *A*. Because it waters their crops, especially in the absence of irrigation (*lit.* water). *B*. I know (*lit.* understood) [my friend] that cotton, corn, and beans only need rain in winter. *A*. You've forgotten the vegetables and that's important, but then you're from Cairo (i.e. a townsman). *B*. True, but anyway, the weather in summer is better in the country than in the towns. *A*. There's no doubt about that (*lit.* that you are speaking the truth), yet the towns are nice in

wáqt iʃʃíta. Ɂismáḫli dilwaqti. *B.* fúrṣa-kwayyísa, Ɂatɣáʃʃim innína
nitqáabil marra tánya. fi ḫífzị̆-lláah. *A.* Ɂalláah yiḫfáz̧ak.

22. Ɂaháali-lqúṭr[1] ilmáṣri

Ɂaháali-lqúṭr ilmáṣri yuskúnu-lmúdun w-ilɁaryáaf. baɣd̬úhum
sakníin fiṣṣiɣíid wi dá filwágh ilqíbli ganúub ilqahíra[2]-w dóol
iṣṣaɣáyda, wi baɣd̬úhum filwágh ilbáḫari ʃamáal ilqahíra, w-innáas
illi sakníin fíih ismúhum baḫárwa.

ɣala d̬affitéen inníil manṭíqa-zraɣíyya dayyáqa w-iṣṣáḫra
timtáddï min báɣd ilmanṭíqa di-lɣáayit ilḫudúud ilmaṣríyya fiʃʃárqị̆
w-ilɣárb. fiʃʃárqị̆-nláaqi ṣáḫra-ssíina-w ṣáḫra-lbáḫr ilɁáḫmar wi
filɣárb iṣṣáḫra-lɣarbíyya, w-innáas illi biyɣíiʃu fiṣṣáḫra ɣadádhum
qalíil w-ismúhum ilbádw.

Ɂáhl iṣṣiɣíid ɣadáthum wi lahgáthum w-iṣṭilaḫáthum tixtílif ɣan
bitáaɣit innáas illi sakníin filmúdun wi ḫátta ɣan bitáaɣit ilbaḫárwa-
lli sakníin filwágh ilbáḫari-w húmma kamáan muxtalifíin ɣan
sukkáan ilmúdun. Ɂilbádw illi-yɣíiʃu fiṣṣáḫra rúḫḫal mitnaqqilíin,
ɣadáthum wi lahgáthum muxtálifa[3] bilmárra ɣan baqíyyit sukkáan
ilqúṭr ilmáṣri, wi dóol qabáayil.

Ɂiṣṣiɣíid biláad ziraɣíyya-w fíiha maṣáaniɣ qalíila, lakin filwágh
ilbáḫari fíih ziraɣáat wi-ṣnaɣáat kitíira ɣalaʃáan ilmuwaṣaláat sáhla.
laḫáz̧na-nnï ɣádad kibíir min Ɂaháali-ṣṣiɣíid ráḫalu min biládhum
lilmúdun ikkibíira-w báɣd ilmúdun ilɁúxra-lli fíiha-ṣnaɣáat zayyï
maṣáaniɣ innasíig w-ilɣázl w-ilɁizáaz w-iṣṣíini w-ilbitróol wi
hakáza.

23. Ɂiddíin ilɁisláami

lilmuslimíin kitáab muqáddas[4] huwwa-lqurɁáan iʃʃaríif, w-ilqur-
Ɂáan Ɂasáas iddíin ilɁisláami-w gamíiɣ ilmuslimíin fi kúll iddínya-
yɁámnu bíih wi yiḫtirmúuh wi-ysaddaqúuh wi yiɣtíqdu-nnu
kaláam alláah.

---

[1] *q* as in 'Classical'.   [2] Or *ilqaahíra*; *q* as in 'Classical'.
[3] Or, 'more colloquially', *mixtílfa*.
[4] Pronounce *q* as in 'Classical'. The word is typical of the whole text which,
given its subject-matter, requires more deliberate utterance and some attention
to 'Classical' form.

wintertime. Would you excuse me now. *B*. It's been nice seeing you (*lit*. happy chance). I hope we shall meet again. Goodbye (*lit*. in the protection of God). *A*. Goodbye.

22. *The people[s] of Egypt*

The people of Egypt live in the towns and countryside. Some, [and they are] the Sa'idi's, live in Upper Egypt, which is the [southern] part south of Cairo, while others, called Baharwa, live in Lower Egypt¹ north of Cairo.

There is a narrow fertile strip on both sides (*lit*. banks) of the Nile, and thereafter (*lit*. after this zone) the desert stretches to the Egyptian borders in both the east and west. In the east we find the Sinai and Red Sea Deserts, and in the west the Western Desert. The people living in the desert are few in number and called Bedouin.

The customs, dialects, and expressions of the people of Upper Egypt differ from those of the town dwellers and also from those of the fellaheen living in the Delta, who in turn differ from the townsfolk. The Bedouin living in the desert are nomads with customs and speech totally different from the rest of the inhabitants of Egypt;² they (live in) tribes.

Upper Egypt is agricultural with few industrial installations, but in the Delta, where communications are easy, there is both agriculture and industry (*lit*. crops and industries) on a considerable scale. We have witnessed many Sa'idi's leaving their villages for the big towns and for certain others where there are (to be found) such industries as textiles (*lit*. weaving and spinning), glass, pottery (*lit*. china), petroleum, &c.

23. *The Muslim religion*

The Holy Book of the Muslims (*lit*. for the Muslims a holy book) is the [Noble] Koran, which is the basis of the Muslim religion. [All] Muslims all over the world trust in it, revere it, believe it, and are sure that it is the word of God.

¹ Or 'the Delta'.
² Notice that the Bedouin is not felt to be Egyptian.

rúknĭ min Ṣarkáan iddíin ilṢisláami ṢilṢimáan w-ittasdíiq bi waḥdaníyyit illáah[1] wi húwwa-nnútqĭ biʃʃahadatéen,[2] yaɣni wáagib ɣala kúllĭ múslim wi muslíma-nnu-yqúul 'Ṣaʃhádu Ṣan láa[3] Ṣiláaha Ṣilla-lláah' wi 'Ṣaʃhádu Ṣanna muḥámmad rasúul alláah'; w-ilṢimáan maɣnáah inn ilwáaḥid yiṢáamin billáah wi malaṢíkatu[4] wi kútubu wi rúsulu w-ilyóom ilṢáaxir w-ilqádar[5] xéeru-w ʃárru(h).

táani rúkn iṣṣála. Ṣilmuslimíin biyṣállu xámas Ṣawqáat finnaháar w-illéel wi húmma-ṣṣúbḥ w-iḍḍúhr w-ilɣáṣr w-ilmáɣrib w-ilɣíʃa.

táalit rúkn izzáka. lazímhum yizákku, yaɣni-yṭalláɣu-zzáka wí da min Ṣamwálhum yiddúuh lilfúqara.

ráabiɣ rúkn iṣṣóom. húmma biyṣúumu ʃáhrĭ fissána-smu ramaḍáan, yaɣni ma yaklúuʃ wala yiʃrabúuʃ ṭúul innaháar milfágrĭ liḥadd ilmáɣrib. wi lámma yáklu filmáɣrib yisámmu-lṢaklĭda-lfuṭúur wi baɣdéen biyáklu baɣdĭ núṣṣ illéel wi-ysámmu-lṢaklĭda-ssuḥúur.

xáamis rúkn ilḥágg,[6] wi maɣnáah innĭ wáagib ɣala-lmuslimíin min kúllĭ dáwla-w min kúllĭ bálad Ṣisláami-lli yiqdáru yirúuḥu-lmákka ɣalaʃáan yiḥíggu-f ʃáhr ismu-lḥúgga.[7]

ɣánd ilmuslimíin ɣidéen diniyyíin rasmiyyíin Ṣismŭhum ɣíid ilfíṭr wí da báɣdĭ ʃáhrĭ ramaḍáan ɣala ṭúul w-innáas biysammúuh ilɣíid iṣṣuɣáyyar, wi ɣíid iddiḥíyya, yikúun baɣd ilḥággĭ-f ʃáhr ismu-lḥúgga w-innáas biysammúuh ilɣíid ikkibíir.

24. Ṣilmuwaṣaláat[8] fi máṣr

ṭúruq ilmuwaṣaláat fi máṣrĭ-ktíir. fíih muwaṣaláat bissíkka-lḥadíid lilmúdun w-ilṢaryáaf. Ṣinnáas biysáfru-ktíir bilwaburáat yaɣni bilquṭuráat, wi fíih muwaṣaláat ziraɣíyya.

Ṣinnáas biyirkábu kamáan Ṣutubisáat wi taksiyyáat, wi fíih kamáan

---

[1] A 'classicism'; colloquial = (waḥdaníyyit) alláah.
[2] For the more typically colloquial ʃahattéen.
[3] Pronounced Ṣalláa.
[4] Strictly malaaṢíkatuh in 'Classical' Arabic. The more colloquial form is malaykítu(h).   [5] See footnote 4 on page 160.
[6] Among less educated speakers, ḥigg.   [7] Or Ṣilḥigga.
[8] Or, among the less sophisticated, muwaṣláat.

One of the pillars of Islam is faith and belief in the Oneness of God. The latter requires (*lit.* is) the utterance of the two acts of faith, for (*lit.* that is) every Muslim man and woman is in duty bound to say, 'I believe that there is no god but God', and, 'I believe that Muhammad is the Prophet of God.' Faith implies (*lit.* its meaning is) that one believes in God, His angels, His writ (*lit.* books), His prophets, the Day of Judgement (*lit.* the last day), and fate, whether good or bad (*lit.* its goodness and its badness).

The second pillar is prayer. Muslims pray five times during the day and night: (these prayers are) the dawn, noon, afternoon, sunset, and evening prayers.

The third pillar is almsdeeds. They must give of their own substance to the poor (*lit* they must give alms, that is bring forth alms [and that] from their possessions to give [it] to the poor).

The fourth pillar is fasting. They fast in the month [of the year] called Ramadan, when (*lit.* that is) they neither eat nor drink all day long from dawn to sunset. The meal eaten at sunset is called 'Sĭlfuṭuur', and that taken later on, after midnight, 'Sĭssuḥuur'[1] (*lit.* and when they eat at sunset, they call that meal, &c.).

The fifth pillar is the pilgrimage, in accordance with which (*lit.* and its meaning is) Muslims of every nationality (*lit.* from every nation) and from all Islamic countries must, if they are able, go to Mecca on pilgrimage during the month of that name.

Muslims have two official religious feasts known as the 'Feast of breaking the fast' which takes place immediately after the month of Ramadan and which is popularly called (*lit.* the people call) the 'Little feast', and the 'Feast of the sacrifice' which occurs after the pilgrimage in the pilgrimage month and is termed the 'Big feast'.

24. *Communications in Egypt*

Means of communication in Egypt are many. There are railways (*lit.* rail communications) serving the towns and country, and people travel a lot by rail (*lit.* by trains). There is also road (*lit.* land) transport.

People also use (*lit.* ride) buses and taxis, and in addition there

---

[1] This meal must be eaten before sunrise.

muwaṣaláat biṭṭayyaráat wi bittalliɣrafáat wi bittilifonáat wi bilbúṣṭa. wi fíih muwaṣaláat nilíyya yaꜧni binníil, w-ilmuwaṣaláat innilíyya-tkun bilmaráakib iʃʃiraꜧíyya.

wi fíih muwaṣaláat kuwayyísa filmúdun ilkubáar zayyĭ máṣrĭ w-iskindiríyya. muwaṣaláat ilmadintéen dóol bitturmayáat walla bilꜤutubisáat walla bittaksiyyáat walla bilꜧarabiyyáat ilmalláaki.

wi kamáan fih ꜧarabiyyáat kibíira-smắha luriyyáat náqlĭ-w ꜧarabiyyáat ṣuɣayyára-smắha kárru-ygurrắha-ḥṣáan[1] walla-ḥmáar[1] li náql ilbaḍáayiꜧ w-ilḥagáat ittiqíila.

wi fíih muwaṣaláat ṣaḥrawíyya-smắha muwaṣaláat iṣṣáḥra zayyĭ síkkit iṣṣáḥra ben máṣrĭ w-issuwées wi ben máṣrĭ w-iskindiríyya-w ben máṣrĭ w-ilfayyúum. w-ilmuwaṣaláat iṣṣaḥrawíyya-tkúun bi ꜧarabiyyáat ilꜤutubisáat wi bittaksiyyáat wi bilꜧarabiyyáat ilmalláaki.

máṣrĭ ṣáꜧba filmuwaṣaláat fiʃʃawáariꜧ wi filmayadíin min kútr izzáḥma-w láazim kullĭ wáaḥid ráakib ꜧarabíyya walla máaʃi ꜧala rigléeh yaxud báalu min ꜧiʃaráat ilmurúur wi ꜧaskári-lmurúur.

ꜧiza kan wáaḥid ꜧawiz yiꜧáddi min ʃáariꜧ li ʃáariꜧ walla ꜧáawiz yiꜧáddi min midáan, ꜧiza káanit issíkka maftúuḥa walla maqfúula, yilzámu-ybúṣṣĭ-ʃmáal wi-ymíin wi kamáan ʃimal táani-w quddáam. wi kamáan muhímmĭ qáwi-nnĭ kúllĭ wáaḥid yítbaꜧ niꜧáam ilmurúur fi máṣrĭ-w yímʃi ꜧarraṣíif. wi lámma-ykun ꜧáawiz yírkab ꜧarabíyyit ꜧutubíis walla turmáay yilzámu yúqaf ꜧalmaḥáṭṭa.

ꜧiza káan waḥid ráakib ꜧarabíyya malláaki walla biskilítta[2]-w máaʃi fi ʃáariꜧ billéel lázmu-ywállaꜧ ilfanúus. ꜧiza ma kánʃĭ yíꜧmil kída-lbulíiṣ yidaffáꜧu-mxálfa. wi lazim kúllĭ wáaḥid yíꜧraf innĭ kúll issayyaráat[3] bitímʃi ꜧalyimíin fiʃʃawáariꜧ.

25. ꜧistixráag izzéet ilxáam

A. ꜧáhlan wi sáhlan. B. ꜧáhlan wi sáhlan bíik. A. bitíꜧmil éeh dilwaqti? B. ꜧana baʃtáɣal fi ʃírkit ilbitróol. A. fíih ʃarikáat fi máṣrĭ-l ꜧináaꜧit ilbitróol? B. ꜧáywa, fíih. / A. ꜧiʃʃarikáat di-btíꜧmil

---

[1] See Part I, Appendix C, 1 (b), note (iii).
[2] Or baskalítta.
[3] sayyáara is sometimes used in educated colloquial for ꜧarabíyya.

are communications by air[craft], telegraph[s], telephone[s], and post, while the Nile is navigated by sailing craft (*lit.* and there are Nile communications, that is by the Nile, and the Nile communications are by sailing-boats).

There are good means of transport in the large towns such as Cairo and Alexandria. Communication[s] in these two towns is by tram[s], bus[es], taxi[s], and private car.

There are also lorries (*lit.* big vehicles called transport lorries) and small horse- or donkey-drawn carts for the transport of merchandise and heavy goods.

There are, too, desert communications like the [desert] road(s) between Cairo and Suez, Cairo and Alexandria, and Cairo and the Fayoum. Desert transport is by bus[es], taxi[s], and private car[s].

Travelling on the roads and in the squares of Cairo is difficult because of the crowds (*lit.* Cairo is difficult in communications, &c.), and everyone driving (*lit.* riding in) a car or walking must pay attention to road signs and the traffic policeman.

If one wants to cross from one street to another or to cross a square, then whether the road is clear or busy (*lit.* open or closed), he must look to the left, then to the right, then left again and in front. It is also very important that one follows the rule of the road (*lit.* arrangement of the traffic) in Cairo and walks on the footpath. Anyone wanting to take a bus or a tram, must wait at the stop.

Anyone driving a car or riding a bicycle [and going along the road] at night should see that his lights are on (*lit.* must light the light of the vehicle). If he does not do so, he will be fined by the police (*lit.* the police will make him pay a fine). Everyone must also know that all vehicles drive (*lit.* go) on the right in the streets.

25. *The production of crude oil*

A. Hullo. *B.* Hullo. *A.* What are you doing now? *B.* I'm working for an oil company. *A.* Are there oil companies (*lit.* for the making of oil) in Egypt? *B.* Yes, indeed (*lit.* there are). / *A.* What do these

éeh? *B.* bitíbḫas ɣan izzéet ilxáam illi biysammúuh ilɣummáal
'kirúud'.¹ *A.* Ɛizzéet ilxáam biyitwígid féen? *B.* Ɛizzéet ilxáam
biyitwígid fi ras ɣáarib w-ilɣardáqa-w ṣúdrĭ-w ɣásal. *A.* wi húmma
féen? *B.* ɣala sáaḫil ilbáḫr ilƐáḫmar. *A.* qúlli ɣalá-smĭ-ʃʃírka-lli-
btíbḫas ɣan izzéet ilxáam hináak. *B.* ʃírkit Ɛabáar izziyúut ilƐin-
giliziyya-lmaṣríyya límitid. *A.* báɣdĭ ma tíwgid iʃʃírka izzéet ilxáam
bitíɣmil éeh? *B.* bitúḫfur Ɛabáar ziyáada. *A.* wi-btíɣmil éeh
fizzéet ilxáam ilmustáxrag? *B.* bitiʃḫínu-f maráakib maxṣúuṣa-
ysammúuha tankárz bitsáafir filbáḫrĭ-w bitwaṣṣálu-l zetíyyit ʃíllĭ
fissuwées. *A.* léeh iʃʃírka-btíʃḫin izzéet lizzetíyya? *B.* ɣalaʃáan
yikarrarúuh wi yistaxrágu mínnu muntagáat muxtálifa. *A.* Ɛis-
máḫli dilwaqti, Ɛana mistáɣgil w-aʃkúrak qáwi. *B.* Ɛilɣáfw. Ɛin
ʃáaƐ alláah aʃúufak marra tánya. maɣa-ssaláama. *A.* Ɛalláah
yisallímak.

26. *takríir izzéet ilxáam*

A. ṣabáaḫ ilxéer. *B.* ṣabáaḫ ilfúll. Ɛizzáyyĭ ṣiḫḫítak? *A.* Ɛilḫámdu
lilláah. Ɛizzáyyĭ ṣiḫḫítak ínta? *B.* lilláah ilḫámd. *A.* bitiʃtáɣal
féen dilwaqti? *B.* Ɛana-tnaqáltĭ lizzetíyya fissuwées. *A.* Ɛizzetíyya
di-kbíira? *B.* Ɛáywa-kbíira ɣalaʃan bitkárrar Ɛáɣlab izzéet ilxáam
ilmáṣri. *A.* Ɛizzetíyya-btistílim izzéet izzáay? *B.* bitistílmu
milmaráakib wi-txazzínu fittunúuk. *A.* wi baɣdéen? *B.* baɣdéen
bitsaxxánu-f Ɛafráan wi-btistáxrag mínnu báɣḍ ilmuntagáat
ilbitrolíyya. *A.* záyyĭ Ɛéeh masalan? *B.* záyy ilmazúut w-ilgáaz
w-ilbanzíin w-ilƐasfáltĭ w-ilbutagáaz. *A.* bássĭ kída? di ḫáaga sáhla
qáwi. *B.* láƐ, múʃ sáhla ɣaʃan fíih ɣamaliyyáat kitíira fizzetíyya-l
takríir izzéet ilxáam. *A.* wi fíih Ɛaqsáam² tánya? *B.* Ɛáywa fíih,
masalan qísm² ilhandása w-ilmáɣmal w-ilmáxzan w-ilḫisabáat wi
ɣéeru(h). *A.* Ɛizzetíyya ɣala sáaḫil ilbáḫr ilƐáḫmar³? *B.* láƐ, hiyya
ɣala-ssáaḫil ilyárbi min xalíig issuwées. *A.* qurayyíba milqanáal²?
B. Ɛáywa-qrayyíba, wi hiyya ɣannáḫya-lqiblíyya milqanáal. *A.* wi
híyya ɣala masáafit káam kilumítrĭ min máṣr? / *B.* míyya xámsa-w

---

¹ You will also hear *kiróod* and *kilóod*, especially in the oilfields.
² *q* is generally pronounced by the educated as in 'Classical' Arabic. Some
speakers use *k* for *q* in *qandal*.
³ Or *Ɛilbáḫrĭ láḫmar*.

companies do? *B.* Search for crude oil [which the workmen call 'crude']. *A.* Where is the crude oil found? *B.* [The crude oil is found] In Ras Gharib, Hurghada, Sudr, and Asl. *A.* Where are they? *B.* On the Red Sea coast. *A.* What's (*lit.* tell me) the name of the company prospecting for crude oil there? *B.* The Anglo-Egyptian Oilfields (*lit.* wells) Limited. *A.* What does the company do after finding crude oil? *B.* It drills more wells. *A.* And what does it do to the crude oil taken out? *B.* It ships it in seagoing tankers (*lit.* special ships called tankers travelling on the sea) [which deliver it] to the Shell Refinery at Suez. *A.* Why does the company take it there (*lit.* the oil to the Refinery)? *B.* For refining and extracting various products from it.

A. Would you excuse me now, I'm in (rather) a hurry. Thank you very much. *B.* Not at all. I hope to see you again. Goodbye. *A.* Goodbye.

26. *Refining the crude oil*

A. Good morning. *B.* Good morning. How are you? *A.* Very well, thank you. How are *you*? *B.* Very well, thanks. *A.* Where are you working now? *B.* I've been transferred to the Refinery at Suez. *A.* Is it a big refinery? *B.* Yes, because it refines most Egyptian crude oil. *A.* How does it get the oil? *B.* It receives it by sea (*lit.* from the ships) and stores it in [the] tanks. *A.* Then what happens (*lit.* and then)? *B.* It heats it in furnaces and extracts from it certain petroleum products. *A.* Such as? *B.* For example, fuel oil, kerosine, benzine, asphalt, and butagaz. *A.* Is that all? That seems very little (*lit.* a very easy thing). *B.* Not at all, because there are many operations [in the Refinery] in the refining of crude oil. *A.* Are there any other departments? *B.* Yes, for example, there's the engineering department, the laboratory, the materials (*lit.* stores), and accounts departments and (others) besides [it]. *A.* Is the Refinery on the Red Sea Coast? *B.* No, it's on the west shore of the Gulf of Suez. *A.* Near the Canal? *B.* Yes, on the south side of the Canal. *A.* And how many kilometres (*lit.* at a distance of how many, &c.) is it from Cairo? / *B.* About a hundred

ɣiʃríin kíilu taqríiban. *A.* w-ilⱭabáar fi ras ɣáarib biɣíida ɣan
issuwées? *B.* zayyï mitéen w-arbiɣíin kíilu missuwées ɣala sáaḥil
ilbáḥr ilⱭáḥmar ilɣárbi. *A.* wi ṣúdr? *B.* ɣannáḥya-ttánya lilbáḥr
ilⱭáḥmar[1] ḥawáali xámsa w-arbiɣíin kíilu missuwées. *A.* múmkin
agíilak búkra filbéet? *B.* Ɑitfáḍḍal, tiʃárraf. *A.* mutaʃákkir. Ɑila-
lliqáaⱭ.[2]

27. *tawzíiɣ wi béeɣ ilmuntagáat ilbitrolíyya*

A. Ɑáhlan wi sáhlan. *B.* Ɑáhlan wi sáhlan bíik. Ɑizzáyyï ḥadrítak?
A. Ɑilḥámdu lilláah, w-izzáyyak w-izzáyy ilɣéela? *B.* Ɑaʃkúrak,
lilláah ilḥámd, bi xéer. *A.* Ɑana-smíɣt innak dilwáqti-f fárɣï ʃírkit
ʃíllï fissuwées. *B.* Ɑáywa, ṣaḥíiḥ. *A.* qúlli, Ɑéeh ilfárqï ben ʃírkit
ʃíllï-w ʃírkit Ɑabáar izziyúut ilⱭingilizíyya-lmaṣríyya? *B.* Ɑilfárq
innï ʃírkit ʃíllï bitwázzaɣ wi bitbíiɣ muntagáat ʃíll. *A.* w-iʃʃírka-
ttánya? *B.* hiyya-btistáxrag izzéet ilxáam wi-tkarráru(h). *A.* Ɑil-
máktab irraⱭíisi-btaɣ ʃírkit ʃíllï féen? *B.* fi máṣr. *A.* wi fih káam
fárɣï filqúṭr ilmáṣri? *B.* fih xámas furúuɣ. *A.* tísmaḥ tiqúlli féen
wi féen. *B.* húmma-f báɣḍ ilmúdun ikkibíira, yaɣni-f máṣrï
nafsáha w-iskindiríyya-w bursaɣíid w-issuwées. *A.* wiláakin
qultíli fih xámas furúuɣ wi sammétl-arbáɣa báss. *B.* Ɑáywa, wi
fáaḍil fárɣ ilⱭaryáaf wi húwwa biybíiɣ wi biywázzaɣ muntagáat
ʃíllï-l báaqi-lqúṭr ilmáṣri. *A.* Ɑilmuntagáat lilbéeɣ bitíigi-mnéen?
B. baɣḍáha-btistaxrágu-zzetíyya bissuwées. *A.* Ɑilmuntagáat
ilmustaxrága mizzéet ilxáam ilmáṣri-btíkfi-lqúṭr ilmáṣri walla láⱭ?
B. láⱭ, kitíir milmuntagáat ilbitrolíyya-lmustaɣmála filqúṭr ilmáṣri
gáyya min bárra. *A.* Ɑéeh iṭṭúruq illi bíiha bitwázzaɣ ʃírkit ʃíll
ilmuntagáat ilmitkarrára fissuwées w-ilmuntagáat ilmustawráda
min bárra. *B.* bitwazzáɣhum bi masúura ben issuwées wi máṣr,
wi mawaɣíin, wi luriyyáat, wi quṭuráat, wi fanaṭíiz, wi kamáan bi
baramíil, wi ṣafáayiḥ. *A.* Ɑilmawaɣíin bitwázzaɣ ilmuntagáat
izzáay? *B.* bitinqílha wi-tsáafir bíiha fittíraɣ / wi-f náhr inníil.

---

[1] See Lesson 2, 1, note (6).
[2] *q* is generally pronounced by the educated as in 'Classical Arabic'.

and twenty-five. *A.* Are the wells at Ras Gharib far from Suez?
B. About two hundred and forty kilometres from Suez on the
west coast of the Red Sea. *A.* And Sudr? *B.* On the other side
of the Red Sea about forty-five kilometres from Suez. *A.* May I
call on (*lit.* come to) you tomorrow at the house? *B.* Certainly,
please do (*lit.* you will honour (me)). *A.* Thank you. Au revoir.

27. *The distribution and marketing of petroleum products*

A. Hullo. *B.* Hullo, how are you? *A.* Very well, thank you, and
how are you and your family? *B.* We're all very well, thank you.
A. I hear you're now in the Shell branch at Suez. *B.* Yes, that's so.
A. Tell me, what is the difference between the Shell Company and
the Anglo-Egyptian Oilfields Limited? *B.* The difference is
that the Shell Company distributes and markets Shell products.
A. And the other company? *B.* It produces and refines crude oil.
A. Where's the head office of the Shell Company? B. In Cairo.
A. How many branches are there in Egypt? *B.* Five. *A.* Could
(*lit.* you forgive)[1] you tell me where they all[2] are? *B.* In certain of
the big towns, that is in Cairo itself, Alexandria, Pord Said, and
Suez. *A.* But you told me there are five and you've named me
only four. *B.* Yes, the remaining one is the Provincial Branch.
It markets and distributes Shell products in the rest of Egypt.
A. Where do the products for marketing come from? *B.* The
Refinery at Suez produces some of them. *A.* Are the products
produced from Egyptian crude oil enough for Egypt('s needs) or
not? *B.* No, many petroleum products used in Egypt come from
elsewhere (*lit.* outside). *A.* How (*lit.* what are the means by which)
does Shell distribute the products refined at Suez and the imported ones? *B.* (In bulk) By pipe line between Suez and Cairo,
as well as by lighter[s], lorry[-ies], train[s], and tank-cart[s], and
also (packed in) drums and tins. *A.* How do the lighters distribute
the products? *B.* They carry [and travel with] them on the canals

---

[1] A much politer way of putting the question than, say, *wi húmma féen?*
[2] This is the force of the repetition.

A. ya tára ʃirkit ʃíllĭ bitbʃíɽ ilkimawiyyáat kamáan? *B.* láʕ, ʕilmuntagáat ilkimawíyya-tbíɽha ʃirka tánya. *A.* ʕismắha ʕéeh?
B. ʕismắha ʃírkit ʃíllĭ-l tawzíiɽ ilkimawiyyáat li mắ ʂrĭ límitid.
A. ʃéeʕ ɣaríib. ʕana ma kúntĭʃ ɽáarif inn iʃʃarikáat kubáar wi
kutáar zayyĭ kída. ʕana mamnúun gíddan. *B.* ʕilɽáfw.

28. ḥuqúul¹ ʕabáar izziyúut

ʕilmuhandisíin iljulujiyyíin² yiɽráfu ḥasab xibríthum ʕanwáaɽ wi
ʕaʃkáal iʂʂuxúur illi yímkin tíxzin izzéet ilxáam. ʕilmuhandisíin
dóol ma yiqdarúuʃ yiqúulu-nnĭ fíih zéet mawgúud wiláakin yiqdáru
yiɽráfu ʕin káanit iʂʂuxúur munásba-l wugúud izzéet walla láʕ.

baɽd ilbáḥsĭ da yímkin iʃʃírka túḥfur bíir w-iza káanit ilbíir di
tíntig zéet túḥfur ʕabáar tánya. ʕilmuhandisíin illi-byuḥfúru-
lʕabáar nisammíihum muhandisíin ḥáfr.

w-ilmuhandisíin ilmasʕulíin ɽan istixráag izzéet ilxáam milʕabáar ilmaḥfúura húmma-mhandisíin ʕintáag wi hína núqta-
mhímma ʕinnĭ ḥawáali tisɽíin filmíyya milʕabáar ilmaḥfúura bitkun
náʃfa yaɽni ma tintígʃĭ zéet.

ʕaḥyáanan biykúun fíih ɣáaz fizzéet wi-qráyyib min magmuɽáat
ilʕabáar ilmuxtálifa biykúun fíih maḥaṭṭáat tunúuk wi saharíig.
ʕissaharíig bitífʂil ilɣáaz mizzéet wi baɽdĭ kída-yrúuḥ izzéet
littunúuk w-ilɣáaz yirúuḥ li bumbáat illi-btídɟaṭ baɽd ilɣáaz
wi-btiɽmílu banzíin. ʕilɣáaz illi fáaḍil biyustáhlak³ filʕafráan wi-f
báɽd ilʕabáar li-msáɽdit ilʕintáag wi filbiyúut liṭṭábx.

wi filmaḥaṭṭáat ilmazkúura bumbáat bitwáʂʂal izzéet ilxáam
littunúuk ɽand irraʃíif w-ilbanzíin ilmazkúur biyíwʂal fi masúura
ben maḥaṭṭáat ittunúuk w-irraʃíif.

náql izzéet ilxáam lizzetíyya-b tankárzĭ-btíigi missuwées biddóor,
yaɽni márkib bitfárray fi-tnúuk izzetíyya filwáqt illi márkib ɣérha-
btíʃḥin milḥuqúul.

manáaṭiq ilḥuqúul muʃ qurayyíba min ʕáyyĭ bálad. kúllĭ

---

¹ ḥuqúul is a 'learned' word in which q is pronounced in its 'Classical' form.
A semi-technical passage of this kind is bound to contain 'classicisms' of lexicon
and pronunciation.
² Pronounce j approximately as j in English 'jeep'.
³ A passive form from the 'Classical' language. The distinction yustáhlak 'is
consumed': yistáhlik 'consumes' is commonly made in educated colloquial.

and the Nile. *A.* I wonder if Shell also markets chemical products?
B. No. They are marketed by another company. *A.* What's that
called? *B.* The Shell Chemical Distributing Company of Egypt
Limited. *A.* It's extraordinary, I didn't realize the companies
were so big and varied (*lit.* many). I'm very grateful. *B.* Not at all.

28. *The oilfields* (lit. *fields of the oilwells*)

Geologists know from [their] experience the rock-types and forma-
tions that are likely to contain (*lit.* store) crude oil. They cannot
say that oil is present but they are able to say (*lit.* know) whether
or not the rocks suggest (*lit.* are suitable for) the presence of oil.

After this investigation the company may drill a well, and if this
[well] produces oil, it will (then) drill others. The engineers who
drill wells are called (*lit.* we call them) drillers (*lit.* engineers of
drilling).

The engineers responsible for the production of crude oil from
the wells when drilled are production engineers. An important
point (to note) here is that about ninety per cent. of drilled wells
are dry, that is they do not produce oil.

Gas is usually present in the oil, and close to groups of [different]
wells there are block stations (*lit.* tank stations and separators).
The separators (*lit.* containers) separate the gas from the oil, after
which the oil goes to the tanks and the gas to pumps that compress
some of it to (*lit.* and make it) benzine. The remaining gas is
consumed in the furnaces and at certain wells in order to assist production, as well as in the houses for cooking.

At the block stations already mentioned pumps deliver the crude
oil to tanks at the jetty, while the benzine [referred to] goes (*lit.*
arrives) by pipe line between the tank stations and the jetty.

Transport of the crude oil to the Refinery is by tankers which
come from Suez in turns, that is to say that a ship is discharging
into the Refinery tanks at the same time as another ship is loading
at the Fields.

[The areas of] The fields are not near any town. Each / area is

manṭíqa bálad bi nafsắha. fíih biyúut lilmuhandisíin w-ilmuwaẓẓafíin w-ilɣummáal wi ɣeláthum. yiɣíiʃu-f náfsï manáaṭiq ilḥuqúul
fa yilzámhum ittashiláat w-ilxadamáat ligtimaɣíyya li tanẕíim
ḥayáthum hináak.

29. Ɛizzetíyya

A. qúlli, Ɛéeh yíḥṣal baɣdï ma túdxul ilmaráakib míinit izzetíyya?
B. bitwáṣṣal izzéet ilxáam littunúuk fizzetíyya bi bumbáat.
A. wiláakin izzáay izzetíyya-btistáxrag ilmuntagáat mizzéet?
B. Ɛáwwil ɣamalíyya-btitɣímil fi qísm[1] ittaqṭíir. *A.* wi Ɛéeh biyíḥṣal
hináak? *B.* hináak Ɛafráan bitsáxxan izzéet liḥáddï ma yíbqa-zzéet
sáaɛil wi ɣáaz wi dóol yikúunu dáaxil sahríig. *A.* wi baɣdéen?
B. baɣdï kída-byáxdu-ssáaɛil min táḥtï wí da húwwa-lmazúut.
A. w-ilɣáaz? *B.* w-ilɣáaz baɣdï ma yíṭlaɣ fissahríig yíbrad wi
báɣdï mínnu yibqa gáaz wi báaqi-lɣáaz yíbrad fi-mbarridáat wi
yibqa banzíin. *A.* fíih bilantáat ɣer kída? *B.* Ɛáywa, fíih. biyistax-
rágu Ɛasfált min mazúut fi-blántï-w banzíin wi butagáaz min
mazúut fi-blántï táani. *A.* baɣdï kída-lmuntagáat dóol yikúunu
gahzíin lilbéeɣ? *B.* láɛ, líssa muʃ kullúhum. ɛilɛasfált w-ilmazúut
gahzíin wiláakin ilbaqyíin lúhum ɣamaliyyáat tánya-xɣuṣíyya-l
tanḍífhum. *A.* míin ilmasɛulíin ɣan ittaksíir w-ilqísmï-btáɣhum
ismu Ɛéeh? *B.* Ɛilmasɛulíin ismǔhum muhandisíin kimawiyyíin
w-ilqísm ismu-lmustaxragáat. *A.* fíih Ɛaqsáam[1] tánya fizzetíyya?
B. Ɛáywa, fíih. másalan qísm ilhandása w-ilḥisabáat w-ilmáxzan
wi qálam ilmustaxdimíin w-ilqísm iṭṭíbbi w-ilmáɣmal. *A.* simíɣt
innï fíih qisméen tanyíin ma ẕakártïʃ[2] ismǔhum wi húmma-
ssikirtárya-w qísm iʃʃáḥnï w-ittaxzíin. *B.* Ɛáywa, ṣaḥíiḥ. *A.*
wi-smíɣt innï-f kúll ilḥuqúul wi kamáan fizzetíyya fih qísmï
handása. *B.* Ɛáywa, w-ilmuhandisíin illi fíih mínhum mitxaṣṣaṣíin[3]

---

[1] q of *qism* in the sense of 'department' is almost invariably pronounced as in
'Classical'.
[2] See Introduction, B (ii).   [3] Or *muta-*.

a town on its own. There are houses for the technical staff, administrative staff, workmen, and their families. They live at the fields themselves so they need facilities and social services for the organization of their life there.

29. *The Refinery*

A. Tell me what happens after the ships enter the Petroleum Basin (*lit.* the Refinery Harbour). *B*. They pump (*lit.* deliver by their pumps) the crude oil into the tanks at the Refinery. *A*. But how does the Refinery extract the products from the oil? *B*. The first operation is undertaken in the Distillation Department. *A*. And what happens there? *B*. Furnaces heat the oil and turn it into (*lit.* until the oil becomes) liquid oil and gas which then go into (*lit.* and they are inside) a separator.[1] *A*. And then? *B*. They take the liquid oil from the bottom, and that's fuel oil. *A*. And the gas? *B*. After it rises (*lit.* comes out) in the separator, it cools. Some of it becomes kerosine while the rest [of the gas] cools in condensers and becomes benzine. *A*. Are there other plants besides? *B*. Yes, there are. They extract asphalt from fuel oil in one plant and benzine and butagaz [from fuel oil] in another. *A*. Are these products then ready for sale? *B*. Not all of them yet. The asphalt and fuel oil are ready but the rest require other special refining operations (*lit.* operations for their cleaning). *A*. Who are responsible for cracking and what is their department called? *B*. They are known as chemical engineers and the department is the Manufacturing Department (*lit.* department of extracts). *A*. Are there other departments in the Refinery? *B*. Yes, there are, such as the Engineering Department, Accounts, Materials, Staff, Medical, and Laboratory. *A*. I've heard that there are two other departments you haven't mentioned [their names], [and they are] the Secretarial, and Stocks (*lit.* loading) and Shipping (*lit.* storage). *B*. Yes, that's true. *A*. I hear too that there are engineering departments at every field and also one at the Refinery. *B*. Yes, and some engineers are (*lit.* and the engineers that there are, among them are, &c.) special-

---

[1] At the Refinery 'column' is also used for the piece of plant termed *sahrīig* in Arabic. *sahrīig* is a general word for 'tank, container'.

filmikaníika w-ilhandása-lmadaníyya w-ilmaṭáafi w-ikkaḥrába, wi
filḫuqúul w-izzetíyya ʕaſyáal ɣer kída ḥasab iḫtiyáag ilɡámal.

30. furúuɡ ſírkit ſíllĭ-l máṣr

A. liḥáddĭ dilwáqti ma-tkallimnáaſ ílla ɡazzéet ilxáam w-istixráag
ilmuntagáat, wiláakin izzáay ṭaríiqit béɡhum? B. ſírkit ſíllĭ bitbíiɡ
ilmuntagáat fi-frúɡha. A. wi féen ilfurúuɡ dóol? B. filmúdun
ikkibíira, yaɡni máṣrĭ-w bursaɡíid w-iskindiríyya w-issuwées wi-f
fárɡ iskindiríyya mawgúud máṣnaɡ li-ṣnáaɡit iſſáḥm, wi máṣnaɡ
li-ṣnáaɡit iſſámɡ, wi-gháaz xuṣúuṣi-l xálṭĭ baɡdĭ-zyúut ittazyíit
ilʕaṣlíyya-l daragáat tánya. A. wiláakin míin illi biybíiɡ ilmuntagáat filʕaryáaf? B. fárɡ ilʕaryáaf yidíir kúll ilʕaryáaf wiláakin
ma-ybíɡſ ilmuntagáat lizzabáayin bi náfsu liʕann ilbéeɡ biykúun
bi wáṣṭit ilwúkala w-ilmutɡahhidíin illi biybíiɡu muntagáat ſíllĭ
lizzabáayin. A. wiláakin filfurúuɡ ittánya-mwaɡɡafíin iſſírka
húmma-lli biybíiɡu-b nafsúhum maɡʕínni fíih wúkala kamáan.
B. ʕáywa, ṣaḥíiḥ, wiláakin iſſírka w-ilwúkala múſ ḍiddĭ báɡḍ.
A. muntagáat izzéet ilxáam ilmáṣri-tkáffi-lqúṭr? B. láʕ, ma-
tkaffíiſ listihláak ilqúṭr ilmáṣri-w baɡḍ ilmuntagáat mustawráda
min dúwal tánya. A. kúll ilmuntagáat ilmustahláka mustaxrága
mizzetíyya bissuwées? B. láʕ, báɡḍ ilmuntagáat múſ mustaxrága-f
máṣrĭ-wláakin ilmustaxrága w-ilmustawráda-btitníqil li maxáazin
ilfurúuɡ. A. ʕizzáay? B. bi masúura maxṣúuṣa ben issuwées wi
máṣrĭ-l náql ilgáaz w-ilbanzíin wi billuriyyáat wi bissíkka-lḥadíid
yaɡni biṭṭaríiqa-lmunásba mizzetíyya w-ilmawáani-lmustawrída.
A. yaɡni kúll ilmaxáazin biyistílmu-lmuntagáat biṭṭúruq dóol?
B. ʕáywa, wi kamáan fiṣṣafáayiḥ w-ilbaramíil. A. ṭáyyib, w-izzáay
biyistílim izzibúun milmáxzan ilmuntagáat ilmaṭlúuba? B. ḥásab
iṭṭalabáat min máktab ilmabiɡáat w-ilmáxzan biysállim iṭṭalabáat
billuriyyáat ʕaw biṭṭaríiqa-lmunásba masalan / issarríiḥa. A. wi

ists in mechanical engineering, civil engineering, fire-fighting, and electrical engineering. There are (moreover) other jobs both in the fields and the Refinery as demanded by the (nature of the) work (*lit.* according to the need of the job).

30. *The branches of the Shell Company of Egypt*

A. Up to now we've only talked about crude oil and the extraction of products, but how are they marketed (*lit.* how is the method of their sale)? *B.* The Shell Company sells the products through its branches. *A.* Where are they? *B.* In the big cities, that is in Cairo, Port Said, Alexandria, and Suez. At the Alexandria branch there are grease- and candle-making factories and special plant for the blending of certain basic lubricating oils to (produce) other grades. *A.* But who sells the products in the provinces? *B.* The Provincial Branch controls all the country area but does not itself sell the products to customers. These sales are made through agents and sub-agents (*lit.* because selling is by means of agents and sub-agents who sell Shell products to the customers). *A.* But at the other branches it is Shell staff who themselves do the selling, though there are also agents. *B.* Yes, that's true, but the Company and the agents are not in opposition (*lit.* against each other). *A.* Are the products of Egyptian crude oil sufficient for (the needs of) the country? *B.* No, they are not enough for Egyptian consumption and some are imported from other countries. *A.* Are all the products consumed refined at the Refinery in Suez? *B.* No, some [of the products] are not refined in Egypt, but those that are, together with those imported, are taken (*lit.* transported) to the Installations (*lit.* the stores of the branches). *A.* How? *B.* By special pipe line between Suez and Cairo which carries kerosine and benzine, as well as by lorry and railway, in fact by any (*lit.* the) suitable means from the Refinery or ports of import. *A.* You mean all installations receive the products by these means? *B.* Yes, and also in tins and drums. *A.* All right, and how does the customer get from the installation the products he wants (*lit.* asked for)? *B.* According to the orders from the Sales Office. The installation delivers the orders by lorry or suitable means, for example, (by)

ˁéeh ӡámal maḥaṭṭáat ilbanzíin? B. dí maḥaṭṭáat li béeӡ ilbanzíin
wi fíiha ӡummáal mitmarraníin ӡattaʃḥíim biyʃaḥḥámu-lӡarabiyyáat
ilmalláaki w-illuriyyáat w-ittaksiyyáat wi hakáza. A. kúll ilmaḥaṭ-
ṭáat di bitdírha[1]-ʃʃírka? B. láˁ, ˁiʃʃírka bitdíir baӡḍúhum wilwúkala
biydíiru-lbáaqi. A. fi kúll ilmúdun? B. láˁ, ˁilmaḥaṭṭáat illi
filmúdun bitdírha-ʃʃírka walla-lwúkala, wi filˁaryáaf ilwúkala
biydíiru-lmaḥaṭṭáat kulláha. A. yíẓhar baqá-nnĭ-f ˁáyyĭ makáan
ṣuɣáyyar walla-kbíir múmkin niʃtíri muntagáat ʃíll. B. náӡam, wi
ma tinsáaʃ innĭ min ḍímnĭ-mwaẓẓafíin iʃʃírka-mhandisíin wi-
mwaẓẓafíin fanniyyíin li-msáӡdit izzabáayin. A. ˁífriḍ innĭ
ˁáyyĭ-zbúun ӡandu muʃkíla-f maṣnáӡu ˁaw ˁáyyĭ ḥáaga tánya
yíqdar yúṭlub istiʃáara fanníyya miʃʃírka? B. ˁáywa, ˁilxúbara[2]-
btuӡ iʃʃírka-f kúll istiӡmaláat ilmuntagáat ilbitrolíyya taḥtĭ xídmit
zabayínha.

31. ˁidáarit iʃʃarikáat fi máṣr

fi máṣrĭ makáatib rúˁasa-ʃʃarikáat ilmaẓkúura filmuḥawráat issábqa.
makáatib ˁidáarit ʃírkit ʃíllĭ-w ʃírkit ˁabáar izziyúut ilˁingilizíyya-
lmaṣríyya mawgúuda-f ӡimáara wáḥda w-ilmáktab irraˁíisi-l
ʃírkit ʃíllĭ-l tawzíiӡ ilkimawiyyáat li máṣr mawgúud fi-ӡmáara yérha.
ˁamma-ʃʃírka-lmasˁúula ӡan istixráag izzéet ilxáam wi munta-
gáatu(h), ˁilˁaqláam[3] ilmawgúuda-f maktábha-rraˁíisi hiyya taqríiban náfs ilˁaqláam ilmawgúuda filḥuqúul w-izzetíyya. ˁis-
múhum qálam ilhandása-w qálam ilḥisabáat wi qálam ilḥáfrĭ-w
qálam iljulújya-w qálam ilmisáaḥa-w qálam ilˁistiɣláal.
bi xuṣúuṣ ʃírkit ʃíllĭ fíiha ˁaqláam[3] fanníyya-l béeӡ muntagáat
ʃíll, wi kamáan ˁaqláam li tawzíiӡ ilmuntagáat, yaӡni qálam ilbitu-
míin wi qálam iṭṭayaráan wi qálam ilyáaz issáaˁil w-ilqálam ilfánni-w
hakáza. ˁamma min gíhat tawzíiӡ ilmuntagáat fíih ˁaqláam handasíyya muxtálifa. fíih kamáan qálam ḥisabáat ӡáamm[4] istiʃáari-l
kúll ilmasáaˁil ilḥisabíyya lilˁaqláam w-ilˁaqsáam[3] ittánya, / wi kúll

---

[1] Pronounced biddírha.
[2] Or xubaráaˁ (see Lesson 32, pattern (vi), note).
[3] Notice not only the 'Classical' pronunciation of q but also that ˁ is not elided;
both features are common in semi-Classical language of this kind.
[4] See Part I, Appendix B, note (c).

pedlars. *A*. And what is the job of the service (*lit.* petrol) stations?
B. They are [stations] for the sale of benzine, while workmen
experienced in greasing (are there to) service private cars, lorries,
taxis, and so on. *A*. Does the Company control all these stations?
B. No, it controls some while agents control the rest. *A*. In every
city? *B*. No, stations in the towns are operated by the Company
or agents, while in the country the agents administer them all.
A. It appears then that one (*lit.* we) can buy Shell products in any
place, large or small. *B*. Yes, and don't forget that among (*lit.*
from the collection of) the Company's staff are engineers and
technical staff to help customers. *A*. Suppose any customer has
a problem in his factory or some such (*lit.* any other) difficulty, can
he ask for technical advice from the Company? *B*. Yes, the Company's experts in all uses of petroleum products are at the service
of its customers.

31. *The administration of the companies in Egypt*

The head offices of the companies mentioned in previous discus-
sions are in Cairo. Those (*lit.* the offices of the management) of the
Shell Company and the Anglo-Egyptian Oilfields are in one building, while that of the Shell Chemical Distributing Company of
Egypt is in another.

As far as the company responsible for the production of crude
oil and its products is concerned,[1] the departments in the head
office are roughly the same as those in the fields and the Refinery.
They are [called] Engineering, Accounts, Drilling, Geology, Sur-
vey, and Exploitation.

Peculiar to the Shell Company are the technical departments for
the sale and distribution of Shell products (*lit.* for the sale of Shell
products, and also for the distribution of the products). These are
the Bitumen, Aviation, Liquid Gas, and Technical Departments,
&c. On the distribution [of the products] side there are various
engineering departments. There is also a general Accounts division
advising other departments and sections on all accounting matters.

[1] i.e. A-E. O.

ilʕaqláam dóol biyiʃtáɣalu-l kúll ilfurúuʒ filmanṭiqá-lli¹ ʕidarítha-f máṣr.

filʒimáara dí fíih kamáan ʕaqláam istiʃaríyya liʃʃirkitéen, zayy ilʕaqláam illi biydírha musáaʒid ilmudíir ilʒáamm lilʕidáara, wi húmma qálam ittadríib wi qálam ilʒalaqáat iṣṣinaʒíyya wi qálam ʕidáarit ilmustaxdimíin wi qálam iṭṭíbbi wi qálam ilʒalaqáat ilʒáamma.²

maʒʕínnĭ qálam ilmaxáazin ilʒáammĭ tábaʒ ʃírkit ʕabáar izziyúut ilʕingilizíyya-lmaṣríyya, ʕilqálam da-stiʃáari kamáan li ʃírkit ʃíllĭ wi-l kúllĭ-frúʒha.

32. ʕistiʒmáal ilmuntagáat ilbitrolíyya

sukkáan ilqúʈr ilmáṣri-byistaʒmílu-lmuntagáat ilbitrolíyya tamálli. biyímʃu ʒala síkak marṣúufa bilʕasfált wi-byirkábu sayyaráat bitistáʒmil máddit³ iddíizil. náfs ilmádda-lli-btitríṣif bíiha-ssíkak filʕaryáaf wi filmúdun marṣúufa bíiha ʕárḍ ilmaṭaráat. figgáwwĭ biyʃúufu-ṭṭayyaráat illi-btistáhlik banzíin min dáraga ʒálya-w báʒḍ iṭṭayyaráat ilʒaʃríyya biṭṭíir bi gáaz maxṣúuṣ. ʕilʒarabiyyáat ilmallúaki w-ilmutsikláat w-ittaksiyyáat wi báʒḍ illuriyyáat bárḍu-btistáhlik banzíin wiláakin darágtu ʕaqállĭ milli-btistaʒmílu-ṭṭayyaráat. kullína níʒraf inn ilgáaz binistahlíku filmáṭbax filʕafráan w-ilwaburáat wiláakin káam wáaḥid yíʒraf inn iggarráara filʒízba-btiʃtáɣal bilgáaz? ʕilyáaz ilmadɣúuṭ issáaʕil ill-ísmu butagáaz húwwa ʕáyḍan mustáʒmal fi ʕafráan iṭṭábx.

ʕilqúʈr ilmáṣri fíih dilwáqti-ṣnaʒáat kitíira-w biyʃayyálu baʒḍĭ ʕaláthum bilbuxáar. zamáan kanu-byiḥráqu-lfáḥmĭ-f ʕafránhum wiláakin filwáqt ilḥáaḍir ilmazúut mustáʒmal fi ʕáktar ilmaṣaaniʒ zayyĭ ma húwwa mustáʒmal kamáan fi waburáat issíkka-lḥadíid wi filmaráakib. muʃ láazim kull ilʕaláat yikúunu ʃayyalíin bilbuxáar wiláakin baʒḍŭhum biyiʃtáɣalu-b ʒídad bitistáhlik mádda bitrolíyya.

listiʒmaláat ilmazkúura ʕaylábha-f ʒídad wi ʕaláat, masalan fiṭṭayyaráat w-ilʕutubisáat w-ilmaráakib w-ilmaṣáaniʒ wi hakáza, wi la búddĭ mittaʃḥíim ben ilmaʒáadin ilmutaḥarríka wi yistaʒmílu fittaʃḥíim ʃáḥmĭ maxṣúuṣ li kúllĭ ʕáala-w ʒídda, wi fíih kamáan / zet

---

¹ Notice the position of the prominent syllable in the junction.
² See Part I, Appendix B, note (c).
³ Or *máaddit* (See Part I, Appendix B, note (c)).

All these departments work on behalf of all branches in the zone whose management is in Cairo.

Also in the building are advisory departments for both companies, such as those under the Assistant General Manager (Admin.), namely Training, Industrial Relations, Personnel Administration, Medical, and Public Relations.

Although the Materials (*lit.* general stores) Department comes under the Anglo-Egyptian Oilfields, this department also advises Shell and all its branches.

32. *The use of petroleum products*

The inhabitants of Egypt are constantly using petroleum products. They walk on roads made with asphalt and ride in vehicles using diesel oil. The same material of which country and town roads are made is used for making airfields (*lit.* the ground of airfields is made from it). In the sky they see aeroplanes using (*lit.* consuming) high-grade benzine, while some modern aircraft fly on special (quality) kerosine. Private cars, motor-cycles, taxis, and some trucks also use benzine but of a lower grade than that used by aircraft. We all know we use kerosine in kitchen ovens and stoves, but how many realize that the tractor on the farm works on kerosine? The compressed liquid gas called Butagaz is also used in cooking-ovens.

Nowadays in Egypt there are many industrial undertakings and the machines for some of them (*lit.* some of their machines) work by steam. They formerly burned coal in their furnaces but at the present time fuel oil is used in most plants in the same way as it is in railway locomotives and ships. All machines do not require to be worked by steam and (*lit.* but) some are driven by engines consuming a petroleum product.

The above-mentioned uses are mostly in engines and machines, for example in aircraft, motor buses, ships, factories, &c., but between moving metals lubrication is essential, and [in lubrication] for every machine and engine an appropriate lubricant is used (*lit.* they use). There is also / lubricating oil for the lubrication of

ʃáḥmĭ-l tazyíit Ṣaláat baꭓd iṣṣinaꭓáat zayy innasíig w-ittallagáat wi
hakáza.

la búddĭ núẓkur kamáan muntagáat ilmawádd[1] ilkimawíyya.
Ṣilmustaꭓmála filmanáazil húmma-ʃʃiltúksĭ w-ittibóol wi fíih
mawáddĭ tánya-xṣuṣíyya lizziráaꭓa wi-l ṣináaꭓit ilbilástik wi-f
ṣináaꭓit ilbúuya-w ꭓérha. filṢáwwil kanit ilmuntagáat ilbitrolíyya
mustaꭓmála lilṢináara w-ittadáawi báss, wiláakin dilwáqti ꭓádad
ilmuntagáat Ṣáktar min Ṣalféen, ḥátta zéet iʃʃáḥmĭ-l wáḥdu Ṣáktar
min mitéen dáraga.

33. máktab ilmustaxdimíin

A. biṣṣúdfa-smíꭓt innĭ-f maṣrufáat istixráag ilmuntagáat ilbitrolíyya
nísba-kbíira maṣrúufa ꭓala makáatib ilmustaxdimíin. *B.* náꭓam,
ṣaḥíiḥ. *A.* Ṣizzáyyĭ dá? *B.* ꭓalaʃan Ṣáyyĭ máktab lilmustaxdimíin
masṢúul ꭓan Ṣaqsáam kitíira. *A.* másalan zayyĭ Ṣéeh? *B.* zayy il-
ꭓalaqáat[2] iṣṣinaꭓíyya w-iṭṭíbb w-ilwiqáaya[2] min ilṢiṣabáat w-il-
maṭáaꭓim w-ittarfíih w-ittadríib. *A.* kúllĭ dá? wiláakin dóol
maxṣuṣíin lilꭓummáal, walla lilmuwaẓẓafíin kamáan? *B.* humma
maxṣuṣíin lilꭓummáal w-ilmuwaẓẓafíin, wiláakin ma tiftikírʃ innĭ
máktab ilmustaxdimíin ꭓawiz yáaxud milmuʃrifíin masṢuliyyáthum.
A. Ṣana muʃ fáahim da biẓẓábṭ. *B.* wugúud máktab ilmustaxdimíin yisáhhil li báꭓd ilmuʃrifíin innŭhum yiḥawwílu lilqismída-
lmaʃáakil illi bénhum wi ben ꭓummálhum. *A.* Ṣummáal iʃʃírka
ꭓámalit éeh? *B.* fíih baráamig maxṣúuṣa lilmuʃrifíin wi-b taṭbíqha
titḥássin Ṣaꭓmálhum wi Ṣaꭓmáal ꭓummálhum wi-mwaẓẓa-
fínhum. *A.* ma fíiʃ baráamig ꭓérha-l tadríib ilmuʃrifíin? *B.* Ṣáywa,
fíih, wi ḥanírgaꭓ lúhum baꭓdéen. *A.* ṭáyyib. wi Ṣéeh ilwiqáaya
min ilṢiṣabáat? *B.* xallíin-aqaddímlak suṢáal. Ṣéeh fíkrak tikun
natíigit ḥádsa tíḥṣal? *A.* Ṣilꭓáamil yitꭓáwwar. *B.* Ṣáywa w-aḥyáanan
yimkin yimúut. wiláakin fih natáaṢig[3] ꭓéer kida w-iza ma kánʃĭ
fíih báḥsĭ ꭓan sábab ilḥádsa yimkin tíḥṣal marra tánya. *A.* yaꭓni-
lqismída masṢúul ꭓan mánꭓ ilḥawáadis? *B.* míʃ bassĭ kída,
liṢann ilṢáḥsan innína nímnaꭓ ilḥawáadis / qablĭ-ḥṣúlha. *A.* dá

---

[1] Or *mawáadd*.
[2] Pronounce *q* as in 'Classical'.
[3] The usual colloquial form is *natáayig*.

machines in certain industries, for example textiles, refrigeration, and so on.

We must also refer to the chemical products. Those used domestically (*lit.* in the homes) are Shell Tox and Teepol. There are, too, other products specially for agriculture, plastics, the paint industry, &c. At first petroleum products were used for lighting and medicine only, but nowadays the number of products exceeds two thousand, lubricating oil alone having more than two hundred grades.

33. *The Personnel Department*

A. I heard by chance that a large percentage of the expense[s] of producing petroleum products is spent on personnel departments. *B.* Yes, that is so. *A.* How is that? *B.* Because any personnel department is responsible for many departments. *A.* Which, for example? *B.* Industrial Relations, Medical (*lit.* medicine), Safety, Canteens, Welfare, and Training. *A.* All those (*lit.* that)! Are they only for (*lit.* special to) the workmen or for the staff as well? *B.* For labour and staff, but don't think that the Personnel Department wants to take their responsibilities away from the supervisors. *A.* I haven't understood that properly. *B.* The existence of a Personnel Department makes it easy for some supervisors to pass to that department the problems (that arise) between them and their men. *A.* What has the Company done (about it), then? *B.* There are special courses (*lit.* programmes) for supervisors designed to improve (*lit.* and by their application they improve) their methods (*lit.* works) and the work[s] of their men and staff. *A.* Aren't there any other courses for the training of supervisors? *B.* Yes, there are. We'll come back to them later. *A.* Good. Now what is Safety? *B.* Let me put a question to you. What do you think is the result of an accident [which happens]? *A.* The man is hurt. *B.* Yes, and sometimes he may die. But there are other effects and if there is no investigation into the reason for the accident, it may happen again. *A.* Does that mean that the department is responsible for the prevention of accidents? *B.* Not only that, but it's (surely) best for us to prevent accidents / before they

ṣaḫíiḫ. wi Ṣéeh ʃuɣl ilqísm iṭṭíbbi? *B.* Ṣilqísm iṭṭíbbi-l wáḥdu(h),
wi fíih Ṣagzaxáana-w filḫuqúul fih mustaʃfayáat taḫtï Ṣidáarit
ilṢaqsáam iṭṭibbíyya. *A.* w-ilɣalaqáat iṣṣinaɣíyya yaɣni Ṣéeh?
B. fíih qawaníin ḫukumíyya zayyï qanúun ɣáqd¹ ilɣámal ilfárdi-w
ɣéeru(h), wi taṭbíiq ilqawaníin ilxuṣuṣíyya lilmustaxdimíin
masṢúul ɣánha qísm ilmustaxdimíin. *A.* mafhúum, wiláakin iza
káanit fíih muʃkíla maɣa-lɣummáal míin biymassílhum? *B.* niqa-
báthum¹ wi fíih Ṣittiḫáad niqabáat ilɣummáal w-ilmuwaẓẓafíin li-
ṣnáaɣit ilbitróol. *A.* w-iza káanit ʃírka wi-nqáaba ma yittifqúuʃ
maɣa báɣḍï-f muʃkíla, biyiɣmílu Ṣéeh? *B.* fíih qawaníin tiḫáddid
iṭṭúruq ilxuṣuṣíyya-l ḫáll ilmaʃáakil wi súuṢ ittafáahum. *A.* ma
qúltïʃ innak ḫatfahhímn-áktar ɣan ittadríib? *B.* Ṣáywa, qúltï kída.
fíih baráamig kitíira-xṣuṣíyya lilmuʃrifíin li ɣalaqáat ilɣámal wi
taḥsíin wasáaṢil ilɣámal wi taɣlíim ilɣámal. *A.* bássï kída? *B.* láṢ,
dóol mufidíin lilmuʃrifíin fi Ṣáyyï dáraga wi-l báɣd ilɣummáal
wiláakin fih baráamig ɣérha lilmuʃrifíin ikkubáar, wi fih baráamig
fanníyya-l míhan baɣd ilmuwaẓẓafíin w-ilɣummáal. *A.* wi fíih
ḫáaga tánya lilɣummáal? *B.* Ṣummáal. báɣd ilbaráamig ilmaẕ-
kúura-mfíida lúhum zayyï ma qultílak wiláakin fíih kamáan wárʃa
maxṣúuṣa littadríib ɣaṣṣinaɣáat w-ilmíhan ittánya-l ɣummáal
ilyomíyya w-iʃʃahríyya-w lilmuwaẓẓafíin. *A.* xaláaṣ baqa? *B.* láṢ,
wilakin ana m-aqdárʃ aqúllak fi wáqtï wáaḥid ɣan kúll iʃʃúɣl
illi-byinɣímil fi qísm ilmustaxdimíin wilakin iza kúntï ɣáawiz
tíɣraf áktar, Ṣáḥsan ṭaríiqa tísṢal raṢíis qísm ilmustaxdimíin figgíha-
btáɣtak.

---

¹ Pronounce *q* as in 'Classical'. This does not apply to ɣ*aqd* in the everyday
sense of 'contract'.

occur (*lit.* their occurrence). *A*. Agreed. And what does the Medical Department do? *B*. The Medical Department is independent
(*lit.* on its own). There are dispensaries and, in the fields, hospitals
under the direction of the medical departments. *A*. And what
about Industrial Relations? *B*. There are statutory (*lit.* governmental) laws such as the Individual Contract of Service Law and
others, and the Personnel Department is responsible for the application of the laws, as far as they concern employees. *A*. I see. Now
if there is a dispute with the workmen, who represents them?
B. Their syndicates, and there is a Federation of Syndicates of
Petroleum Workers. *A*. If a company and a syndicate do not agree
[together] on a matter, what do they do? *B*. There are laws
defining the proper means for the solution of problems and dis-
agreements (*lit.* badness of understanding). *A*. Didn't you say
you'd tell (*lit.* explain to) me more about training? *B*. Yes, I did.
There are a number of special supervisors' courses on Job Relations, on the improvement of working methods and on the giving
of instruction (*lit.* teaching the job). *A*. Is that all? *B*. No, those
are useful to supervisors of any grade and to certain of the workmen, but there are other courses for senior supervisors as well as
technical courses in the trades of certain staff and workmen. *A*. Is
there anything else for the workmen? *B*. Certainly. As I've told
you, some of the courses I've mentioned are useful to them, but
there's also a special workshop for industrial training and other
occupations, (available to) (*lit.* for) daily- and monthly-paid workmen and (also) to staff. *A*. Is that all now? *B*. No, but I can't tell
you all at once about all the jobs undertaken in the Personnel
Department, [but] if you want to know more, the best way is to
ask the head of the Personnel Department in your (own) zone.

APPENDIX A

Greetings (taḥiyyáat)

Most of us do what is expected of us, and what we say is usually determined by the situation and by what is said to us. This general feature of language is nowhere better illustrated than by Arabic in which many expressions 'trigger off' fixed formulaic responses, both 'question' and 'answer' being in turn bound to the situation. Here and there in the examples below 'classicisms' are evident, for example in the common greeting ʕissaláamu ɣaléekum.

(*a*) The following provides in sequence the necessary 'gambits' for the encounter of two friends or acquaintances, host and guest, &c.

A. ʕissaláamu ɣaléekum[1]   lit. *Peace be on you* (said by newcomer)

B. ɣaléekumu-ssaláam wi raḥmátu-   lit. *Peace be on you, the*
lláah wi barakáatu(h)   *mercy of God and his blessings*

Note

This is the usual greeting between Muslims and may be used to a Muslim at any time. Notice the plural -**kum**, a fairly common feature of the language of personal address and greetings.

or

A. ʕáhlan wi sáhlan   *Greetings* (by host)
B. ʕáhlan wi sáhlan bíik   *Greetings*

Note

Rather less formal than ʕissaláamu ɣaléekum. Used, for example, when passing an acquaintance in the street, it may be translated *hello*. ʕáhlan, used alone, is still less formal.

or

A. saɣíida   *Greetings* (by new-comer)

B. saɣíida-mbáarak (or mbárka)   *Greetings*

[1] Rarely used by women.

Note

sa؟iida and its response are not used between Muslims.

A. ؟itfáḍḍal istaráyyaḫ.   ؟izzáyyï   *Please sit down. How*
   ḫaḍrítak (or ؟izzáyyï ṣiḫḫítak   *are you?*
   or simply, ؟izzáyyak)?

Note

؟izzáyyï ḫaḍrítak i̇s the most formal, and ؟izzáyyak the most friendly of the
alternatives. ؟izzáyy ilḫáal is yet a fourth possibility.

B. ؟ilḫámdu lilláah, ؟alláah yiḫfá-   *Very well, thank you* (lit.
   ẓak (or ṣiḫḫíti-kwayyísa). ؟iz-   *praise be to God, may*
   záyyï ḫaḍrítak ínta?   *God protect you* (or
                                          my health is good)).
                                          How are YOU?

A. ؟ilḫámdu lilláah   *Very well, thank you.*

A. ؟izzáyy ilẓéela?   *How is the family?*
B. ؟ilḫámdu lilláah, kuwayyisíin   *Fine, thank you.*

A. ؟izzáyyï-wláadak?   *How are the children?*
B. kullŭhum bi xéer wi-ybúusu   *They are all well* (lit. *all*
   ؟idéek   *of them are well and*
                                          kiss your hands).

A. ʃarraftína   lit. *You have honoured*
                                          us (i.e. *I'm very pleased*
                                          to see you).

B. ؟alláah yiʃárraf qádrak (or   lit. *May God honour*
   ؟alláah yiʃarráfak)   *you.*

or

A. nawwártï bétna (or nawwartína)   lit. *You have given our*
                                          house light.

B. ؟alláah yináwwar ẓaléek   lit. *God give you light!*

or

A. ؟anistína   lit. *You have cheered us.*
B. ؟alláah yi؟áṅsak   lit. *May God cheer you!*

or

A. ḥáṣalit ilbáraka   lit. *Blessing has come.*
B. ʕalláah yibáarik fíik   lit. *God bless you!*

Notes

  (i) Notice how frequently a given root is repeated in both 'question' and 'answer'.
  (ii) ʕanistína and especially ḥáṣalit ilbáraka, are commonly used at the end of a visit.

A. ʕitfáḍḍal fingáan qáhwa   *Do have a cup of coffee.*
B (when coffee has been drunk). qáhwa   lit. *May you always*
   dáyman   *have coffee!*
A. dáamit ḥayáatak   lit. *May your life be everlasting!*

B (when leaving). ʕaḥíbb astáʕzin or   *Please excuse me, I have*
   ʕastáʕzin baqa or ʕismáḥli,   *an appointment.*
   ɤándi maɤáad
A. xallíik ʃuwáyya, lissa bádri   *Stay a while, it is still early.*

B. ʕaʃkúrak   *Thank you* (sc. *but I must go*).

A. sallímli ɤala-lʕawláad   *Remember me to the children.*

B. ʕalláah yisallímak   *Thank you, I will* (lit. *God give you peace*).

A. maɤa-ssaláama   *Good-bye!*
B. ʕalláah yisallímak   *Good-bye!*

(*b*) Passing the time of day.

The above greetings ʕissaláamu ɤaléekum, ʕáhlan wi sáhlan, and saɤíida together with their responses are used as general greetings at any time of day. In addition, learn the following:

A. ṣabáaḥ ilxéer (or innúur)   *Good-morning!*
B. ṣabáaḥ ilxéer (or innúur) ɤaléek   *Good-morning!*
   or ʕalláah yiṣabbáḥak bilxéer

Note

ṣabáaḥ innúur, which may also be used as a response to ṣabáaḥ ilxéer, is somewhat formal. From less sophisticated speakers, you will also hear ṣabáaḥ ilfúll and ṣabáaḥ ilqíʃṭa.

A. naháarak saƗíid	*Good-day !*
B. naháarak saƗíid mubáarak	*Good-day !*

Note

This exchange is chiefly used between Christians, or Christian and Muslim.

A. misáaʕ ilxéer (or mísa-lxéer)	*Good-evening !*
B. misáaʕ ilxéer (or mísa-lxéer) Ɨaléek or ʕalláah yimassíik bil-xéer	*Good-evening !*

Note

ʕásƗad alláahu misáak with the response ʕalláah yimassíik bilxéer is sometimes used by the educated.

or

A. léltak saƗíida	*Good-evening !*
B. léltak saƗíida-mbáarak (or mbár-ka)	*Good-evening !*

Note

Again unlikely to be used between Muslims.

A. tíṣbaḥ Ɨala xéer	*Good-night !* (on parting at night)
B. ʕalláah yiṣabbáḥak bilxéer or w-ínta min ʕáhl-ilxéer or w-ínta min ʕáhlu(h)	*Good-night !*

(*c*) More specific occasions.

A. ʕin ʃáaʕ alláah issána-ggáyya tikun Ɨala gábal Ɨarafáat	Good wishes on the occasion of the big
B. (ʕíḥna w-íntu) gámƗan, ʕin ʃáaʕ alláah	feast Ɨíid ilʕáḍḥa or Qurban Bairam.
A. kúllï sána w-inta ṭáyyib or kúllï Ɨáam w-antum bi xéer	On the occasion of other feasts, including the

B. w-ínta ṭáyyib or w-ínta biṣṣíḥḥa
w-issaláama

important Ramadan
Bairam.

A. ḥággĭ mabrúuk (or mabrúur) or
ḥággĭ mabrúur wi zámbĭ may-
fúur
B (pilgrim). ɣuqbáal ɣandŭkum or
ʕalláah yibáarik fíik

To pilgrim returning
from Mecca.

A. mabrúuk. ɣuqbáal ilbakáari
or mabrúuk. ʕin ʃáaʕ alláah
zurríyya ṣálḥa
B (groom or bride). ʕalláah yibáarik
fíik

To groom or bride after
wedding.

A (the eater). ʕilḥámdu lilláah
B. bilhána w-iʃʃífa or (after drink only)
haníyyan (or haníiʕan)
A. ʕalláah yihanníik or hannáak
alláah

After meal or drink.

A (the sneezer). ʕilḥámdu lilláah
B. yarḥámkumu-lláah or ráḥamak
alláah

After a sneeze.

A. naɣíiman
B (the bather). ʕánɣam alláah ɣaléek

To one after he has
bathed or shaved.

A. ʃíddĭ ḥéelak. ʕilbaqíyya-f ḥayáatak
B (the bereaved). w-ilbaqíyya-f ḥayáatak

After a death.

A. ʕin ʃáaʕ alláah tikun ríḥla-kwayyísa
B. ʕin ʃáaʕ alláah, wi-nʃúuf wiʃʃŭ-
kum bi xéer

To one about to go on a
journey.

A. ḥamdílla bissaláama (or ɣas-
saláama)
B (the traveller). ʕalláah yisallímak

To one returning from
a journey.

A (the beggar). ḥásana lilláah A request for alms.

B. Sálláah yiɛṭíik or ɛal-alláah or (Refusal)
   ɛal-álla

A. ʃíddi̇ ḥéelak Encouragement to one

B. Siʃʃídda ɛal-alláah whose spirits are flag-
ging.

A. rabbína yústur To reassure one who

B. Sin ʃáaS alláah has expressed anxiety.

A. salámtak When visiting a sick

B (the invalid). Sálláah yisallímak person.

A. mabrúuk Congratulations.

B. Sálláah yibáarik fíik

or

A. Sahanníik . . . (e.g. bi nagáaḥak on
   your success)

B. Saʃkúrak

A. Sitfáddal Invitation to join you

B (refusing the invitation). láS, muta- (eating, drinking, &c.).
   ʃákkir or ɛiʃt

(d) General expressions of politeness (no response involved).

   ɛan íznak or Sismáḥli Excuse me !
   káttar xéerak or mutaʃákkir or Thank you.
   mutaʃakkiríin or Saʃkúrak or
   maɛa-ʃʃúkr or ʃúkran

Note

In this case, the response Silɛáfw Don't mention it is very common.

   min fádlak . . . Please . . .
   Siɛmil maɛrúuf . . .
   walláahi tiɛmílli-lxídma di . . .[1]
   walláahi tixdímni . . .[1]

   [1] Notice this use of the 'oath'. Cf. wi-ḥyáatak (see p. 203, fn. 1).

Note

An imperative usually follows: e.g. **min fáḍlak iddíini kubbáayit máyya**
Please give me a glass of water.

ʕargúuk . . .

Note

The imperfect (2nd person) follows: e.g. **ʕargúuk tirúuḥ** *Please go.*

ʕana líyya ɣandak rága   *I have a favour to ask you.*

APPENDIX B

Exclamations and 'Oaths'

(*a*) The following exclamations **(kilmáat ilʕistiɣráab)** are common:

> **subḫáan alláah!**
> ⎧**(ʃéeʕ) ɣaríib!**
> ⎨**(ʃéeʕ) ɣagíib!**
> ⎩**(ʃéeʕ) múdhiʃ!**
> **yáa saláam!**
> **ʕálla(h)!**
> **ʕéhda!** or **déhda!**

Although the above are given in approximately ascending order of emphasis, the English equivalent of a given example will depend on the context and, to a lesser extent, on individual taste. Selection may be made from the following: 'What!', 'Well!', 'Indeed!', 'Well, I never!', 'Fancy!', 'Good heavens!', 'Great Scott!', 'Good Lord!', 'Bless my soul!', &c.

Other common exclamations are:

ɣáal, ɣáal! *Excellent!*
wálla(h)! or **láʕ, ya ʃéex!** *Really!, You don't say!*
ya-xṣáara! *What a pity!*
ya ḫáwl lilláah! *What a loss!* (e.g. on hearing of death of one highly respected)
ɣéeb ɣaléek! *Shame on you!*

ḥaráam ɣaléek!   *Shame on you !* (religious matter)
ʕamma ráagil!   *What a man !*

Note

Other nouns may be substituted for **ráagil**, e.g. **ʕamma ḥárr** *Isn't it hot !*

ʕaɣúuzu billáah!   *Oh, Lord !*

Note

The translation is approximate. **ʕaɣúuzu billáah** is used when anything displeases you.

ʕiʃmíɣna (kida)!   *Why do you do that ?*

Note

ʕiʃmíɣna implies disapproval or surprise, and is equivalent to **léeh baqa!** Both may often be translated *How can you say that !*

Notice also the exclamatory **ya réet** as, for example, in **ya rétni rúḥt!** *If only I had gone !*

(*b*) The 'oaths' (see Part I, Lesson 13, 3) are often used for exclamation or emphasis, e.g. **walláahi-lɣaẓíim!** *Good Lord !*, **walláahi-nta muʃ kuwáyyis!** *How very unpleasant you are !*, **walláah-ana ɣándi ḥáẓẓ!** *I am indeed lucky !*

The 'oaths' as such, i.e. used, for example, to vouch for the truth of what is said as in **walláahi-lɣaẓíim ma ʃúftu(h)** *By God (the Mighty), I did not see him*, vary according to the educational standard of the speaker. Educated speakers use **walláahi-lɣaẓíim, walláahi,** and **winnábi,** but the unsophisticated have a greater range. They may, for example, swear to divorce or on the life of a member of the family as in **wi-ḥyáat íbni** or **wi-ḥyáat abúuya,** or local saints may be invoked as, for example, in the Cairene **wi-ḥyáat sayyídna-lḥuséen** or **wi-ḥyáat issayyída zéenab.**

The oaths are not, of course, used indiscriminately without reference to the personal background of the speaker. Only a married man with a son may swear by his son's life. Similarly, swearing to divorce or on the good name of one's family are only used by married men as in the strong oaths **ɣaláyya-ṭṭaláaq bittaláata** or **ɣaláyya-lḥaráam min béeti.** For the single man, **walláahi-lɣaẓíim** is the strongest oath.

The oaths as such have virtually no binding force among educated people today. In contrast, however, if the Bedouin swears to divorce his wife unless his guest continues to eat, then he may well do so in the event of the guest's refusal. The student should not himself attempt to use the oaths except in their exclamatory function: he is otherwise almost certain to offend or, at best, to amuse the Arabic speaker.[1]

[1] See also p. 189, fn. 1.

PART III
VOCABULARY

The following vocabulary of approximately 2,000 words covers the lexical material used in this book —with the exception of the greetings, exclamations, and similar material presented in some detail in Part II, Appendixes A and B—with the addition of a small number of useful, everyday words.

Blank pages are provided at the end of both sections (Arabic–English and English–Arabic) for the student's use in extending his vocabulary and meeting his individual needs.

VOCABULARY
ARABIC-ENGLISH

Order of alphabet

The alphabetical order employed is as far as possible that of the roman alphabet, with ḍ, ḥ, ṣ, ṭ, ẓ following d, h, s, t, z respectively, and the four 'unusual' shapes ʕ, ʃ, ɛ, and ɣ placed in that order at the end. j has been omitted (see Introduction, p. 8). The complete order is, therefore, *a*, b, d, ḍ, *e*, f, g, h, ḥ, *i*, k, l, m, n, *o*, q, r, s, ṣ, t, ṭ, *u*, w, x, y, z, ẓ, ʕ, ʃ, ɛ, ɣ, of which a, e, i, o, u have been printed in italic to underline the fact that no entry begins with a vowel.

Method of entry

   (i) Verbs are entered in the 3rd pers. sing. masc. perfect, followed by the corresponding person of the imperfect and translated by the English infinitive.

 (ii) **ʕit-** and **ʕin-** passive forms of the verb have not been included when the simple form has already been entered.

(iii) Verbal nouns have been entered separately.

(iv) Participles which are immediately relatable to verbal forms (see Lesson 33) have not been included as a general rule. They have been separately entered, however, when

    (*a*) they are not immediately relatable to a given verbal form, e.g. **ʃáaɣil** *worrying*, **mafṣúul** *sold (after bargaining)*; **mifáaṣil** (cf. **fáaṣil, yifáaṣil** *to bargain*) will not be entered;

    (*b*) a corresponding verbal form occurs in the language but has not been included in the Vocabulary, e.g. **mádɛi** *invited, asked*; **dáɣa, yídɛi** does occur but has not been used in the book and in any case is less frequent in this sense than **ɛázam, yíɛzim** *to invite*;

    (*c*) the common English translation of the participle is not at once suggested by that of the related verbal form, e.g. **láabis** *wearing, dressed* (cf. **líbis, yílbis** *to put on, wear*), **masʕúul** *responsible* (cf. **sáʕal, yísʕal** *to ask*);

    (*d*) they occur in the Arabic-English exercises of Part I before Lesson 33.

(v) Those non-verbal forms for which gender and number distinctions are made, i.e. nouns, adjectives, participles, certain numerals, &c., are treated as in Part I. Nouns are entered in the singular, followed by the plural form, if any; plurals are not entered separately, except for the relatively few broken plurals which occur in the Arabic–English exercises of Part I before Lesson 32. Adjectives, participles, demonstratives, &c., as well as those nouns with both masculine and feminine forms in the singular, are entered under the masculine singular, followed by the corresponding feminine and plural forms. Similarly, the 'masculine' form of numerals ('1' and '3–10') is given pride of place.

(vi) Collective nouns are entered in the collective form, followed by their 'unit' and 'counted' forms; corresponding broken plural forms, if any, are included after 'counted' forms.

(vii) Comparative forms of adjectives have not been entered except in the rare case of a consonantal difference between the positive and comparative forms, e.g. **muhímm** *important*, **ʕahámm** *more important*.

Abbreviations and diacritics

The following abbreviations are used:

v.	verb	m.	masculine
n.	noun	f.	feminine
v.n.	verbal noun	pl.	plural
adj.	adjective	s.	singular
a.p.	active participle	c.	collective
p.s.	pronominal suffix	tr.	transitive
pf.	perfect	intr.	intransitive
impf.	imperfect		

(with reference to English translation) — applies to tr. transitive / intr. intransitive

Two diacritics are also used as follows:

* —with words containing **r,** to indicate where necessary that the vowel **a** preceding or following the consonant must be of 'back' quality (see Introduction, p. 9, (ii), (*b*)).

† —with words containing **q,** to indicate that the consonant is usually pronounced by educated speakers as in 'Classical' Arabic.

ARABIC-ENGLISH

b

baab, Sabwáab (or Sibwáab) or bibáan door, gate

baal thought; care

xad, yaaxud baal + p.s. to take care

báaliy, yibáaliy to exaggerate

báaqi, báqya, baqyíin remaining

báaqi remainder, change (money)

baar*, baráat* bar

báarik, yibáarik to bless

baat, batáat armpit

báayin

baayin gala + p.s. or n. . . . to look . . .

báayix, báyxa, bayxíin disagreeable

báafa, bafawáat pasha

baag, yibíig to sell

bádal (or badal min) + n.
bádal ma + v. } instead of

bádana, badanáat tribe

bádawi, badawíyya, bádw Bedouin

bádla, bídal suit

bádri early

báddag, yibáddag to shop

báhari, baharíyya, bahariyyíin northern, northerner

Silwágh ilbáhari Lower Egypt, the Delta

báhas, yíbhas to investigate, inquire, study

bahháar*, bahháara* sailor

bahr*, biháar* sea

Silbáhr ilSáhmar* the Red Sea

Silbáhr ilSábyad ilmutawáşşit the Mediterranean Sea

bahráawi*, bahrawíyya*, bahárwa* inhabitant of Behera province

bahárwa fallahíin peasants of the Delta

bahríyya navy

bahs (v.n.) research, inquiry

báka, yíbki to cry, weep

baláat (c.), baláata, balatáat tiles; tiled floor

baláaf without; gratis

bálad (f.), biláad town, village; country

báladi, baladíyya local, native; vulgar, low-class

baladíyya, baladiyyáat town-council

bálag, yíblag to swallow

ball, yibíll to wet

bállay, yibállay to forward, dispatch; inform

bálta, baltáat axe

báltu, baláati overcoat, raincoat

bándar*, banáadir town

bank, bunúuk (or binúuk) bank

bantalóon, bantalonáat trousers

banzíin petrol

báqa, yíbqa to be, become, remain

baqáalu filmustáffa múdda he's been in hospital for some time

báqa then, well

baqíyya remainder

baqq (c.), baqqáaya, baqqáat bugs

baqqáal, baqqalíin grocer

baqfíif tip, baksheesh

bára*, yíbri to sharpen

báraka*, barakáat* blessing

bard cold

xad, yaaxud bard to catch cold

bárdu still, also

baríid post, mail

barmíil, baramíil barrel, drum

barníita* (or burnéeta), baraníit* hat

barr* land (opposed to 'sea'); country

bárra* outside

barráad*, barradíin* fitter

barráad*, barariíd* teapot

barráani*, barraníyya*, barraniyyíin* outer

baskalítta, baskalittáat bicycle

bass only, just

básal (c.), básala or başaláaya, başaláat onions

bášbaş, yibáşbaş to ogle

başíit, başíita, buşáat[1] small, trifling

batáatiş (c.), batatşáaya, batatşáat potatoes

batn (f.), butúun stomach

---

[1] Plural rare

battáal, battáala, battalíin bad; unemployed

báttal, yibáttal to give up

baxíil, baxíila, búxala miser, miserly

baxt luck

    ɣándak báxt you are lucky

bayáada, bayadáat pillow-case, sheet

bayyáaɣ, bayyáaɣa, bayyaɣíin seller

báyyad, yibáyyad to paint (white or cream); polish (brass)

baʃkáatib chief clerk

báɣat, yíbɣat to send

baɣd after

baɣdéen afterwards, later

    wi baɣdéen wayyáak baqa! what's the matter with you!

báɣdi ma + v. after

baɣd some; each other

    záyyi báɣd, gámbi báɣd, &c. like each other, next to each other, &c.

baɣúud (c.), **baɣúuda, baɣudáat** mosquitoes

beed (c.), **béeda, bedáat** eggs

    béed madrúub scrambled eggs

been between

beet, biyúut house

beeɣ (v.n.) selling, sale

    lilbéeɣ for sale

bi by, with, in

    biẕẕábt exactly, properly

bidd + p.s. + v. to be keen to

bidúun without

bidáaɣa, badáayiɣ merchandise, goods

bihíima, baháayim animal

(ʔil)bihéera Behera province

bíiba, bibáat pipe (smoking)

biir, ʕabáar* *or* **ʕabyáar*** well

bíira beer

bilánt, bilantáat plant (industrial)

bilástik plastic, plastics

bináaya, binayáat building

bint, banáat girl, daughter

bírid, yíbrad* to (become) cool

birnáamig, baráamig programme, course, curriculum

bisílla (c.), **ḥabbáayit b., ḥabbáat b.** peas

biskilítta (*see* **baskalítta**)

bitáaɣ, bitáɣt, bitúuɣ of, belonging to

bitíllu *or* **láḥma-btíllu** veal

bitróol petroleum

bitróoli, bitrolíyya petroleum (*adj.*)

bitumíin bitumen

bitáaqa, bitaqáat *or* **batáayiq** card

biʃwéeʃ slowly

biɣíid, biɣíida, buɣáad far, distant

buféeh, bufeháat buffet

búkra* tomorrow

    báɣdi búkra the day after tomorrow

    báɣdi báɣdi búkra in two days' time

bulíiṣ police

    ɣaskári bulíiṣ policeman

búmba, bumbáat pump

buqq mouth

bursaɣíid Port Said

burtuqáan (c.), **burtuqáana, burtuqanáat** oranges

búṣta post

buṣtági, busṭagíyya postman

butagáaz Butagaz

búuya, buyáat paint

buxáar* steam

buɣd distance

d

da, di (díyya, díyyat), dool this, that, these, those

daar*, duur house

daar*, yidíir to administer, direct

daar*, yidúur to go around

daas, yidúus to slip, stumble

dáawa, yidáawi to prescribe medicine for

dáaxil inside

dáfaɣ, yídfaɣ to pay

dáffaɣ, yidáffaɣ to charge, make pay

dafɣ (v.n.) payment, paying

daháan (v.n.) painting

dáhab gold

dáhan, yídhin to paint

dálaq, yúdluq to spill

dall, yidíll to guide, show

damm blood

    ɣáawiz agárri dámmi I want to stretch my legs (*lit.* make my blood flow)

dámya

    wáraqit dámya fiscal stamp

daqíiq, daqíiqa delicate, fine

daqíiqa, daqáayiq minute

daqn (f.), **duqúun** chin, beard

daqq, yidúqq to knock; press (switch); ring (of bell)

dáraga*, daragáat* degree, class, rank; step, rung

dáras, yídris to study, learn

dárris (or dárras), yidárris (or yidárras) to teach

dars, durúus lesson

dásta, dísat dozen

dáwa (m.), ʕadwíya medicine

dáwla, dúwal nation

dáwwar*, yidáwwar* to look for (+ ʒala); go round

dáwʃa trouble, noise, commotion

dawʃági, dawʃagíyya troublesome, noisy

dáxal, yúdxul to enter

daxlíyya

  wizáarit iddaxlíyya Ministry of the Interior

dáyman always

dáyyaq, dayyáqa, dayyaqíin narrow

déhda! what! indeed!

dibbáan (c.), dibbáana, dibbanáat flies

diib, diyáaba jackal, wolf

díik (or dáak) innaháar* the other day, some days ago

diik, diyúuk cockerel

  díik rúumi turkey

diin (or diyáana), ʕadwáan (or diyanáat) religion

díini, diníyya, diniyyíin religious

díizil diesel

dilwáqti now

dimáay brain, head

dínya world

  ʕiddínya dálma it is dark

  ʕiddínya malyáana náas there are people everywhere

diqíiq flour

diráaʒ, ʕadríʒa arm

disímbir December

diwáan, dawawíin office; compartment

(ya) dóobak just, only

door, ʕadwáar* turn; floor, story

  biddóor in turn

dubáara* string

dúkha, díkha, dúkham that, those

dukkáan, dakakíin shop

duktúur, dakátra doctor

duláab, dawalíib cupboard

durg, ʕadráag* drawer

duséeh, duseháat file, record, dossier

duxúul (v.n.) entering

  mamnúuʒ idduxúul no entry!

duxxáan smoke, tobacco

dúyri straight, straight away

ḍ

ḍáani mutton

  fáxda (or fáxdit) ḍáani leg of mutton

ḍaaʒ, yiḍíiʒ to be lost

ḍabʒ, ḍubúʒa hyena

ḍáffa, ḍifáaf bank (river)

ḍahr, ḍuhúur[1] back

ḍaláam darkness

ḍall, yiḍíll to lose one's way

ḍall shade

ḍállim, yiḍállim to become dark

  ʕiddínya bitḍállim it is getting dark

ḍálma darkness

ḍárab, yíḍrab to hit; multiply

ḍarb (v.n.) hitting; multiplying

ḍárba, ḍarbáat blow

ḍarúuri, ḍaruríyya essential, inevitable

ḍáyyaʒ, yiḍáyyaʒ to waste: lose

ḍáyaṭ, yíḍyaṭ to press, compress; oblige, compel

ḍeef, ḍiyúuf or ḍuyúuf guest

ḍidd against

ḍíḥik, yíḍḥak to laugh; (+ ʒala) to laugh at, cheat

ḍiḥíyya (see ʒiid)

ḍiḥk (v.n.) laughing, laughter

ḍimn

  min ḍimn . . . from among . . .

ḍiyúuf (see ḍeef)

ḍuhr noon

  báʒd idḍúhr (in the) afternoon

  qábl idḍúhr (in the) morning

f

fa and

fáadi, fádya, faḍyíin empty, free, unoccupied

---

[1] Plural rare.

fáaḍil, fáḍla, faḍlíin remaining
fáahim, fáhma, fahmíin understanding, having understood
fáakir, fákra, fakríin remembering, having remembered
faaq, yifúuq to sober up
faar*, firáan mouse
faar*, yifúur to rise (of milk), boil
fáaris, firsáan horseman
fáariy, fárya, faryíin empty
  kaláam fáariy nonsense
fáaṣil, yifáaṣil to bargain
faat, yifúut to pass, pass by
  ʕilqáṭrï fáatu(h) he missed the train
faddáan, fadadíin acre
faḍḍ, yifúḍḍ to mediate (in dispute); disperse
fáḍḍa silver
fáḍḍa, yifáḍḍi to empty
fáḍḍal, yifáḍḍal to prefer
faḍl
  min fáḍlak please
fáḍla remains (e.g. of meal)
fagr dawn
fáhhim, yifáhhim to explain
faḥm (c.), **faḥmáaya, faḥmáat** coal, charcoal
fakaháani, fakahaníyya fruiterer
fákha, fawáakih fruit
fakk, yifúkk to change (money); undo
fákka (small) change
fákkar*, yifákkar* to remind; think, ponder
faláafil condiments
falláaḥ, falláaḥa, fallaḥíin peasant
fann, funúun art, skill, technique
fannáan, fannáana, fannaníin artist, actor
fánni, fanníyya, fanniyyíin technical; skilled
fanúus, fawaníis lamp, headlight
faqíir, faqíira, fúqara* poor (person)
fáraḍ, yífriḍ to suppose; compel, bind
faránsa* France
fansáawi*, faransawíyya*, faransawiyyíin* French(man)
farárgi, farargíyya poulterer, chicken farmer
fáraz, yífriz to separate, sort out
fáraʃ, yífriʃ to furnish
fárda, fírad (single) one

fárdi, fardíyya individual (adj.)
  masʕála fardíyya personal matter
farḍ, faráaʕiḍ* (or **faráayiḍ***) condition, tenet
farq, furúuq difference
farráaʃ*, farraʃíin* messenger
fárrag*, yifárrag* to show round
fárraq, yifárraq to distribute
fárray, yifárray to empty; fire (rifle)
fárxa, firáax chicken
farʃ furniture; (v.n.) furnishing
farᴄ*, furúuᴄ branch
farᴄúuni, farᴄuníyya, faráᴄna* Pharaonic
fáṣal, yífṣil to separate
faṣl, fuṣúul chapter; season
faṣúlya (c.), **ḥabbáayit f., ḥabbáat f.** beans
fátaḥ, yíftaḥ to open
fátla, fítal string, thread
fáttaḥ, yifáttaḥ to open (of flower, eye, &c.)
  lazim tifattáḥi ᴄéenik you (f.) must have your wits about you
fáttiʃ, yifáttiʃ to inspect
fatúura, fawaṭíir bill
fawáakih (see **fákha**)
fáxda, ʕifxáad thigh
fáyda, fawáayid advantage
  ma fíiʃ fáyda there's no point
(ʕil)fayyúum Fayoum
fayyúumi, fayyumíyya from Fayoum
feen where
fi in, among
fibráayir (or **fab-**) February
fíḍi, yífḍa to (become) empty, be unoccupied
fíḍil, yífḍal to continue to; be left over
figl (c.), **fígla, figláat** radishes
fíhim, yífham to understand
fihranháyt* Fahrenheit
fiih there is/are
fiil, ʕafyáal elephant
fikr, ʕafkáar* opinion, thought
filfil (c.), **filfíla, filfiláat** pepper, pepper-plants
  qárnï* filfil (pl. **qurúun f.**) chilli
filúus (f.) money
fingáal, fanagíil cup
fingáan, fanagíin (see **fingáal**)
finṭáaz, fanaṭíiz cart

fiṣáal (*v.n.*), fiṣaláat bargaining
fíṭir, yíftar to breakfast
fiṭr (*v.n.*)
 ҫíid ilfíṭr feast of Ramadan Bairam
fíyya, fiyyáat value
fiҫl, ʕafҫáal deed, doing
fooq above, over; upstairs
foqáani, foqaníyya, foqaniyyíin upper
fulúuka, faláayik sailing-boat
furn, ʕafráan* oven
fúrṣa, fúraṣ chance, opportunity
fúsḥa pleasure, holiday; stroll
fustáan, fasatíin dress
fuṭúur breakfast
fuul (*c.*), ḥábbit *or* ḥabbáayit f., ḥabbáat f. beans
 fúul sudáani peanuts
fúuṭa, fúwaṭ towel

g

gaab, yigíib to bring; get
gáadil, yigáadil to argue with
gáahil, gáhla, gahlíin ignorant
gáahiz, gáhza, gahzíin ready
gáamiҫ, gawáamiҫ mosque
gaar*, giráan neighbour
gáawib, yigáawib to answer
gaay (*a.p. of* geh, yíigi) *or* gayy, gáaya *or* gáyya, gayíin *or* gayyíin coming; next
gáayiz + li + *p.s.* to be allowed to
gaaz kerosine
gábal, gibáal mountain, hill
gáhhiz, yigáhhiz to prepare
gamáaҫa[1] people, assembly
gámal, gimáal camel
gámaҫ, yígmaҫ to collect
gamb, ʕignáab side
gamb beside
 humma sakníin gambína they live next door to us
gambári (*c.*), gambaríyya, gambariyyáat prawns
gamíil, gamíila, gumáal beautiful
gamíiҫ all
gamúus (*c.*), gamúusa, gamusáat, gawamíis buffaloes

---

[1] Usually with vocative particle *ya*.

gamҫ (*v.n.*) collection, collecting
 gámҫ ilmaḥṣúul harvest
gámҫa, gamҫáat university
ganáab (+ *p.s.*) polite term of address
gánnin, yigánnin to drive mad
ganúub south (of)
gára* (*or* yígra*) ʕéeh! what's the matter, what's up!
gára (*or* gíri), yígri to run
gáraḥ, yígraḥ to hurt, wound, injure
gáras*, ʕagráas* bell
gárdal, garáadil bucket
garíida, garáayid newspaper; frond, leaf (of palm)
garr*, yigúrr to pull
garráara*, garraráat* tractor
gawáab, gawabáat letter
gawáab, ʕagwíba answer
gaww air, weather
gázma, gízam pair of shoes
gazmági, gazmagíyya shoemaker
gáẓar (*c.*), gáẓara *or* gaẓaráaya, gaẓaráat carrots
gaẓẓáar, gaẓẓaríin butcher
gaҫáan, gaҫáana, gaҫaníin *or* gawáaҫa hungry
geeb, giyúub pocket
geeʃ, giyúuʃ army
geh, yíigi to come
 law géet lilḥáqq in fact (*lit.* if you come to the truth)
gíbna cheese
gidd, gudúud grandfather
gídda, giddáat grandmother
gíddan very
gidíid, gidíida, gudáad new
gíha, giháat side; aspect; neighbourhood
 min gíhat ... in regard to ...
giháaz, gihazáat *or* ʕaghíza plant (industrial)
(ʕil)gíiza (*or* Gigg-) Giza
ginéeh, gineháat pound
ginéena, ganáayin garden
gooz, ʕigwáaz husband
góoza, gíwaz hookah
gulf golf
gulúus (*v.n.*) sitting
 ʕóḍt iggulúus lounge, sitting-room
gúmruk, gamáarik Customs, Customs building
 marréet* bilgúmruk I passed through the Customs

gurnáal,[1] garaníil* newspaper, journal
gúuɤa hunger
guwánti, guwantiyyáat pair of gloves
gúwwa inside
guwwáani, guwwaníyya, guwwaniyyíin inner, interior

ḥ

ḥáadi, ḥádya, ḥadyíin calm
(ya) ḥáanim polite term of address to young woman
ḥaat, ḥáati, ḥáatu bring, fetch!
ḥáayig, ḥáyga, ḥaygíin rough (sea); out-of-temper
ḥábhab, yiḥábhab[2] to bark
ḥadíyya, ḥadáaya gift
(wi) ḥakáza and so on
ḥandása engineering
ḥandási, ḥandasíyya engineering (adj.)
ḥáram* or Ɂahráam*, Ɂahramáat* pyramid
ḥáwa air
ḥáwwa, yiḥáwwi to ventilate
ḥéeṣa clamour
ḥídma, ḥudúum garment
ḥiláal crescent
ḥína here
ḥináak there
ḥíndi, ḥindíyya, ḥanádwa Indian
ḥíyya she, it
ḥudúum (see ḥídma) clothes
ḥúmma they
ḥúwwa he, it

ḫ

ḫáaḍir certainly
ḫáaḍir, ḫáḍra, ḫaḍríin present
filwáqt ilḫáaḍir at present
ḫáafi, ḫáfya, ḫafyíin barefooted
ḫáaga, ḫagáat thing
ḫáakim, yiḫáakim to be strict with
ḫaal, Ɂaḥwáal condition, state
Ɂizzáyy ilḫáal? how are you?
ɤala kúlli ḫáal in any case

háala (as ḫaal)
ḫáalan soon, at once
ḫáami, ḫámya, ḫamyíin sharp (of thing or person)
ḫáara*, ḫawáari side-street, lane
ḫáawil, yiḫáawil to try
ḫaaʃ, yiḫúuʃ to stop, prevent
ḫabb, yiḫíbb to like (to), be fond of
ḫábba, ḫabbáat grain, seed; handful, some; while (n.)
ḫabbáaya, ḫabbayáat or ḫabbáat grain, seed
ḫabíib, ḫabíiba, ḫabáayib friend; lover
ḫadd anyone
ḫadd, ḫudúud limit, boundary, frontier
ḫáddid, yiḫáddid to limit, fix
ḫadíid iron
ḫádsa, ḫawáadis accident, incident
ḫáḍar, yíḫḍar to be present at
ḫáḍḍar, yiḫáḍḍar to prepare; bring
ḫáḍrit (usually+ak/ik/ku(m)) polite term of address
ḫáfar*, yúḫfur to dig, drill (well)
ḫáfaḍ, yíḫfaḍ to learn by heart
ḫáfaẓ, yíḫfaẓ (see ḫáfaḍ)
ḫáfla, ḫafaláat party, celebration
ḫafr* (v.n.) digging, drilling
ḫáfẓa, ḫawáafiẓ receipt-book; receipt
ḫágar* (c.), ḫágara*, ḫagaráat*, ḫigáara* or Ɂaḥgáar* stone
ḫágaz, yíḫgiz to book, reserve
ḫagg (see ḫigg)
ḫagg, ḫuggáag (or ḫiggáag) pilgrim
ḫagg, yiḫígg to make the pilgrimage
ḫagm, Ɂaḥgáam or ḫugúum size
ḫáka, yíḫki to talk, narrate
ḫakíim, ḫúkama doctor
ḫakíim ilɁasnáan (or lisnáan) dentist
ḫaláal righteousness
ḫaláawa, ḫalawiyyáat sweet, sweetmeat
ḫálaq, yíḫlaq to cut (hair), get hair cut, shave
ḫalawáani, ḫalawaníyya confectioner
ḫall, yiḫíll to solve; undo
ḫall (v.n.), ḫulúul solution
ḫálla, yiḫálli to sweeten; eat as sweet
ḫálla, ḫílal pot

---

[1] With 'back' aa in the final syllable.
[2] 'Back' a's.

ḥallúuf, ḥalalíif pig, pork
ḥámad, yíḥmid to praise (God)
ḥámal, yíḥmil to carry, bear; be pregnant
ḥamd (*v.n.*) praise (of God)
ḥaml (*v.n.*) pregnancy
ḥammáam, ḥammamáat bath, bathroom
ḥámmil, yiḥámmil to load
ḥanafíyya, ḥanafiyyáat tap
ḥanṭúur, ḥanaṭíir gharry
ḥaqíiqa
  ʕilḥaqiiqa-nn … the fact is that …
ḥaql†, ḥuqúul† field
ḥaqq, ḥuqúuq right
  ɤándak ḥáqq you are right
  bilḥáqq true, exactly
ḥáqqaq, yiḥáqqaq to verify
ḥaráam* unrighteousness
ḥaráami*, ḥaramíyya* thief
ḥaráara* temperature, heat
ḥáraq, yíḥraq to burn
ḥarb*, ḥurúub war
ḥarf*, ḥurúuf letter (of alphabet)
ḥaríim women
ḥaríiq fire
ḥaríiqa, ḥaráayiq fire
ḥaríir silk
ḥarr* heat
ḥarr*, ḥárra* hot
ḥárrak*, yiḥárrak* to move
ḥásab, yíḥsib to calculate, reckon, consider
ḥásab according to
ḥásana, ḥasanáat alms
ḥássin, yiḥássin to improve
ḥáṣal, yíḥṣal to happen
ḥáṣba measles
ḥáṣṣal, yiḥáṣṣal to obtain
ḥátta even
ḥaṭṭ, yiḥúṭṭ to put
ḥawáali about, approximately
ḥawaléen around, surrounding
ḥáwwid, yiḥáwwid to turn, take a turning
ḥáwwil, yiḥáwwil to transfer
ḥáwwiʃ, yiḥáwwiʃ to save (up)
ḥayáah (*f.*) life
  wi-ḥyáatak[1] please (*lit.* 'and your life')

ḥayawáan, ḥayawanáat animal
ḥayy, ʕaḥyáaʕ quarter (of town)
ḥazẓ good fortune
  ɤándu ḥázẓ he is lucky
ḥáʃara*, ḥaʃaráat* insect
ḥaʃíiʃ grass; hashish
ḥaʃʃáaʃ, ḥaʃʃaʃíin hashish-addict
ḥáʃʃiʃ, yiḥáʃʃiʃ to take hashish
ḥeeṭ, ḥeṭáan wall
ḥibr ink
ḥidáaʃar* eleven
ḥifẓ protection (of God)
  fi ḥífẓi-lláah goodbye
ḥigg pilgrimage
(ʕil)ḥígga the pilgrimage month
ḥíila, ḥíyal trick
ḥikáaya, ḥikayáat story
ḥikimḍáar, ḥikimḍaríyya hakimdar, police chief
ḥiláaqa (*v.n.*) shaving
ḥilm, ʕaḥláam dream
ḥilw, ḥílwa, ḥilwíin sweet, delightful
ḥiml, ʕiḥmáal load
ḥisáab, ḥisabáat bill, account
ḥisáabi, ḥisabíyya financial
ḥítta, ḥítat bit, piece; while (*n.*)
ḥíyali, ḥiyalíyya, ḥiyaliyyíin tricky, trickster
ḥizb, ʕaḥzáab party (political)
ḥúfra*, ḥúfar* hole
(ʕil)ḥúgga (*see* (ʕil)ḥígga)
ḥukm judgement; wisdom
ḥukúuma, ḥukumáat government
ḥukúumi, ḥukumíyya, ḥukumiyyíin governmental
ḥumáar*, ḥimíir donkey
ḥurr, ḥúrra*, ʕaḥráar* free
ḥurríyya freedom
ḥuṣáan, ḥiṣína[2] horse
ḥuṣúul (*v.n.*) taking place

k

kaam how much, how many
  káam wáaḥid how many
káamil, kámla, kamlíin complete
kaan, yikúun to be
káatib, kátaba clerk
káatim, kátma close (weather)
kabb, yikúbb to pour

----

[1] Chiefly used between friends when a favour is asked.

[2] Plural rarely used (see *xeel*).

kabinéeh, kabinehaat lavatory
kabríit matches
kaddáab, kaddáaba, kaddabíin liar
káfa, yíkfi to be enough
káffa, yikáffi to be enough; (+ ʒan) to desist from
kahrába* electricity; electrical engineering
kahrabáaʕi*, kahrabaʕiyyíin* electrician
kahramáan* amber
kal, yáakul to eat
kaláam speech
kalb, kiláab dog
kállif, yikállif to cost
kállim, yikállim to speak to
kamáan also
kámmil, yikámmil to finish, complete
kánas (or kínis), yíknis (or yúknus) to sweep
kaníisa, kanáayis church
karakóon*, karakonáat* police station
káram* generosity
karíim, karíima, kúrama* generous
kárkib, yikárkib to turn upside down
kárrar*, yikárrar* to refine; repeat
(ʒarabíyya*) karru* cart
kasaróona*, kasaronáat* saucepan
kasláan, kasláana, kaslaníin or kasáala lazy
kássar*, yikássar* to smash
kátab, yíktib to write
katkúut, katakíit chicken
káttar*, yikáttar* to make plentiful
káttar xéerak thank you
káwa, yíkwi to iron
kawy or kayy (v.n.) ironing
kazzáab (see kaddáab)
kaʕínn as if
káʃaf, yíkʃif (+ ʒala) to examine; look up, find, discover
kibíir, kibíira, kubáar* big, large; old
kíbir, yíkbar* to grow up
kída thus, so
  kuwáyyis kida that's fine
  míʃ bi súrʒa kída not so fast
  ʒala kída therefore
kidb (v.n.) lying, telling lies
kídib, yíkdib to lie, tell lies
kifáaya enough

kíilu (or kéelu), kiluwáat kilogram; kilometre
kiis, kiyáas cover; purse
kilíim, ʕiklíma mat
kílma, kilmáat word
kilumítr, kilumitráat kilometre
kimáawi, kimawíyya, kimawiyyíin chemical (adj.); chemist
kimawíyya, kimawiyyáat chemical, chemical product
kímil, yíkmal to finish (intr.)
kísib, yíksab to make a profit
kíswa, kasáawi suit; drapery
kitáab, kútub book
kitáaba (v.n.) writing
kitf, ʕaktáaf or ʕiktífa shoulder
kitíir, kitíira, kutáar* much, many
kízib (see kídib)
kommítra (c.), kommitráaya, kommitráat pears
kóora,* kúwar* (or kíwar*) ball
kubbáaya, kubbayáat glass (drinking)
kúbri, kabáari bridge
kull all, every
kúlli ma + v. whenever
kúrsi, karáasi chair; stand
kurúmb (c.), kurúmba or kurumbáaya, kurumbáat cabbage
kusúuf shame, embarrassment
kutr abundance
kutubxáana Literary Museum
kuwáyyis, kuwayyísa, kuwayyisíin good, nice
kuʃk, ʕikʃáak kiosk

l

la . . . wala neither . . . nor
láabis, lábsa, labsíin wearing, dressed
láakin but
láaqa, yiláaqi to find
láazim necessary; must, have to
lában milk
lábbis, yilábbis to dress, clothe
la búdd must
laff, yilíff to wind round, wrap up; go around
lafẓ, ʕalfáaẓ pronunciation; word; way of speaking
láhga, lahgáat dialect; way of speaking
láḥaẓ, yílḥaẓ to note, notice

láḥma *or* laḥm (*c.*), ḥíttit láḥma, ḥítat láḥm, liḥúum meat
láḥẓa, laḥaẓáat moment; look
lámaɣ, yílmaɣ to shine
lámma when; if
lamúun (*c.*), lamúuna, lamunáat lemons
lándan London
láqa, yílqa to meet; find
laṭiif, laṭíifa, luṭáaf pleasant
law if
láxbaṭ, yiláxbaṭ to muddle
laxbáṭa (*v.n.*) muddling
laziiz, laziiza, luzáaz tasty
laʕ (*or* laa) no
leeh why
leel night, darkness
  billéel at night
léela, layáali night
  ʕilléela *or* ʕilleláadi tonight
li to, for
libáas, libísa (*or* ʕilbísa) *or* libasáat underpants
líbis, yílbis to wear, put on
libnáan (*f.*) Lebanon
libs (*v.n.*) wearing; clothes, way of dressing
liḥádd up to, until
liḥáddĭ ma + *v.* until
líḥiq, yílḥaq to catch (train, &c.)
líssa (not) yet; still
  líssa ma gáaʃ he hasn't come yet
  líssa ɣándu(h) he still has it
'liyyámdi (*see* yoom)
liʕánn because
líɣba, líɣab toy
líɣba, ʕalɣáab game
líɣib, yílɣab to play
liɣáayit . . . (*see* ɣáaya)
loon, ʕalwáan colour
lukánda, lukandáat hotel
lúqma, lúqam piece, morsel
lúqṣur Luxor
luṭf niceness
lúuri, luriyyáat lorry
luzúum need, necessity
lúɣa, luɣáat language

m

ma negative, conjunctive, exclamatory, &c., particles
  ma ʃuftúuʃ I haven't seen him

maníiʃ ráayiḥ I'm not going
wáqtĭ ma, kúllĭ ma, &c. at the time that, whenever, &c.
ma titkállim! speak up!
máalu(h)? what's the matter with him?; what of it!
máaḍi, máḍya, maḍyíin past
maal, ʕamwáal property, possession
máaniɣ
  ɣándak máaniɣ inn . . .? do you mind if . . .?
  ma fíiʃ máaniɣ there's no objection
máaris March
máasik, máska, maskíin holding
maat, yimúut to die
máayu May
máaʃi, máʃya, maʃyíin walking
  máaʃi ! all right, agreed!
  máaʃi-kwáyyis it's going fine
mabíiɣ, mabiɣáat sale, auction
máblaɣ, mabáaliɣ amount
mabrúuk !* congratulations!
mabṣúuṭ, mabṣúuṭa, mabṣuṭíin happy, well
madáam since, because
mádani, madaníyya, madaniyyíin townsman
  ʕilhandása-lmadaníyya civil engineering
máadaɣ, yúmduɣ to chew
madd, yimídd to stretch (out)
mádda *or* máadda,[1] mawádd *or* mawáadd[1] product, material
  ʕilmawáadd ilxáam raw materials
madíina, múdun city
madíina Medina
madrása, madáaris school
  madrása sanawíyya secondary school
  madrása-btidaʕíyya primary school
mádɣi, madɣíyya, madɣiyyíin invited, guest
mádɣu, madɣúwwa, madɣuwwíin (*see* mádɣi)
máḍa, yímḍi to sign
mafhúum of course (*lit.* understood)
máfraʃ*, mafáariʃ covering, cloth, counterpane
máfraʃ ṣúfra* table-cloth

---

[1] See Part I, Appendix B, note (*c*).

mafrúuḍ, mafrúuḍa (+ẓala) imposed (on) (i.e. as condition)
ṣiḥna mafrúuḍ ẓaléena nízmil kída we are in duty bound to do so
mafṣúul, mafṣúula, mafṣulíin sold (after bargaining); rejected
magálla, magalláat magazine
maggáanan free, gratis
máglis, magáalis council
magmúuẓ, magmuẓáat or magamíiẓ collection, group
magnúun, magnúuna, maganíin mad
mahíyya, maháaya or mahiyyáat pay, salary
maḥáll, maḥalláat place; home
maḥáṭṭa, maḥaṭṭáat station; stop (bus, tram, &c.)
maḥdúud, maḥdúuda, maḥdudíin limited, fixed
máḥḍar, maḥáaḍir report; procès-verbal
maḥfáẓa, maḥáafiẓ purse, wallet
maḥfúuẓ, maḥfúuẓa, maḥfuẓíin protected; learnt by heart
maḥkúum
    maḥkúum ẓaléeh bi . . . he has been sentenced to . . .
makáan, ṣamáakin place
mákana, makanáat machine
makaróona* macaroni
mákka Mecca
makkáar*, makkáara*, makkaríin* cunning
maknása, makáanis broom
maksúuf, maksúufa, maksufíin embarrassed, ashamed, confused
máktab, makáatib office; desk
maktába, maktabáat library
maktába, makáatib bookshop
mákwa, makáawi iron
makwági, makwagíyya laundryman
mála, yímla to fill
maláak, maláyka or mala(a)ṣíka angel
málbas, maláabis article of clothing
málha, maláahi amusement
malḥ salt
málik, mulúuk king
málika, malikáat queen
málla, yímálli to dictate (letter)
malláaki
    ẓarabíyya* malláaki private car

mallíim, malalíim milleme
malyáan, malyáana, malyaníin full
malzúum, malzúuma, malzumíin bound, obliged
mamnuníyya gratitude
mamnúun, mamnúuna, mamnuníin grateful
mánaẓ, yímnaẓ to prevent; forbid
mandíil, manadíil handkerchief
mánga (c.), mangáaya, mangáat mangoes
manṭíqa, manáaṭiq area, zone
mánzil, manáazil home, dwelling
mánẓar, manáaẓir sight, view
manẓúur, manẓúura, manẓuríin seen
míʃ manẓúur unlikely
manẓ (v.n.) prevention, preventing; forbidding
maqáas, maqasáat size
maqáṣṣ, maqaṣṣáat scissors
mára* woman, wife
máraḍ, ṣamráaḍ illness, disease
máraḍi,* maraḍíyya* pertaining to illness
ṣagáaza maraḍíyya sick leave
máraqa, maraqáat soup, broth, gravy
maríiḍ*, maríiḍá*, márḍa* ill
márkaz, maráakiz position; centre, station
márkib (f.), maráakib ship
marr*, yimúrr to pass (by)
márra*, marráat* time, occasion
bilmárra completely
marṣúuf, marṣúufa, marṣufíin made-up (of road), compounded
marwáḥa*, maráawiḥ* fan
masáafa, masafáat distance
masáaṣan in the evening, p.m.
másaḥ, yímsaḥ to wipe
másal, ṣamsáal proverb, saying
másal, ṣamsíla example
másalan for example
maskíin, maskíina, masakíin poor, unfortunate
mássil, yimássil to act, represent
masúura*, mawasíir pipe
masṣála, masáaṣil matter, problem
masṣulíyya, masṣuliyyáat responsibility

masʕúul, masʕúula, masʕulíin (ʒan) responsible (for)

maṣáalíḥ (*see* maṣláḥa)

maṣláḥa, maṣáaliḥ department (especially of government)

máṣnaʒ, maṣáaniʒ factory

maṣr (*f.*) Cairo; Egypt

máṣraf, maṣáarif drain; exchange-bank

máṣri, maṣríyya, maṣriyyíin Cairene; Egyptian

maṣrúuf, maṣrufáat *or* maṣaríif expense, expenditure; fees

maṣṭára, maṣáaṭir ruler

matíin, matíina, mutáan[1] strong, durable

maṭáafi firefighting

maṭáafi-lḥaríiq fire-station; fire-service

maṭáar, maṭaráat airport

máṭar rain

máṭbax, maṭáabix kitchen

máṭli, maṭlíyya, maṭliyyíin plated

máṭli bilfádda silver-plated

máṭraḥ, maṭáariḥ place; room

máṭʒam, maṭáaʒim restaurant, canteen

mawḍúuʒ, mawaḍíiʒ matter, subject

mawgúud, mawgúuda, mawgudíin present

mawlúud, mawlúuda, mawludíin born

máwqif, mawáaqif stand, rank

maxṣúuṣ, maxṣúuṣa, maxṣuṣíin special

máxzan, maxáazin store

máyya[2] water

máyyit, mayyíta, mayyitíin *or* ʕamwáat dead

mazúut fuel oil

mázza 'mezzy' (i.e. titbits of food taken with drinks)

mazbúuṭ, mazbúuṭa, mazbuṭíin correct

mazbúuṭ! exactly!

maʕmúur, maʕamíir Mamur (police official)

maʃy (*v.n.*) walking, going; conduct

maʃyúul, maʃyúula, maʃyulíin busy

[1] Plural rare.

[2] 'Back' *a* in first syllable.

máʒa with

maʒa-lʕásaf I'm sorry

maʒa-ssaláama goodbye

maʒa záalik nevertheless

maʒáad, mawaʒíid appointment

filmaʒáad on time

maʒáaʃ, maʒaʃáat pension

máʒbad, maʒáabid tomb

máʒdan, maʒáadin metal

maʒíiʃa, maʒáayiʃ cost of living, standard of living

maʒláqa, maʒáaliq spoon

maʒlúum of course (*lit.* learnt)

máʒmal, maʒáamil laboratory

máʒna, maʒáani meaning

maʒrúuf* of course (*lit.* known)

maʒúun, mawaʒíin lighter (boat); container

maʒzúum, maʒzúuma, maʒazíim guest, invited

maʒʕínn although

máyrib evening, sunset

biláad ilmáyrib the Maghrib

mibarrída, mibarridáat cooler

midáan, mayadíin square

mifáddad, mifaddáda, mifaddadíin silvered

mifállis, mifallísa, mifallisíin penniless, bankrupt

miggáwwiz (*see* mitgáwwiz)

migíyy (*v.n.* of geh, yíigi) coming

mígra, magáari drain

mihándis, mihandisíin engineer

míhna, míhan trade, occupation

miḥáafiẓ, miḥafẓíin governor

miḥáfẓa (*or* mu-), miḥafẓáat governorate

miḥáwra (see muḥáwra)

miḥtáag, miḥtáaga, miḥtagíin (+li) needing, in need of

miil, ʕamyáal mile

miin who?

míina, mawáani harbour, port

mikaníika mechanics, mechanical engineering

mikaníiki, mikanikíyya mechanic

miláad, mawalíid birth

miláaya, milayáat sheet

miláff, milaffáat file, folder

milk, ʕamláak property, possession

milyóon (*or* malyóon), malayíin million

min from, of
mínéen whence?
minádya (v.n.) calling
mináfsa (v.n.) rivalry
mináqʃa (v.n.), minaqʃáat discussion
miqáabil
  bidúun miqáabil without obligation (*lit.* without exchange)
miqyáas†
  miqyáas inníil nilometer
miráahin*, miráhna*, mirahníin* having bet
miráaya, mirayáat mirror
mirábba*, mirabbáat* jam
mísa evening
misáᵹda (v.n.) help
mísik, yímsik to hold, grasp
mistáᵹgil (*or* mu-), mistaᵹgíla, mistaᵹgilíin urgent; in a hurry
mistáᵹmil (*or* mu-), mistaᵹmíla, mistaᵹmilíin used; second-hand
mistíwi, mistiwíyya, mistiwiyyíin ripe
miswádda, miswaddáat draft copy
miṣóogar* (*or* mu-), miṣógra*, miṣogríin registered
mitgáwwil (*or* muta-), mitgawwíla, mitgawwilíin migrant; itinerant
mitgáwwiz, mitgawwíza, mitgawwizíin married
mitmarran* (*or* muta-), mitmarrána*, mitmarraníin* experienced
mitnáqqil, mitnaqqíla, mitnaqqilíin nomadic
mitr, ʕamtáar* *or* ʕimtáar* metre
mitráahin*, mitráhna*, mitrahníin* (wayya) having bet (with)
mitsámma, mitsammíya, mitsammiyíin called, named
mittífiq, mittífqa, mittifqíin having agreed, in agreement
mitwáṣṣaṭ, mitwaṣṣáṭa, mitwaṣṣaṭíin medium, average
mitxáṣṣaṣ (*or* muta-), specialized, specialist
mitʕákkid (*or* muta-), mitʕakkída, mitʕakkidíin sure
mitʕássif (*or* muta-), mitʕassífa, mitʕassifíin sorry
mitʕáxxar*, mitʕaxxára*, mitʕaxxaríin* late, delayed

mitᵹállaq, mitᵹalláqa, mitᵹallaqíin hanging, suspended
mitᵹáwwid, mitᵹawwída, mitᵹawwidíin (ᵹala) accustomed (to)
mityáddi, mityaddíya, mityaddiyíin having lunched
mityáyyar*, mityayyára*, mityayyaríin* changed
miṭáᵹᵹam (*or* mu-), miṭaᵹᵹáma, miṭaᵹᵹamíin inlaid
miṭmaʕínn (*or* mu-),[1] miṭmaʕínna, miṭmaʕinníin assured, free from worry.
mixádda, mixaddáat pillow, cushion
mixálfa (v.n.), mixalfáat fine
mixállil (c.), mixallíla, mixalliláat pickles
míyya, miyyáat hundred
  tisᵹíin filmíyya ninety per cent.
mizáan, mawazíin balance, scales
miʃ not
míʃi, yímʃi to walk, go
míʃmiʃ (c.), miʃmíʃa *or* miʃmiʃáaya, miʃmiʃáat apricots
miᵹáawin (*or* mu-), miᵹáwna, miᵹawníin assistant
miᵹáksa (v.n.), miᵹaksáat argument, dispute
miᵹmáari, miᵹmariyyíin civil engineer
miᵹtímid, miᵹtímda, miᵹtimdíin (ᵹala) depending on, trusting in
miɣlawáani, miɣlawaníyya, miɣlawaniyyíin profiteer
móoḍa, moḍáat fashion
moot death
mooz (c.), móoza *or* mozáaya, mozáat bananas
  ṣubáaᵹ *or* ṣáabiᵹ móoz banana
mubílya, mubilyáat furniture, piece of furniture
mudárris, mudarrísa, mudarrisíin teacher
múdda, múdad period
  min múdda for some time
múdhiʃ, mudhíʃa, mudhiʃíi ₁ wonderful
mudíir, mudiríin director, manager; Mudir

---

[1] *miṭṭámmin* among less sophisticated speakers.

mudiríyya, mudiriyyáat director-
ate; province; Mudir's office
mufakkíra* (or mifakkára*), mufakkiráat* diary
mufáttiʃ, mufattíʃa, mufattiʃíin
inspector
mufíid, mufíida useful
múfriḥ, mufríḥa, mufriḥíin auspicious
muftáaḥ, mafatíiḥ key
muhímm, muhímma, muhim-
míin important, interesting
múhmil, muhmíla, muhmilíin
lazy, slothful
muḥáḍra (v.n.), muḥaḍráat lecture
muḥáwra*, muḥawráat* discussion, conversation; dialogue
muḥtámal
min ilmuḥtámal likely, probable
múmkin possible
munáasib, munásba, munasbíin
suitable
munáwra*, munawráat* manœuvre
munfáɣil, munfáɣila, munfaɣilíin
upset, angry
muntagáat (pl. only) products
muntáʃir, muntáʃira*, muntaʃiríin
widespread, spread out
munxáar*, manaxíir nose
muqáabil† (see miqáabil)
muqábla (v.n.), muqabláat appointment; meeting
muqáddas†, muqaddása†, muqad-
dasíin† holy, sacred
murúur traffic
musáaɣid, musáɣda, musaɣdíin
assistant
múslim, muslíma, muslimíin
Muslim
mustáqbal
filmustáqbal in (the) future
mustáwrad*, mustawráda*, mus-
tawradíin* imported
mustáwrid, mustawrída, mustaw-
ridíin importing
mustáxdim, mustaxdíma, mustaxdimíin employee
mustáɣmal (see mistáɣmil)
mustáɣmar*, mustaɣmára*, mus-
taɣmaríin* colonized
mustáɣmir, mustaɣmíra*, mus-
taɣmiríin colonizing, colonist
muṣṭárḍa mustard

mutaḥárrik (or mitḥárrak), muta-
ḥarríka, mutaḥarrikíin moving
mutállag (or mitállig), mutallága,
mutallagíin iced
máyya-mtallága or -mtallíga
iced water
mutawáṣṣiṭ (see mitwáṣṣaṭ)
mutaʃákkir, mutaʃakkíra*, mutaʃakkiríin thank you
mútqan, mutqána well-made
mutsíkl (or mutusíkl), mutsikláat
motor-cycle
mutɣáhhid, mutɣahhidíin agent,
sub-agent
mútɣib, mutɣíba, mutɣibíin tiring,
tiresome
mutmaʕínn (see miṭmaʕínn)
múulid, mawáalid birthday (of
saint)
muwáṣla, muwaṣaláat or muwaṣláat communication, link
muwáẓẓaf, muwaẓẓáfa, muwaẓẓafíin employee
muxtálif, muxtálifa, muxtalifíin
different
muxx, ʕimxáax brains, intelligence
muʕáddab, muʕaddába, muʕad-
dabíin polite, well-mannered
muʕtámar*, muʕtamaráat* conference
muʃ not
muʃáwra* (v.n.), muʃawráat* advice, consultation
muʃkíla, maʃáakil problem, difficulty
múʃrif, muʃrifíin supervisor
muɣállim, muɣallíma, muɣalli-
míin teacher
muɣáskar*, muɣaskaráat* (military) camp
múɣdi, muɣdíya, muɣdiyíin infectious
muɣtámid (see miɣtímid)

n

náada, yináadi to call
náadi, nawáadi or ʕandíya club
náakif, yináakif to argue, ask impor-
tunately
naam, yináam to sleep
náaqir, yináaqir to squabble; answer
back

náaqiṣ, náqṣa, naqṣíin missing
náaqiʃ, yináaqiʃ to discuss
naar* (f.), niráan* fire
naas people
náatig, nawáatig total (arithmetic)
náawi, náwya, nawyíin
  n. + impf. to intend to . . .
náaʃif, náʃfa, nawáaʃif or naʃfíin
  dried up, dry
nábi, ʕanbíya prophet
náḍḍaf, yináḍḍaf to clean
náfaʒ, yínfaʒ to be of use
náffaḍ, yináffaḍ to shake, beat (carpet)
nafs (or nifs)
  n. + p.s. + impf. to want to . . .
  n. + p.s. or n., e.g. nafsáha, náfs
  innáḥya self, same, e.g. herself,
  the same side
naggáar*, naggaríin* carpenter
naháar* day
  ʕinnahárḍa today
náhhaq, yináhhaq to bray
nahr*, ʕanháar* river
naḥl (c.), náḥla, naḥláat bees
náḥya, nawáaḥi side, bank
namusíyya, namusiyyáat mosquito-net
namúus (c.), namúusa, namusáat
  mosquitoes
náqal, yínqil to transport; copy
naql (v.n.) transport, conveying;
  copying
náqqa, yináqqi to choose
náqqaṣ, yináqqaṣ to decrease
naqʃ (v.n.) decoration, decorating
nasiig (v.n.) weaving
náṣaḥ, yínṣaḥ to advise
naṣíib share, portion
naṣṣáab, naṣṣáaba, naṣṣabíin
  swindler
nátag, yíntig to extract
natíiga, natáayig or natáaʕig result,
  outcome
naxl (c.), náxla, naxláat, naxíil
  palm-trees
názzil, yinázzil to bring or take
  down; take hemp
naʃʃáal, naʃʃalíin pickpocket
náʃʃif, yináʃʃif to dry
náʒam yes
  ʕáynaʒam yes
náʒga, naʒgáat or niʒáag sheep

niḍíif, niḍíifa, nuḍáaf clean
nígma, nugúum or nigúum star
niḥáas copper, brass
  niḥáas áṣfar* brass
  niḥáas áḥmar* copper
(ʕin)níil Nile
níili, nilíyya of the Nile
nímra, nímar number
niqáabaṭ, niqabáatṭ union, trade-union, syndicate
nísba, nísab percentage
  binnisba li . . . in comparison
  with . . .
nísi, yínsa to forget
níyya disposition; appetite
nízil, yínzil to descend; stay (e.g. at
  hotel)
niẓáam arrangement, organization
niʃáan, nayaʃíin badge, medal
niʒnáaʒ mint
noom sleep
  ʕóḍt innóom bedroom
nooʒ, ʕanwáaʒ kind, sort
nufímbir November
nufúuz influence
nugúum (see nígma)
núkta, núkat or nikáat joke
núqṭa, núqaṭ dot, stop
nuṣṣ, ʕanṣáaṣ or ʕinṣáaṣ half
  núṣṣ illéel midnight
nuṭq (v.n.) pronunciation, utterance
núubi, nubíyya, nubiyyíin Nubian
nuur, ʕanwáar* light

q

qáabil, yiqáabil to meet
qáabil
  qáabil littagdíid subject to renewal
qáadir, qádra, qadríin able to
  miʃ qáadir ásmaʒ I can't hear
qáafil, qáfla, qaflíin having closed
qaal, yiqúul to say, tell
qaam, yiqúum to stand (up)
  qaam + pf. to start to, suddenly
  to . . .
qáaʒid, qáʒda, qaʒdíin sitting
  q. + impf. to be -ing
qábaḍ, yíqbaḍ to receive (pay);
  (+ ʒala) to arrest
qabíiḥ, qabíiḥa, qúbaḥa or qabáayiḥ
  uncouth
qabíila, qabáayil tribe

qabl before
qábl iḍḍúhr in the morning, a.m.
qáblï ma + *v.* before
qádam, ʕiqdáam foot
qádar*† fate, destiny
qadd extent, size
  qaddï ʕéeh? to what extent, how far, how long?
  múʃ qaddï kída not so much
  geh, yiigi ɣala qadd . . . to fit
  ɣala qáddï ma yíqdar* as far as he can
qáddim, yiqáddim to bring; come quickly
qadíim, qadíima, qudáam old, ancient
qáfal, yíqfil to lock, close, turn off
(ʕil)qahíra*† Cairo
qáhwa coffee
qáhwa, qaháawi café
qála, yíqli to fry
qálab (*or* **qílib**), **yíqlib** to overturn
qálam, ʕiqláam pen
  qálam ḥíbr fountain pen
  qálam ruṣáaṣ (lead) pencil
qálam†, ʕaqláam† department
qalíil, qalíila, quláal few, little
  qalíil ilʕádab (*f.* **qalílt ilʕádab**) ill mannered
qall, yiqíll to be less; lessen
qálɣa citadel
qámar* moon
qamḥ wheat
qamíiṣ, qumṣáan shirt
(ʕil)qanáal† the Canal
qanṭára, qanáaṭir footbridge
qanúun†, qawaníin† law
qára*, yíqra* to read; study
qaráayib* (*see* **qaríib**)
qáraf* strain, stress
  qáraf iʃʃúɣl overwork
qaríib, qaráayib* relative
qarnabíiṭ* (*c.*), **qarnabíiṭa*, qarnabiṭáat*** cauliflower
qárrab*, yiqárrab* to approach; bring near
  q. + impf. to be about to . . .
qárya†, qúra*† village
qásam (*or* **qísim**), **yíqsim** to divide
qássim, yiqássim to divide
qaṣd intention
  qaṣd + p.s. + impf. to be determined to . . .

qaṣr, quṣúur palace
qaṣṣ, yiqúṣṣ to cut (with scissors or shears)
qátal (*or* **qítil**), **yíqtil** to kill
qáṭam, yúqṭum to bite
qáṭaɣ, yíqṭaɣ to cut
  q. tazkára* to get a ticket
qaṭr, quṭuráat* *or* **qúṭura*** train
qáwi very
qáwi, qawíyya, qawiyyíin strong
qáwwim, yiqáwwim to start (car, train, &c.); (make) stand
qáɣad, yúqɣud to sit down; stay
  q. + impf. to continue -ing
qaɣádtï¹-f máṣrï múddit usbúuɣ I stayed in Cairo for a week
qíbli, qiblíyya, qibliyyíin southern, southerner
qídir, yíqdar* to be able to
qifl, ʕiqfáal lock
qiráaya (*v.n.*), **qirayáat** reading
qirʃ, qurúuʃ piastre
  qírʃï sáaɣ piastre
  qírʃï taɣriifa half-piastre
  qírʃ ábyaḍ half-piastre
qism†, ʕaqsáam† part, division; department, section
qiyáam (*v.n.*) departure (of train, &c.); standing
qíʃṭa, qíʃaṭ cream
quddáam in front (of)
quddamáani, quddamaníyya, quddamaniyyíin front, facing
qumáaʃ material, cloth
quráyyib*, qurayyíba*, qurayyibíin* near
qurúuʃ (*see* **qirʃ**)
(ʕil)qurʕáan† the Koran
quṣáad opposite
quṣáyyar*, quṣayyára*, quṣayyaríin* small, short
quṭn, ʕaqṭáan cotton
quṭr†, ʕaqṭáar† country
  ʕilqúṭr ilmáṣri Egypt
qúuṭa (*c.*), **quṭáaya, quṭáat** *or* **quṭayáat** tomatoes
quɣáad (*v.n.*) sitting

r

ráabiɣ*, rábɣa* fourth
ráaḍi, ráḍya, raḍyíin pleased

¹ Pronounced *qaɣáttï*.

ráagil*, riggáala man
raah*, yirúuh to go
  ráah mínni I've lost it
ráaha* rest
  béet irráaha lavatory
ráahil*, rúhhàl nomad
ráakib, rákba, rakbíin riding
raas* (f.), ruus head
ráayih, ráyha, rayhíin going
rábat*, yúrbut to tie (up); bandage
rabb* Lord
rabííჳ* spring
rábta, rúbat bundle
radd*, yirúdd (+ ჳala) to answer;
  return
  ráddi gúჳtu-b . . . he took the edge
    off his appetite with . . .
radd* (v.n.), rudúud answer(ing);
  return(ing)
rádyu, radyuháat wireless (set)
ráda, yírdi to please, satisfy
ráfad, yírfid to dismiss, discharge
ráfaჳ*, yírfaჳ to lift
  ჳírfaჳ ṣóotak! speak up!
raff*, rufúuf shelf
rággaჳ, yirággaჳ to bring back, return
ráhal*, yírhal to go away; migrate
ráhhab*, yiráhhab* (+ bi) to welcome
ráhma* mercy
ráma, yírmi to throw
ramadáan* Muslim (fasting) month;
  proper name
raml*, rimáal sand
rámli*, ramlíyya* sandy
rásmi, rasmíyya, rasmiyyíin official
rasúul*, rúsul messenger, prophet
raṣíif, ჳarṣífa pavement; platform
raṣṣ, yirúṣṣ to arrange, stack, draw up
ráttib, yiráttib to tidy, put in order
ratb, rátba damp
ratl, ჳirtáal ¾ pound (weight)
ráwa, yírwi to water, irrigate
ráwwah*, yiráwwah* to return
  (home)
rayy* (v.n. of ráwa, yírwi) watering,
  irrigation
rayy*, ráyya*, rayyíin* watered (of
  land); in flood (river)
ráyyis*, rúyasa ganger
raჳíis, rúჳasa chief, head

raჳíisi*, raჳisíyya*, raჳisiyyíin*
  principal, chief
raჳy* opinion
reet (see ya)
rídi, yírda to be pleased, satisfied;
  agree
rígiჳ, yírgaჳ to come back
rigl (f.) foot, leg
ríhla, rihláat journey
riih, ჳaryáah wind
ríiha, rawáayih* smell
riiq saliva
ríiʃa, ríyaʃ feather
ríkib, yírkab to mount, ride
rixíiṣ, rixíiṣa, ruxáaṣ cheap
ríxiṣ, yírxaṣ to be (or become) cheap
riyáada sport, athletics; mathematics
riyíif, ჳaryífa loaf
rubჳ, ჳarbáaჳ or ჳirbáaჳ quarter
  rúbჳi sáaჳa quarter of an hour
rufáyyaჳ, rufayyáჳa, rufayyaჳíin
  thin, flimsy
rugúuჳ (v.n.) return(ing)
rukn, ჳarkáan* corner; tenet
rukúub (v.n.) riding
  ჳúgrit irrukúub fare
rumáani, rumaníyya, rumaniyyíin
  Roman
rutúuba dampness, humidity
ruuh, ჳarwáah* soul
  máat ჳala rúuhu middíhk he
    died of laughing
  biykállim rúuhu(h) he talks to
    himself
rúuma Rome
rúumi, rumíyya, rumiyyíin or
  ჳarwáam* European
  díik rúumi turkey

S

saab, yisíib to leave
sáabiq, sábqa, sabqíin preceding,
  former
sáabiჳ, sábჳa seventh
sáada unsweetened, plain
  qáhwa sáada coffee without sugar
sáadiq, yisáadiq
  s. ჳalჳáqd to sign a contract
sáadis, sádsa sixth
sáafir, yisáafir to depart, travel
sáahil, sawáahil shore

sáakin, sákna, sukkáan inhabitant

sáakit, sákta, saktíin silent, of few words

sáamiḥ, yisáamiḥ to forgive

saaq, yisúuq to drive

sáatit, sátta sixth

sáawa, yisáawi to equal

sáaҁil or sáayil, saҁíla or sáyla, sawáaҁil or sawáayil liquid, flowing

sáaɤa, saɤáat hour; clock, watch

saɤítha at that time

ҁissáaɤa káam? what time is it?

sáaɤi, suɤáah postman

sáaɤid, yisáaɤid to help

sáaɤit ma + v. at the time that . . .

saaɤ piastre

sábab, ҁasbáab reason, cause

sábaq, yísbaq to precede, go on ahead

sábat, ҁisbíta basket

sábaɤ, sábɤa seven

sabaɤṭáaʃar* seventeen

sabb, yisíbb to curse, swear

sabɤ, subúɤa lion

sabɤíin seventy

sádaq, yísdaq to tell the truth

sadd, yisídd to block; pay (bill or debt)

sáddaq, yisáddaq to believe

sáfar*, ҁasfáar* journey

sagáayir (see sigáara*)

sággil, yisággil to record, register

sáhhil, yisáhhil to facilitate

sahl, sáhla, sahlíin easy

sahríig, saharíig tank, container

sahúula ease, easiness

saḥáab (c.), saḥáaba, saḥabáat, súḥub clouds

sákan (v.n.) living, inhabiting

sakráan*, sakráana*, sakraníin* drunk

saláam peace, tranquillity

saláama safety

salamítha I hope she gets well

maɤa-ssaláama goodbye

sálaf debt

xad, yaaxud salaf to incur a debt

salafíyya, salafiyyáat loan

sállif, yisállif to lend

sállim, yisállim to deliver, hand over

sallímli ɤala . . . remember me to . . .

sáma sky

sámaḥ, yísmaḥ (+ʾli) to excuse

sámak (c.), sámaka, samakáat, ҁasmáak fish

sámma, yisámmi to call, name

sammáak, sammakíin fishmonger

sána, siníin or sanawáat year

ҁissána or ҁissanáadi this year

ҁissána-lli fáatit last year

sanáawi, sanawíyya, sanawiyyíin annual

madrása sanawíyya secondary school

sandawítʃ, sandawitʃáat sandwich

sandúuq, sanadíiq box

sánna, yisánni to support, second (motion)

sánya, sawáani second (of time)

saqqáara* Sakkaara

sáqɤa cold (weather)

sáraq, yísraq to steal

sardíin (c.), sardíina, sardináat sardines

saríiɤ, saríiɤa, sariɤíin fast, speedy

sarríiḥ, sarríiḥa pedlar, hawker

sáwa simultaneously, together

sawwáaḥ, sawwáaḥa, sawwaḥíin tourist

sawwáaq, sawwaqíin driver

sáxxan, yisáxxan to heat

sayyáara*, sayyaráat* vehicle

sayyída, sayyidáat (female) saint; lady

sáҁal, yísҁal to ask

seef, siyúuf sword

sibáaḥa (v.n.) swimming

síbḥa, síbaḥ rosary

sibtímbir September

sidr (see ṣadr)

sigáara*, sagáayir cigarette

sigáara zanúbya cigar

siggáada, sagagíid carpet

sign, sugúun prison

(ya) síidi (pl. ҁasyáadi) term of address; saint

síina Sinai

síira conduct, behaviour; reputation

gaab, yigiib siira ɤan to mention

síkin (or sákan), yúskun to live, inhabit; settle (down)

sikirtárya (or sikirtaríyya) secretariat

sikirtéer, sikirtéera, sikirteriyyíin secretary

síkit (or sákat), yúskut to stop talking, be quiet

síkka, síkak road, way

síkka ḥadíid railway, railroad

sikkíina, sakakíin knife

síllim, saláalim ladder

sillíma, saláalim step, stair

simíin, simíina, sumáan fat

símiɛ, yísmaɛ to hear, listen

siníin (see sána)

sínima, sinimáat cinema

sinn, ʕasnáan tooth; age

  ṭabíib or ḥakíim ilʕasnáan dentist

siríir, saráayir bed

síriɛ, yísriɛ to hurry

sírqa theft

sitáara*, satáayir curtain

sitt, sítta six

sitt, sittáat woman

sittíin sixty

siṭṭáaʃar* sixteen

síxin (or súxun), yísxan to be (or become) hot

siyáasa politics; policy

siyáasi, siyasíyya, siyasiyyíin political

siɛr, ʕasɛaar* price

subɛ, ʕasbáaɛ or ʕisbáaɛ one-seventh

subɛumíyya seven hundred

suds, ʕasdáas or ʕisdáas one-sixth

suḥúur meal taken before daybreak in Ramadan

súkkar* (c.), ḥíttit súkkar, ḥítat súkkar sugar

  qáhwa súkkar ziyáada well-sweetened coffee

sukúndu

  dáraga*-skúndu second class

súlfa, súlaf loan

surúur pleasure

súrɛa speed

  bi súrɛa fast, quickly

suttumíyya six hundred

suuq, ʕaswáaq market

suuʕ evil

  súuʕ ittafáahum misunderstanding, disagreement

(ʕis)suwées (f.) Suez

suxn, súxna, suxníin hot

suxuníyya fever

suʕáal, ʕasʕíla question

ṣ

ṣáadif, yiṣáadif to meet by chance

ṣáafi, ṣáfya, ṣafyíin clear

ṣáaḥib, ʕaṣḥáab friend; owner

  ṣáaḥib ɛiyáal father, family man

ṣáala, ṣaláat hall, entrance-hall

  ṣáalit irráqṣ dance-hall

ṣáaliḥ, ṣálḥa, ṣalḥíin fit; wholesome; righteous

ṣaam, yiṣúum to fast

ṣaar, yiṣíir to become

(ʕiṣ)ṣáaɣa jewel-market in Cairo

ṣabáaḥ

  ṣabáaḥ ilxéer good morning

  ṣabáaḥ innúur good morning

  ṣabáaḥ ilfúll good morning

  ṣabáaḥ ilqíʃṭa good morning

ṣabáaḥan a.m.

ṣabb, yiṣúbb to pour (out)

ṣábi, ṣabíyya, ṣubyáan young boy or girl

ṣabr patience

ṣádaf (c.), ṣádafa, ṣadafáat seashells

ṣadr (or sidr) chest

ṣaff, ṣufúuf row, line

ṣafíiḥa, ṣafáayiḥ (large) tin, can, drum

ṣaḥḥ, yiṣáḥḥ to be correct; be possible

ṣáḥḥa, yiṣáḥḥi to wake up

ṣaḥíiḥ, ṣaḥíiḥa correct

ṣaḥn, ṣuḥúun plaṭe, dish, platter

ṣáḥra*, ṣaḥáara* desert

ṣaḥráawi, ṣaḥrawíyya, ṣaḥrawiyyíin of the desert

ṣaḥw, ṣáḥwa clear (of weather)

ṣála, ṣalawáat prayer

ṣálaṭa salad

ṣálla, yiṣálli to pray

ṣánaɛ, yíṣnaɛ to manufacture

ṣaníyya, ṣawáani tray

ṣantigráad* Centigrade

ṣantimítr, ṣantimitráat* centimetre

ṣaráaḥa* frankness

ṣáraf*, yíṣrif to spend

ṣarráaf*, ṣarrafíin* or ṣayárfa* cashier

ṣaṭḥ, ṣuṭúuḥ roof

ṣaṭr, ṣuṭúur line

ṣáwwar*, yiṣáwwar* to photograph

ṣaxr, ṣuxúur rock

ṣáyyif, yiṣáyyif to spend the summer
ṣaᵹb, ṣáᵹba, ṣaᵹbíin difficult
(ˁiṣ)ṣaᵹíid (or ˁiṣṣiᵹíid) Upper
  Egypt
ṣaᵹíidi (or ṣiᵹíidi), ṣaᵹidíyya,
  ṣaᵹáyda Upper Egyptian
ṣeef summer
ṣíḥḥa health
  ˁizzáyy iṣṣíḥḥa? how are you?
ṣíini china, porcelain
ṣíini, ṣiníyya, ṣiniyyíin Chinese
ṣináaᵹa, ṣinaᵹáat industry
ṣináaᵹi (or ṣanáyᵹi), ṣinaᵹíyya,
  ṣinaᵹiyyíin industrial
ṣiníyya (see ṣaníyya)
ṣirf, ṣírfa only, just, alone
ṣóogar*, yiṣóogar* to register
ṣoom (v.n.) fasting
ṣoot, ˁaṣwáat voice
ṣubáaᵹ (or ṣáabiᵹ), ṣawáabiᵹ finger
  ṣubáaᵹ móoz banana
ṣubḥ morning
  ˁiṣṣúbḥ this morning
ṣúdfa chance
  biṣṣúdfa by chance, suddenly
  ṣúdfa ɣaríiba-w saᵹíida! well
  met!
ṣudr place name
ṣuffáara*, ṣafafíir whistle
ṣúfra*, ṣúfar* dining-table
ṣufrági*, ṣufragíyya* waiter
ṣulḥ peace (opposed to war)
ṣulṭáan, ṣalaṭíin sultan
ṣúura*, ṣúwar* picture, photograph
ṣuᵹúuba, ṣuᵹubáat difficulty
ṣuɣáyyar*, ṣuɣayyára*, ṣuɣayyaríin* small; young

t

taag, tigáan crown
táagir, tuggáar* merchant
taah, yitúuh to be lost
táalit, tálta third
táamin, támna eighth
táani again
táani, tánya second
táani, tánya, tanyíin other; next
táasiᵹ, tásᵹa ninth
táayih, táyha, tayhíin lost
tábaᵹ (invariable) belonging to, under
  the direction of

tábaᵹ, yítbaᵹ to follow
tabyíiḍ (v.n.) painting (white or
  cream)
tadáawi (v.n.) medical treatment
tadríib (v.n.) training
tadxíin (v.n.) smoking
  mamnúuᵹ ittadxíin no smoking
tafáahum (v.n.) understanding
tafkíir (v.n.) thinking; reminding
tafṣíil (v.n.)
  bittafṣíil in detail
tagdíid (v.n.) renewal
tahwíya (v.n.) ventilation
taḥqíiq (v.n.) investigation
  taḥqíiq iʃʃaxṣíyya identity card
taḥsíin (v.n.) improvement
taḥt under(neath); downstairs
taḥtáani, taḥtaníyya, taḥtaniyyíin
  lower
taḥwíida, taḥawíid turning
takábbur (v.n.) pride, haughtiness
takmíla completion
takríir (v.n.) repetition; refining
taks, taksáat (see táksi)
táksi, taksiyyáat taxi
taksíir (v.n.) cracking (i.e. processing
  oil)
tálaf, yítlif to damage, harm
tálat, taláata three
talatíin thirty
talaṭṭáaʃar* thirteen
talg ice
talláaga, tallagáat refrigerator
talliɣráaf*, talliɣrafáat* telegram
tamáam exactly; completely
tamálli always
táman, ˁatmáan price
táman, tamánya eight
tamaníin eighty
tamanṭáaʃar* eighteen
tanḍíif (v.n.) cleaning
tank, tunúuk or tankáat tank
tanzíim (v.n.) organizing, arrangement
taqríiban approximately
taqríir (v.n.), taqaríir report
taqṭíir (v.n.) distillation
tára
  ya tára . . . I wonder . . .
tarfíih* (v.n.) welfare
tárgim, yitárgim to translate
targumáan*, tarágma interpreter,
  dragoman

taríix, tawaríix date; history
taríixi, tarixíyya, tarixiyyíin historical
tarqíya (v.n.) promotion
tartíib (v.n.) arrangement
tasdíiq (v.n.) believing; contracting
tasgíil (v.n.) registration
tashíil (v.n.), tashiláat facilitating, facility
tasníya (v.n.) supporting, seconding
tasɣiira official price-list
taṣríih (v.n.), taṣaríih declaration; permission; duty-slip
taṭbíiq (v.n.) application, putting into practice
tawbíix (v.n.) blaming, rebuking
tawzíiɣ (v.n.) distribution
taxzíin (v.n.) storing
tazkára*, tazáakir ticket
tazkárgi, tazkargíyya ticket-clerk
tazyíit (v.n.) oiling, lubrication
taʃdíid (v.n.) strengthening
taʃḥíim (v.n.) greasing
taɣáala, taɣáali, taɣáalu come (here)!
táɣab fatigue; tedium
taɣbáan, taɣbáana, taɣbaníin tired; unwell
táɣlab, taɣáalib fox
taɣlíim (v.n.), taɣlimáat instruction, teaching
taɣríifa half-piastre
  qirʃi taɣríifa half-piastre
tiffáaḥ (c.), tiffáaḥa, tiffaḥáat apples
tigáara* business
tiin (c.), tíina, tináat figs
tilifóon, tilifonáat telephone
  ʕittilifóon ḍárab the phone rang
  ɣáamil ittilifóon telephone operator
tilitwáar*, tilitwaráat* pavement
tilt, ʕatláat or ʕitláat one-third
tínis tennis
tiqíil, tiqíila, tuqáal heavy
tírɣa, tíraɣ channel, canal
tísaɣ, tísɣa nine
tisaɣṭáaʃar nineteen
tisɣíin ninety
tiɣdáad counting, census
tíɣib, yítɣab to be (or become) tired
toom (c.), tomáaya, tomáat garlic
  ráas* tóom garlic plant
tultumíyya three hundred

tumn, ʕatmáan or ʕitmáan one-eighth
tumnumíyya eight hundred
turáab* dust
túrki, turkíyya, ʕatráak* or tarákwa* Turk, Turkish
turmáay,[1] turmayáat tram
tust toast
tusɣ, ʕatsáaɣ or ʕitsáaɣ one-ninth
tusɣumíyya nine hundred

t

ṭaab, yiṭíib to be (or become) ripe; recover (from illness)
ṭáabiɣ, ṭawáabiɣ stamp
ṭáalib, ṭálaba student
ṭaar, yiṭíir to fly
ṭáaza fresh
ṭábaq, ʕaṭbáaq plate
ṭábax, yúṭbux to cook
ṭabbáax, ṭabbaxíin cook
ṭabíib, ʕaṭibbáaʕ doctor
ṭabíix (cooked) food
ṭabx (v.n.) cooking
ṭábɣan of course
ṭáfa, yíṭfi to extinguish, put out
ṭáfa, yíṭfa to float
ṭálab, yúṭlub to ask for
ṭálab, ṭalabáat request, demand, application
ṭállaq, yiṭállaq to divorce
ṭállaɣ, yiṭállaɣ to take out, bring out; (+ li) look at
ṭalyáani (or ṭul-), ṭalyaníyya, ṭaláyna Italian
ṭámaɣ greed
ṭammáaɣ, ṭammáaɣa, ṭammaɣíin greedy
ṭaqíyya, ṭawáaqi skull-cap
ṭaqs climate, weather
ṭaqṭúuqa, ṭaqaṭíiq ash-tray
  ṭaqṭúuqit sagáayir ash-tray
ṭaráawa* fresh air, freshness
ṭarabéeza, ṭarabezáat table
ṭárad, yúṭrud to expel, eject
ṭáraḥ, yíṭraḥ to subtract
ṭarbúuʃ, ṭarabíiʃ tarboosh
ṭard, ṭurúud parcel
ṭaríiq (m. or f.), ṭúruq way, road
ṭaríiqa, ṭúruq means, method

---

[1] With 'back' aa.

ṭárra, yiṭárri to cool down
ṭawáabiʒ (see ṭáabiʒ)
ṭawíil, ṭawíila, ṭuwáal long, tall
ṭáwwil, yiṭáwwil to lengthen
ṭayaráan* (v.n.) aviation, flying
ṭayyáara*, ṭayyaráat* aeroplane
ṭáyyar*, yiṭáyyar* to make fly
ṭáyyib all right
ṭáyyib, ṭayyíba, ṭayyibíin good
ṭeer, ṭuyúur bird
ṭibb medicine, medical faculty
ṭíbbi, ṭibbíyya medical
ṭiin (c.), ṭíina or ḫíttit ṭ., ṭináat or ḫítat ṭ. clay, mud
ṭíliʒ, yíṭlaʒ to go out, come out; go, drive
ṭúrba, ṭúrab tomb
ṭuul, ʕaṭwáal length
  ʒala ṭúul straight away
  ṭúul innaháar* all day long
  bi ṭúul (or miṭáwla) lengthwise

W

wáagib
  wáagib ʒaláyya-nn . . . it is my duty to . . .
wáaḥid, wáḥda one
  kúlli wáaḥid everyone, each one
  fi wáqti wáaḥid at the same time
  wáaḥid táani another one
wáakil, wákla, waklíin having eaten (a.p. of kal, yáakul)
wáaqif, wáqfa, waqfíin standing
  ʕissúuq wáaqif business is quiet
wáaqiʒ†
  filwáaqiʒ in fact
wáasiʒ, wásʒa, wasʒíin spacious, wide
wáaṭi, wáṭya, waṭyíin low
wáaxid, wáxda, waxdíin having taken (a.p. of xad, yáaxud)
wabúur, waburáat* primus-stove; locomotive; engine
wádda, yiwáddi to take away
wáffar*, yiwáffar* to save
wágad, yíwgid to find
wágaʒ, yíwgaʒ to hurt, ache
  ráasi*-btiwgáʒni I have a headache
wagh, wugúuh face, side
waḥd + p.s.
  (li) wáḥdu(h) on his own

waḥdaníyya oneness
wakíil, wakíila, wúkala deputy
(la . . .) wala (neither . . .) nor
  ma ʒandíiʃ wála wáaḥid I haven't a single one
wálad, wiláad or ʕawláad boy, child
wálla or
wálla[1] by God
walláaʒa, wallaʒáat lighter (cigarette-)
wállaʒ, yiwállaʒ to light
wáqqaf, yiwáqqaf to stop
waqt, ʕawqáat time
  ʕilwáqt ilḫáaḍir the present (time)
  filwaqtída at that time
  dilwáqti now
  wáqti ma + v. at the time that
wára* behind
wáraq (c.), wáraqa, waraqáat, ʕawráaq paper
  wáraqit dámʒa fiscal stamp
wárra, yiwárri to show
warráani*, warraníyya*, warraniyyíin* rearmost
wárʃa, wíraʃ workshop
wasáaxa dirt, dirtiness
wasíila, wasáaʕil method
waṣl, wuṣuláat receipt
  wáṣl ittasgíil receipt
wáṣṣa, yiwáṣṣi to bequeath; (+ ʒala) enjoin (someone)
wáṣṣal, yiwáṣṣal to deliver
wáṣṭa, waṣáayiṭ means; mediation; subterfuge
wáṭan, ʕawṭáan birthplace, native country
wáṭani, waṭaníyya, waṭaniyyíin native, indigenous
wáxri, waxríyya, waxriyyíin late
wáyya with
  wáyya báʒḍ together, with each other
  wi baʒdéen wayyáak! what's the matter with you!
wázan, yíwzin to weigh
wazíir, wúzara* minister
wázzaʒ, yiwázzaʒ to distribute
wáʃwiʃ, yiwáʃwiʃ to whisper
wáʒad, yíwʒid to promise
wi and; while

[1] 'Back' a's.

widn (f.), widáan ear

wíḥiʃ, wíḥʃa, wiḥʃíin bad, unpleasant

wiláakin but, however

wíldit, tíwlid (f. only) to bear, give birth

wiqáaya† safety

wiqáayit issaláama safety

wíqif, yúqaf to stop

wíqiʒ, yúqaʒ to fall

wíqqa, wíqaq oke (measure)

wísix, wísxa, wisxíin dirty

wíṣil (or wáṣal), yíwṣal to arrive

wiṣṭ (see wusṭ)

wiẓáara ministry

raʕíis* ilwiẓáara prime minister

wiẓáarit iddaxlíyya Ministry of the Interior

wiʃʃ, wuʃúuʃ face

wugúud (v.n.) presence

wusṭ, ʕawṣáaṭ middle, centre

wuṣúul (v.n.) arrival

X

xaaf, yixáaf to fear, be afraid

xaal, xiláan uncle (maternal)

ʕíbnï xáali my cousin (maternal)

xáala, xaláat aunt (maternal)

xáaliṣ very, completely

xaam raw, crude

ʕizzéet ilxáam crude oil

ʕilmawáadd ilxáam raw materials

xáamis, xámsa fifth

xáaniq, yixáaniq to dispute, quarrel

xáarig outside

xáaṭir, xawáaṭir idea, mind

ʒaʃan xáṭrak for your sake

xábar*, ʕaxbáar* news, information

ma ʒandíiʃ ʕaxbáar I know nothing about it

xábbar*, yixábbar* to inform

xábbaṭ, yixábbaṭ to knock

xabíir, xúbara* expert

xad, yáaxud to take

qaddï ʕéeh xadítak ʒaʃan ... how long did it take you to ...?

xádam, yíxdim to serve

xadd, xudúud cheek

xaddáam, xaddáama, xaddamíin servant

xaḍḍ, yixáḍḍ to frighten

xaff, yixíff to recover (from illness)

xafíif, xafíifa, xufáaf light

xaláaṣ that's all!

xalíifa, xúlafa caliph

xalíig, xulgáan gulf

xalíig issuwées the Gulf of Suez

xall vinegar

xálla, yixálli to let, allow; leave

xallíik ʒarraṣíiʃ! keep on the pavement!

xallíik ráagil! be a man!

xállaṣ, yixállaṣ to finish, use up

yixalláṣak tídfaʒ káam? how much are you prepared to pay?

xalláʃhum min báʒḍ he separated them, stopped them quarrelling

xállif, yixállif to beget

xámas, xámsa five

xamasṭáaʃar* fifteen

xámra* wine

xamsíin fifty

xárag*, yúxrug to go out

xáraṭ, yúxruṭ to slice, cut; turn (wood)

xárbiʃ, yixárbiʃ to scratch

xaríif autumn

xaríiṭa*, xaráayiṭ* map

xárraf*, yixárraf* to wander in one's mind

xarúuf*, xirfáan sheep

xárʃim, yixárʃim to draw blood from (by inflicting wound)

xáṣam, yíxṣim to deduct

xaṣṣ (c.), xaṣṣáaya, xaṣṣayáat lettuces

xaṣṣ (or xaaṣṣ¹), xáṣṣa (or xáaṣṣa¹) special; private

xáṣṣar, yixáṣṣar to make lose

xátam (or xítim), yíxtim to stamp, frank

xáṭar, ʕaxṭáar danger

xaṭíib, xúṭaba speaker, orator

xaṭṭ, xuṭúuṭ line; writing, calligraphy

xawáaga, xawagáat gentleman

xáwta noise, commotion

xáyri, xayríyya, xayriyyíin pertaining to welfare, well-doing

xazáana, xazáayin or xazanáat safe

xázan, yíxzin to store

xázzin, yixázzin to store

xáʃab (c.), xáʃaba or xaʃabáaya, xaʃabáat wood

¹ See Part I, Appendix B, note (c).

xáʃabi, xaʃabíyya wooden
xaʃʃ, yixúʃʃ to enter
xeel (f.) horses
xeer well-being; goodness
  ṣabáaḥ ilxéer good morning
  mísa-lxéer or misáaʕ ilxéer good
    evening
  kullína-b xéer we are all well
  káttar* xéerak thank you
xíbra* experience
xídma, xadamáat service
  ʕáyyi xídma? what can I do for
  you?
  ʕana-f xidmítak I am at your service
xígil, yíxgal to be ashamed, confused
xíli, yíxla to be (or become) empty
xíliṣ, yíxlaṣ to be finished; (+ min)
  finish with
xílqa, xílaq face, countenance
xináaqa (v.n.), xinaqáat quarrel
xíriṣ (or xúruṣ), yíxraṣ to become
  dumb
xírqa, xíraq rag
xíṣir, yíxṣar to lose
xiyáar*(c.), xiyáara* or xiyaráaya*,
  xiyaráat* cucumbers
xoox (c.), xóoxa, xoxáat peaches
xúḍari, xuḍaríyya greengrocer
xúḍra, xuḍáar vegetable
xums, ʕaxmáas or ʕixmáas one-
  fifth
xumsumíyya five hundred
xuṣáara*, xasáayir loss
  ya-xṣáara! what a pity!
xuṣúuṣ concern
  bi xuṣúuṣ in regard to; belonging
  to
xuṣúuṣan especially
xuṣúuṣi, xuṣuṣíyya, xuṣuṣiyyíin
  special
xúṭba, xúṭab speech, oration

y

ya vocative particle
  ya réet if only
  ya tára* I wonder
ya . . . ya either . . . or
yadd or ʕiid (f.), ʕayáadi hand;
  handle
yágib (+ ʕinn) it is inevitable (that)
yahúudi, yahudíyya, yahúud Jew

yalla!¹ come on!
  yálla bíina! let's go!
  yall-áʃrab!* drink up!
yanáayir January
yáʑni that is (to say)
(ma-)yhímmiʃ it's of no importance
yígra* (or gára*) ʕéeh? what's the
  matter? what's happened?
yigúuz (+li) to be able, permitted
yílzam
  yilzámni-gnéeh I need a pound
yimíin right
  ʕilʕiid ilyimíin the right hand
  ʕáwwil taḥwíida ʑalyimíin the
  first turning on the right
yímkin perhaps
yíʑhar inn . . . it seems that, apparently
yoom, ʕayyáam or ʕiyyáam day
  liyyámdi nowadays
  ʕilyoméen dóol these days
  fi yóom milʕayyáam once upon a
  time
  fi yóom min záat ilʕayyáam once
  upon a time
  fi yóom min dóol once upon a
  time
  yóom ilḥádd Sunday
  yóom litnéen Monday
  yóom ittaláat Tuesday
  yóom lárbaʑ* Wednesday
  yóom ilxamíis Thursday
  yóom iggúmʑa Friday
  yóom issábt Saturday
(ma-)yṣáḥḥiʃ it's unlikely, impossible
yúlya July
(ʕil)yunáan (f.) Greece
yunáani, yunaníyya, yunaniyyíin
  Greek
yúnya June
yusafándi (c.), yusafandíyya,
  yusafandiyyáat tangerines

z

záaḥim, yizáaḥim to crowd (upon)
záakir, yizáakir to learn, study
záalik
  maʑa záalik nevertheless
zaat (see yoom)

¹ 'Back' a's.

zaat self

  huwwa géh bi záatu(h) he came himself

(ʕiz)záay how

záayir, záyra, zuwwáar* (*see* ʐaar) visitor

záḥma crowd

záka alms, almsdeeds

zákka, yizákki to give alms

zamáan long time; of old

  min zamáan for a long time

  zamáan kanu biyʃayyálu bil-buxáar* formerly they worked by steam

  zamánhum míʃyu they must have gone

zaqq, yizúqq to push

záraʐ, yízraʐ to plant, grow, cultivate

zawbáʐa, zawáabiʐ storm, sandstorm

záwwid, yizáwwid to increase

zayy like

  záyyĭ báʕḍ alike, like each other

  záyyĭ wíqqa about an oke

  záyyĭ ḥalátna like us

(ʕiz)záyy

  ʕizzáyy ilḥáal? how are you?

záyyĭ ma + v. just as, in the way that

záyyin, yizáyyin to decorate

záyyit, yizáyyit to oil, grease, lubricate

záʐal anger

zaʐláan, zaʐláana, zaʐlaníin angry

záʐʐaq, yizáʐʐaq to shout

zeet, ziyúut oil

  zéet iʃʃáḥm lubricating oil

zetíyya oil refinery

zíbda butter

zibúun, zibúuna, zabáayin customer

zift tar

  záyy izzíft terrible, awful

  zíftĭ-f zíft unbearable

zíhiq, yízhaq to be tired of

zíina, zináat ornament

zi-lḥígga (*or* zu-lḥúgga) month of pilgrimage

ziráaʐa[1] (*v.n.*), **ziraʐáat**[1] cultivation; crop, field of crops

ziráaʐi,[1] **ziraʐíyya**[1] agricultural; cultivated; fertile

[1] Either 'back' or 'front' *a*.

muwaṣaláat ziraʐíyya land communications

ziyáada, ziyadáat increase; a lot of

  qáhwa súkkar* ziyáada well-sweetened coffee

  kifáaya wi-zyáada more than enough

ziyáara*, ziyaráat* (*see* ʐaar) visit

  géh ziyáara li . . . to visit, go on a visit to

zíʐil, yízʐal to become angry

zuhríyya, zuhriyyáat flower-vase

zukáam cold (in the head)

ʐ

ʐáabiṭ (*or* ḍáabiṭ), **ʐubbáaṭ** officer

ʐáahir, ʐáhra*, ʐahríin clear

ʐáalim, ʐálma, ʐalmíin cruel

ʐaar, yizʐúur to visit

ʐábaṭ, yízbuṭ to control

ʐábaṭ mud

ʐabṭ

  bizʐábṭ exactly

ʐahr (*c.*), **ʐáhra*, ʐahráat*, ʐuhúur** flowers

ʐákar, yúzkur to mention

ʐambaléeṭa uproar

ʐann, yizʐúnn to think

ʐáqṭaṭ, yizʐáqṭaṭ to be overjoyed

ʐarf, ʐurúuf envelope

  ʐárfĭ gawáab envelope

ʐaríif, ʐaríifa, ʐuráaf nice, pleasant

ʐulm oppression, cruelty

ʕ

ʕáadi here/there is/are

ʕáala, ʕaláat machine

  ʕáala kátba typewriter

  kátab, yíktib ʐalʕáala-lkátba to type

ʕáamin, yiʕáamin (bi) to trust (in)

ʕáasif, ʕásfa, ʕasfíin sorry

ʕáaxar*, ʕúxra* other

ʕáaxir last

ʕábadan ever, never

ʕabb, ʕabbaháat father

ʕábu-lhóol the Sphinx

  ṭawáabiʐ min ʕábu qirʃéen two-piastre stamps

ʕábu galámbu crab

ʕabríil (*or* ʕibríil) April

ʕabríiq, ʕabaríiq jug

ʔábyaḍ, béeḍa, biiḍ white
ʔádab politeness
ʔaḍáaf, yuḍíif to add
ʔafándi, ʔafandíyya efendi
ʔafándim? I beg your pardon (on failing to hear what is said)
ʔafrángi*, ʔafrangíyya*, ʔafráng* foreign
ʔagáaza, ʔagazáat leave
ʔagnábi, ʔagnabíyya, ʔagáanib foreign, foreigner
ʔagzaxáana, ʔagzaxanáat dispensary
ʔaháamm more (or most) important
ʔahl, ʔaháali people
ʔáhlan or ʔáhlan wi sáhlan hullo
ʔáhli, ʔahlíyya national, native
ʔahó(h), ʔahé(h), ʔahúm here/there is/are
ʔahráam* (see háram*)
ʔáḥmar*, ḥámra*, ḥumr red
ʔáḥsan better, best; otherwise
ʔaḥyáanan sometimes
ʔakl (v.n.) meal, food; eating
ʔalf, ʔaláaf thousand
ʔalláah God
ʔálla(h) good heavens!
ʔámar*, yúʔmur to order
ʔamíin, ʔamíina, ʔúmana trustworthy
ʔamíir, ʔúmara* prince
ʔámma but; let; as for
    ʔámma ráagil*! what a man!
    ʔámma ḥárr*! isn't it hot!
ʔámmin, yiʔámmin (ʕala) to insure
ʔamr*, ʔawáamir order
ʔamrikáani (or ʔamríiki), ʔamrik(an)íyya, ʔamrik(an)iyyíin (or ʔamrikáan) American
ʔan¹ that (conjunction)
ʔána I
ʔanf, ʔunúuf nose
ʔánhu, ʔánhi, ʔánhum which?
ʔánna¹ that (conjunction)
ʔánsab more (or most) suitable
ʔantíika, ʔantikáat antique, objet d'art
ʔantikxáana, ʔantikxanáat museum
ʔaqáll less, least
    ʕalʔaqáll at least
ʔárbaʕ*, ʔarbáʕa* four

¹ 'Classical' Arabic.

ʔarbaʕtáaʃar* fourteen
ʔarbiʕíin forty
ʔarḍ (f.), ʔaráaḍi earth, land; floor
ʔárḍa, yírḍi to please, satisfy
ʔárnab, ʔaráanib rabbit
ʔársal, yírsil² to send
(ʔil)ʔaryáaf (s. riif) country(side), provinces
ʔasáas, ʔúsus base, foundation
ʔasáasi, ʔasasíyya, ʔasasiyyíin basic
ʔásad, ʔusúud or ʔusúda lion
ʔásaf sorrow
ʔásar*, ʔasáar* trace; (ancient) monument
ʔasári, ʔasaríyya historical, ancient
ʔasfált asphalt
ʔásraʕ* faster, fastest
    bi ʔásraʕ ma yúmkin as quickly as possible
ʔássis, yiʔássis to base
ʔastíika, ʔasatíik rubber, eraser
ʔasanséer, ʔasanseráat* lift
ʔáṣfar*, ṣáfra*, ṣufr yellow
ʔaṣl, ʔuṣúul origin
ʔaṣl ... the fact is that ...
ʔáṣli, ʔaṣlíyya, ʔaṣliyyíin basic, original; of good family
ʔatámm more (or most) complete
    fi ʔatámm ilʔistiʕdáad completely ready, quite prepared
ʔáṭraʃ, ṭárʃa, ṭurʃ deaf
ʔaw or
ʔáwwal, ʔúula first
ʔawwaláani, ʔawwalaníyya, ʔawwalaniyyíin first
ʔáwwil first
ʔáwwil ma + v. as soon as
ʔaxbáar* (see xábar*)
ʔáxḍar, xáḍra, xuḍr green
ʔaxíir, ʔaxíira last
ʔaxíiran at last, finally
ʔaxráani, ʔaxraníyya, ʔaxraniyyíin last
ʔáxraṣ, xárṣa, xurṣ dumb
ʔaxx, ʔixwáat brother
ʔáxxar*, yiʔáxxar* to delay
ʔáyḍan also
ʔáynaʕam³ (see náʕam)
ʔáywa yes
ʔayy any; which?

² 'Classical' Arabic.
³ 'Back' a in first syllable.

ʕázraq, zárqa, zurq blue
ʕázyad more
ʕáɣma, ɣámya, ɣumy blind
ʕáɣrag*, ɣárga, ɣurg lame
ʕáɣwar*, ɣóora*, ɣuur one-eyed
ʕaɣyáan (ilbálad) notables (of the village)
ʕáɣlab most (of)
ʕaɣlabíyya majority
ʕaɣúsṭus August
ʕeeh what?
ʕibn, ʕabnáaʕ son
  ʕíbni ɣámm (or xáal) cousin
ʕibtáda, yibtídi to begin
ʕibtída (v.n.) beginning
ʕibyáḍḍ, yibyáḍḍ to be (or become) white
ʕidáara* administration
ʕídda, yíddi to give
  ʕídda, yíddi kílma to promise, vow
ʕiftákar*, yiftíkir to think; remember
ʕigtáhad, yigtíhid to struggle, strive hard
ʕigtimáaɣi, ʕigtimaɣíyya, ʕigtimaɣiyyíin social; sociable
ʕiḥáala, ʕiḥaláat retirement, resignation
ʕiḥláww, yiḥláww to be (or become) sweet
ʕiḥmárr*, yiḥmárr* to be (or become) red; blush
ʕiḥmiráar* (v.n.) reddening; blushing
ʕíḥna we
ʕiḥtáag, yiḥtáag (li) to need
ʕiḥtáram*, yiḥtírim to revere
ʕiḥtifáal (v.n.), ʕiḥtifaláat celebration
ʕiḥtiyáag (v.n.), ʕiḥtiyagáat need
ʕiid (f.), ʕayáadi hand
ʕiktáʃaf, yiktíʃif to discover
ʕil the
ʕiláah god
ʕilla except
ʕilléela (see léela)
ʕílli who, which (relative)
ʕimáan faith
ʕimbáariḥ yesterday
  ʕáwwil imbáariḥ the day before yesterday
ʕímta when?
ʕimtáar (see mitr)

ʕimtádd, yimtádd to stretch (intr.)
ʕimtiḥáan (v.n.), ʕimtiḥanáat examination
ʕin (kaan) if
  ʕin ʃáaʕ alláah I hope (lit. if God willed)
ʕináara* lighting
ʕinbásaṭ,[1] yinbísiṭ to be pleased
ʕindáhal, yindíhil to be shocked (by unexpected event)
ʕindáhaʃ, yindíhiʃ to be surprised
ʕinfágar*, yinfígir to explode
ʕinfátaḥ, yinfítiḥ to open (intr.)
ʕinfigáar* (v.n.), ʕinfigaráat* explosion
ʕingilíizi, ʕingiliziyya, ʕingiliziyyíin, ʕingilíiz English, Englishman
ʕingiltíra* England
ʕinkásar*, yinkísir to be broken, break
ʕinn that
ʕinnahárda today
ʕinnáma but, nevertheless
ʕinsáan man, human being
ʕínta (m.s.) you
ʕintáag (v.n.) production
ʕintáha, yintíhi to end
ʕintáqal, yintíqil (see ʕitnáqal)
ʕintáxab, yintíxib to elect
ʕintázar, yintízir to expect
ʕínti (f.s.) you
ʕintiháaʕ (v.n.) end
ʕintizáar (v.n.) expectancy
ʕíntu (pl.) you
ʕinʃálla[2] I hope
ʕiqtiṣáad† economics
ʕiqtiṣáadi†, ʕiqtiṣadíyya†, ʕiqtiṣadiyyíin† economic; economist
ʕiskindiríyya Alexandria
ʕisláam Islam
ʕisláami, ʕislamíyya, ʕislamiyyíin Islamic
ʕism, ʕasáami name
ʕisraʕíil* (f.) Israel
ʕisraʕíili*, ʕisraʕilíyya*, ʕisraʕiliyyíin* Israeli
ʕistáahil, yistáahil to be worthy of
ʕistábʃar*, yistábʃar* to be delighted at

---

[1] Pronounced ʕimb-.
[2] 'Back' a's. See also under ʕin.

Ɂistáfham, yistáfham to inquire
Ɂistáhlak, yustáhlak to be consumed
Ɂistáhlik, yistáhlik to consume
Ɂistaḥámma, yistaḥámma to bathe, take a bath
Ɂistaḥáqq, yistaḥáqq to deserve
Ɂistákfa, yistákfa to be satisfied
Ɂistálam, yistílim to receive
Ɂistamárr*, yistamírr to continue
Ɂistánna, yistánna to wait
Ɂistaqáal, yistaqíil to resign
Ɂistaráyyaḥ, yistaráyyaḥ to rest
Ɂistáxdim, yistáxdim to employ
Ɂistáxrag, yistáxrag to extract
Ɂistáʕzin, yistáʕzin to ask permission
  ʕastáʕzin excuse me
Ɂistaɤádd, yistaɤídd to be ready
Ɂistáɤgil, yistáɤgil to hurry
Ɂistáɤlim, yistáɤlim to inquire
Ɂistáɤmil, yistáɤmil to use
Ɂistáɤrab*, yistáɤrab* to be surprised
Ɂistíbna, Ɂistibnáat spare wheel
Ɂistihláak (v.n.) consumption
Ɂistimáara*, Ɂistimaráat* application form
Ɂistiqláal independence
Ɂistixráag* (v.n.) extraction
Ɂistiʃáara*, Ɂistiʃaráat* advice, consultation
Ɂistiʃáari, Ɂistiʃaríyya, Ɂistiʃariyyíin advisory
Ɂistiɤdáad (v.n.) readiness
Ɂistiɤláam (v.n.), Ɂistiɤlamáat inquiry
Ɂistiɤmáal (v.n.), Ɂistiɤmaláat use
Ɂiswádd, yiswádd to be (or become) black
Ɂiswid, sóoda, ṣuud black
Ɂiṣáaba, Ɂiṣabáat injury
Ɂiṣmárr, yiṣmárr to be (or become) brown
Ɂiṣṭáad, yiṣṭáad to hunt
  Ɂiṣṭaad samak to fish
Ɂiṣṭiláaḥ, Ɂiṣṭilaḥáat expression
Ɂitdáawa, yitdáawa (pron. Ɂidd-) to be treated (medically)
Ɂitfáahim, yitfáahim to come to an understanding
Ɂitfáḍḍal, Ɂitfaḍḍáli, Ɂitfaḍḍálu please (as invitation)
Ɂitfárrag*, yitfárrag* to go around (the sights)

Ɂitfáṣal, yitfíṣil to be discharged
Ɂitgánnin, yitgánnin (pron. Ɂidg- or Ɂigg-) to go mad
Ɂitgáwwiz, yitgáwwiz (pron. Ɂidg- or Ɂigg-) to be married
Ɂitḥáal, yitḥáal (ɤalmaɤáaʃ) to retire
Ɂitḥábas, yitḥíbis to be imprisoned
Ɂitḥássin, yitḥássin to improve (intr.)
Ɂitkábbar*, yitkábbar* to be proud, self-opinionated
Ɂitkállim, yitkállim to speak
Ɂitlámm, yitlámm to assemble (intr.)
Ɂitláxbaṭ, yitláxbaṭ to be confused
Ɂitmáttaɤ, yitmáttaɤ (bi) to enjoy
Ɂitmáʃʃa, yitmáʃʃa to go for a walk
Ɂitnáaqiʃ, yitnáaqiʃ to discuss
Ɂitnéen two
Ɂitqáddim, yitqáddim to make progress; be brought
Ɂitqáwwa, yitqáwwa to become strong; make progress
Ɂitráaḍa, yitráaḍa to be satisfied, reconciled, to agree
Ɂitráqqa, yitráqqa to get on, progress
Ɂitráṣaf, yitríṣif to be made up (e.g. road)
Ɂitsáahil, yitsáahil (pron. Ɂits- or Ɂiss-) to be easy-going, tolerant
Ɂitságan, yitsígin (pron. Ɂits- or Ɂiss-) to be imprisoned
Ɂitsálax, yitsílix (pron. Ɂits- or Ɂiss-) to be skinned
Ɂittáakil, yittáakil to be edible; be eaten
Ɂittáfaq, yittífiq to agree
Ɂittákal, yittíkil (ɤala) to rely (on)
Ɂittiḥáad, Ɂittiḥadáat union
Ɂittállaɤ, yittállaɤ (pron. Ɂiṭṭ-) to peer
Ɂitwáffa, yitwáffa to die, pass away
Ɂitxáaniq, yitxáaniq to quarrel
Ɂitxálla, yitxálla (ɤan) to give up
Ɂitzábaṭ, yitzíbiṭ (pron. Ɂidẓ- or Ɂizẓ-) to be caught (out)
Ɂitʃáɤlil, yitʃáɤlil (pron. Ɂitʃ- or Ɂiʃʃ-) to flare up (fire)
Ɂitɤállim, yitɤállim to learn
Ɂitɤáʃʃa, yitɤáʃʃa to dine
Ɂitɤáʃʃim, yitɤáʃʃim to hope
Ɂityádda, yityádda (pron. Ɂidy-) to lunch
Ɂiṭálya Italy

ʕíwᶻa, ʕíwᶻi, ʕíwᶻu take care!
ʕixtáar*, yixtáar* to choose, elect
ʕixtálaf, yixtílif to differ
ʕixtiláaf (v.n.) difference
ʕixtiṣáaṣ, ʕixtiṣaṣáat responsibility
ʕixtiyáar* (v.n.) selection, choice
ʕixtizáal (v.n.) shorthand
ʕiyyáak, ʕiyyáaki, ʕiyyáaku beware
  . . . !; perhaps
ʕiza (kaan) if
ʕizáaz glass
ʕizáaᶻa broadcasting
ʕizn permission
  ʕíznĭ baríid (pl. ʕuzunáat b.)
  postal order
ʕiʃáara*, ʕiʃaráat* sign
ʕiʃtára*, yiʃtíri to buy
ʕiʃtáɤal, yiʃtáɤal to work
ʕiᵹtáqad, yiᵹtíqid to be sure, con-
  vinced
ʕiᵹtáraf*, yiᵹtírif to confess
ʕiᵹtidáal mildness
ʕiᵹtiráaf* (v.n.), ʕiᵹtirafáat* confession
ʕóoḍa, ʕúwaḍ or ʕíwaḍ room
ʕúgra* rate, rate of pay; hire
ʕuktóobar* October
ʕumm, ʕummaháat mother
ʕummáal[1] certainly; then, so
ʕumnubúus, ʕumnubusáat (see
  ʕutubíis)
ʕurúbba Europe
ʕurúbbi, ʕurubbíyya, ʕurubbiyyíin
  European
ʕusbúuᵹ (or ʕisbúuᵹ), ʕasabíiᵹ week
ʕúsra*, ʕúsar* family
ʕustáaz, ʕasádza learned man, professor
ʕúṣṭa, ʕuṣṭawáat artisan; term of
  address
ʕutubíis, ʕutubisáat bus
ʕúxra* (see ʕáaxar)
ʕuxt, ʕixwáat sister
ʕuɤníya (or ʕuɤníyya), ʕaɤáani song

ʃ

ʃaaf, yiʃúuf to see
ʃaal, yiʃíil to carry, take away
ʃáara*, ʃaráat* badge, emblem
ʃáariᵹ, ʃawáariᵹ street
ʃáaṭir, ʃáṭra, ʃuṭṭáar clever

ʃaay tea
(ʕin) ʃáaʕ alláah (see ʕin)
ʃáaɤil, ʃáɤla, ʃaɤlíin worrying
ʃababíik (see ʃibbáak)
ʃábaka, ʃabakáat or ʕiʃbíka net
ʃabbúura* mist, haze
ʃadd, yiʃídd to pull
ʃáfa, yíʃfi to recover (from illness)
ʃágar* (c.), ʃágara*, ʃagaráat*,
  ʃaʃgáar* trees
ʃaháada, ʃahadáat certificate; testimony
ʃáhhil, yiʃáhhil to hurry up
ʃahíyya appetite
ʃahr*, ʃuhúur or ʕáʃhur month
  ʕiʃʃáhr illi fáat/gáay last/next
  month
ʃáhri, ʃahríyya, ʃahriyyíin monthly
  (adj.)
ʃahríyyan monthly (adv.)
ʃáḥan, yíʃḥin to load
ʃáḥat, yíʃḥat to beg
ʃaḥḥáat, ʃaḥḥatíin beggar
ʃáḥḥat, yiʃáḥḥat to give (to beggar)
ʃáḥḥim, yiʃáḥḥim to grease
ʃaḥm, ʃuḥumáat grease
ʃaḥn (v.n.) loading
ʃákar*, yúʃkur to thank
  ʃaʃkúrak* thank you
ʃakk, ʃukúuk doubt
  ma fíiʃ ʃákk doubtless
ʃakl, ʕaʃkáal shape; type
ʃákwa, ʃakáawi complaint
ʃamáal north (of)
ʃamm, yiʃímm to smell
ʃammáaᶻa, ʃammaᶻáat (clothes-)
  hanger
ʃams (f.) sun
  ɤurúub iʃʃáms sunset
  ṭulúuᵹ iʃʃáms sunrise
ʃámsi, ʃamsíyya sunny
ʃamsíyya, ʃamáasi parasol
ʃámᶻa, ʃamᶻáat candle
ʃánab, ʕaʃnáab moustache
ʃánṭa, ʃúnaṭ bag, case; (car-)boot
ʃáqi, ʃaqíyya, ʃaʃqíya rude, naughty;
  criminal
ʃaqíiq, ʃúqaqa blood brother
ʃáqqa, ʃúqaq flat
ʃaráab*, ʃarabáat* pair of socks,
  stockings
ʃariif, ʃariifa, ʕaʃráaf* or ʃúrafa*
  unsullied; of good character

----
[1] 'Back' aa.

ʃaríik, ʃúraka* partner
ʃarq east
  ʔiʃʃárq† ilʕáwṣaṭ the Middle East
  ʔiʃʃárq† ilʕádna the Near East
ʃárqi, ʃarqíyya, ʃarqiyyíin eastern, easterner
ʃarr*, ʃurúur evil
ʃárraf*, yiʃárraf* to honour
ʃarṭ, ʃurúuṭ condition
  ɣala ʃárṭi ʔinn . . . on condition that
ʃaṭáara* cleverness
ʃáxaṭ, yíʃxuṭ (fi) to shout at
ʃaxṣ, ʕaʃxáaṣ person
ʃáxṣi, ʃaxṣíyya personal, private
  biṭáaqit taḥqíiq iʃʃaxṣíyya identity card
ʃawíiʃ, ʃawiʃíyya sergeant; policeman
ʃayyáal, ʃayyalíin porter
ʃayɣáal, ʃayɣáala, ʃayɣalíin hard-working; working (of machine)
ʃáyɣal, yiʃáyɣal to work, operate
ʃeex, ʃiyúux sheikh
ʃeeʕ, ʕáʃya thing
  ʃéeʕ yaríib! extraordinary!
  kúlli ʃéeʕ everything
ʃibbáak, ʃababíik window
ʃíbiɣ, yíʃbaɣ to have enough, be satisfied
ʃidíid, ʃidíida, ʃudáad strong
ʃíhid, yíʃhad to bear witness
ʃiik, ʃikáat cheque
ʃimáal left
ʃíra (v.n.) buying
ʃiráaɣi*, ʃiraɣíyya* sailing (of ship)
ʃírib, yíʃrab* to drink
ʃírka, ʃarikáat company
ʃíta winter
ʃóoka, ʃúwak fork
ʃukr (v.n.) thanks
  maɣa-ʃʃúkr thank you
ʃúkran* thank you
ʃurb (v.n.) drinking
ʃúrba soup
ʃuwáyya a little, rather
ʃuyl, ʕaʃɣáal work
ʃúyla, ʃúyal job

ع

ɣáada, ɣadáat custom, habit
  filɣáada usually

ɣaag ivory
ɣáahid, yiɣáahid to vow, promise
ɣáakis, yiɣáakis to quarrel; argue
ɣaal! fine!
ɣáali, ɣálya, ɣalyíin high
ɣaam, yiɣúum to swim
ɣaam, ʕaɣwáam year
ɣáamil, ɣummáal workman
ɣáaṣif, ɣawáaṣif storm
ɣáawiz, ɣáwza, ɣawzíin wanting (to)
ɣáayiz, ɣáyza, ɣayzíin (see ɣáawiz)
ɣa(a)ʕíli,¹ ɣa(a)ʕilíyya family (adj.)
ɣaaʃ, yiɣíiʃ to live
ɣáaʃir, ɣáʃra tenth
ɣáda, yíɣdi to infect
ɣádad, ʕaɣdáad number
ɣádam
  fi (or li) ɣádam wugúud . . . in the absence of . . .
ɣadátan usually
ɣadd, yiɣídd to count
ɣádda, yiɣáddi to cross; lead (animal)
ɣaddáad, ɣaddadáat meter
ɣaḍḍ, yiɣúḍḍ to bite (usually of animal)
ɣaḍm (c.), ɣáḍma, ɣaḍmáat bone
ɣafw
  ʔilɣáfw don't mention it
ɣafʃ luggage, kit; furniture
ɣágab, yíɣgib to please
  ʕanhú-lli ɣágabak? which one did you like?
ɣágal
  bilɣágal fast, quickly
ɣágala, ɣagaláat or ɣágal wheel; bicycle
ɣágalit issiwáaqa steering-wheel
ɣágami, ɣagamíyya, ɣágam Persian
ɣagúuz, ɣagúuza, ɣagáayiz old
ɣála on
  ɣala féen? where are you going?
  ɣala kída therefore
  ɣala kúllï ḥáal in any case
  ɣala máhlak slowly
  ɣala ṭúul at once, straight away
  ɣaláyya-lḥisáab the bill's on me
  ɣaléek tirúuḥ you ought to go
  ɣalʕaqáll at least
  ma ɣaléhʃ never mind, it doesn't matter

_____
¹ See Part I, Appendix B, note (c).

ɛaláaqat, ɛalaqáatǂ relation, correlation

ʕilɛalaqáat iṣṣinaɛíyya industrial relations

ʕilɛalaqáat iddaxlíyya interior relations

ʕilɛalaqáat ilɛáamma public relations

ɛálam, ʕaɛláam flag

ɛalaʃáan for; in order to; because

ɛalaʃáanak since it's you, for your sake

ɛállaq, yiɛállaq to hang, suspend

ɛállim, yiɛállim to teach; mark

ɛámal, yíɛmil to do, make

ɛámal (v.n.) doing

ɛámal, ʕaɛmáal work

ɛamalíyya, ɛamaliyyáat operation, procedure

ɛá(a)mm,[1] ɛá(a)mma[1] public, general

ɛamm, ʕaɛmáam (paternal) uncle

ʕíbnĭ ɛámmĭ my cousin (paternal)

ɛámma, ɛammáat (paternal) aunt

ɛammáal

ɛammáal yiʃtáɣal he is working

ɛá(a)mmi,[1] ɛammíyya, ɛawá(a)mm[1] or ɛammiyyíin ignorant

ɛan concerning; from; than

yixtílfu ɛan báɛḍ they differ from each other

ʕinnahárḍa-kwáyyis ɛan imbáariḥ it's nicer today than yesterday

ɛand with, in the possession of

ɛándak báxt (or ḥáẓẓ) you are lucky

ɛándak ḥáqq you are right

ʕilkóora* ɛand-ahámmĭ mittínis I prefer football to tennis

ɛándĭ ma + v. as soon as, at the time that

ɛaqd, ɛuqúud contract

ɛaql, ɛuqúul mind

ɛáqrab*, ɛaqáarib spider

ɛárabi*, ɛarabíyya*, ɛárab* Bedouin, Arab

ʕilḥurúuf ilɛarabíyya the Arabic alphabet

(ʕil)ɛárabi* Arabic

[1] See Part I, Appendix B, note (c).

ɛarabíyya*, ɛarabiyyáat* car, vehicle

ɛarabíyya malláaki private car

ɛáraq sweat; dampness

ɛarbági*, ɛarbagíyya* gharry-driver

ɛardiḥáal, ɛardiḥaláat petition

ɛardiḥálgi, ɛardiḥalgíyya scribe

ɛaríiḍ*, ɛaríiḍa*, ɛuráaḍ broad

ɛaríiḍa*, ɛaráayiḍ* petition

ɛárraf*, yiɛárraf* to explain

ɛasáakir (see ɛaskári)

ɛásal honey

ɛaskári, ɛasáakir soldier; policeman

ɛáṣab, ʕaɛṣáab muscle

ɛaṣr, ɛuṣúur era, age

ɛáṣri, ɛaṣríyya, ɛaṣriyyíin modern

(ma) ɛatʃ, no longer

ma ɛátʃĭ fíih there isn't any more

ɛátaʃ thirst

ɛáṭṭal, yiɛáṭṭal to delay, keep waiting

ɛaṭʃáan (or ɛaṭʃáan), ɛaṭʃáana, ɛaṭʃaníin thirsty

ɛáwwaḍ, yiɛáwwaḍ to compensate

ɛáwwar*, yiɛáwwar* to injure

ɛáyli (see ɛa(a)ʕíli)

ɛayyáan, ɛayyáana, ɛayyaníin ill

ɛáyyaṭ, yiɛáyyaṭ to cry, wail

ɛáyyid, yiɛáyyid to feast, make merry

ɛáyyil, ɛayyíla, ɛiyáal child

ṣáaḥib ɛiyáal family man

ɛáyyin, yiɛáyyin to appoint

ɛayzíin (see ɛáayiz)

ɛázam, yíɛzim to invite

ɛaẓíim, ɛaẓíima, ɛuẓamáaʕ mighty, wonderful, extraordinary

ɛaʕíli (see ɛa(a)ʕíli)

ɛáʃa dinner

ɛaʃáan (see ɛalaʃáan)

ɛáʃar*, ɛáʃara* ten

ɛeeb, ɛuyúub shame, shameful act

ɛéeb ɛaléek! shame on you!

ɛéela, ɛeláat family

ɛeen (f.), ɛiyúun eye

ɛeeʃ bread

lúqmit ɛéeʃ a piece of bread

ɛéeʃ báladi local bread

ɛéeʃ afrángi* European bread

ɛídda, ɛídad engine

ɛiid, ʕaɛyáad feast, festival

ɛíid iddiḥíyya or ʕilɛíid ikkibíir Qurban Bairam

ɛíid ilfíṭr or ʕilɛíid iṣṣuɣáyyar* Ramadan Bairam

ɡílba, ɡílab packet, small box
ɡimáara*, ɡimaráat* building
ɡínab (c.), ḥabbáayit ɡ., ḥabbáat ɡ.
   grapes
ɡírif, yíɡraf* to know
ɡiyáada, ɡiyadáat (doctor's) surgery
ɡízba, ɡízab farm
(ʕil)ɡíʃa evening(-prayer)
ɡiʃríin twenty
ɡoom (v.n.) swimming
ɡudw, ʕaɡdáaʕ member; part (of
   body)
ɡúmda, ɡúmad headman
ɡummáal (see ɡáamil)
ɡumr life; age
   ɡumri ma ... ʃ I have never ...
ɡumúumi, ɡumumíyya, ɡumu-
   miyyíin general, public
ɡurd̟ (or ɡard̟) breadth, width
ɡuzúuma, ɡazáayim party
ɡuʃr, ʕaɡʃáar* or ʕiɡʃáar* one-
   tenth

ɣ

ɣaab, yiɣíib to be absent, go away
ɣáali, ɣálya, ɣalyíin dear
   ɣáali ɡaláyya too dear for me
ɣáamid̟, ɣámd̟a not clear, illegible
ɣáaya, ɣayáat purpose, aim
   lilɣáaya extremely
   liɣáayit ma + v. until
   liɣáayit + n. as far as, up to
ɣáayib, ɣáyba, ɣaybíin absent
ɣaaz gas
ɣáda lunch
ɣafíir, ɣúfara* watchman
ɣála expense, high cost of living
ɣála, yíɣli to boil
ɣálab, yíɣlib to beat, defeat

ɣalt̟áan, ɣalt̟áana, ɣalt̟aníin mistaken
ɣáni, ɣaníyya, ʕayníya rich
ɣánna, yiɣánni to sing
ɣaráaba*
   ʕilɣaráaba-nn ... the strange thing
   is that ...
ɣárad̟, ʕaɣráad̟ object, purpose
ɣarb* west
ɣárbi*, ɣarbíyya*, ɣarbiyyíin*
   western, westerner
(ʕil)ɣardáqa Hurghada (place name)
ɣaríib, ɣaríiba, ɣúraba* strange,
   stranger
ɣásal, yíɣsil to wash
ɣasíil (v.n.) washing; things for washing
ɣáṣbin ɡan + p.s. willy-nilly, in spite
   of
ɣát̟a, yut̟ɣáan cover
ɣáyyar*, yiɣáyyar* to change
ɣazáal, ɣizláan gazelle
ɣázal, yíɣzil to spin
ɣazl (v.n.) spinning
ɣaʃíim, ɣaʃíima, ɣuʃm silly, simpleton
ɣaʃʃ, yiɣíʃʃ to swindle
ɣaʃʃáaʃ, ɣaʃʃáaʃa, ɣaʃʃaʃíin swindler
ɣeer just, only; other
   márkib ɣérha a different ship
   ma ʃúfti ɣer húwwa I only saw
   him
   min ɣéer without
   min ɣéer ma + v. without
ɣeet̟, ɣet̟áan field
ɣíd̟ib, yíɣd̟ab to be(come) angry
ɣíli, yíɣla to be(come) expensive
ɣílit̟, yíɣlat̟ to (make a) mistake
ɣubáar* dust
ɣuráab*, ɣiríba (or ʕiɣríba) or
   ɣirbáan crow

VOCABULARY
ENGLISH–ARABIC

Note. See introductory notes to Arabic–English
section for order of Arabic entries, abbreviations
used, &c.

ENGLISH-ARABIC

a

able *to* qáadir, qádra, qadríin
to be able qídir, yíqdar*
about (concerning) ʒan; (surrounding) ḥawaléen; (approximately) ḥawáali, taqríiban, zayy
to be about *to* qárrab* (+ *impf.*)
above fooq
in the absence *of* fi (*or* li) ʒádam wugúud ...
absent ɣáayib, ɣáyba, ɣaybíin
to be absent ɣaab, yiɣíib
accident ḥádsa, ḥawáadis
according to ḥásab
account ḥisáab, ḥisabáat
accustomed (to) mitʒáwwid, mitʒawwída, mitʒawwidíin (ʒala)
to ache wágaʒ, yíwgaʒ
I've a headache ráasi*-btiwgáʒni
acre faddáan, fadadíin
to add ʕaḍáaf, yuḍíif
to administer daar*, yidíir
administration ʕidáara*
advantage fáyda, fawáayid
advice ʕistiʃáara*, ʕistiʃaráat*; muʃáwra*, muʃawráat*
to advise náṣaḥ, yínṣaḥ
advisory ʕistiʃáari, ʕistiʃaríyya, ʕistiʃariyyíin
aeroplane ṭayyáara*, ṭayyaráat*
to be afraid xaaf, yixáaf
after baʒd; báʒdi ma (+ *v.*)
(*this*) afternoon baʒd iḍḍúhr
afterwards baʒdéen
again táani, márra* tánya
against ḍidd; (beside) gamb
age sinn; ʒumr; (era) ʒaṣr, ʒuṣúur
agent wakíil, wúkala; mutʒáhhid, mutʒahhidíin
ago
  two hours ago min (múddit) saʒtéen
  she went to the market two hours ago híyya fissúuq láha saʒtéen
to agree ʕittáfaq, yittífiq
agricultural ziráaʒi,[1] ziraʒíyya[1]
agriculture ziráaʒa[1]

[1] 'Back' or 'front' *aa.*

air gaww; háwa
airfield maṭáar, maṭaráat
Alexandria ʕiskindiríyya
alike záyyi báʒḍ
all kull; gamíiʒ
  all of it kúllu(h)
  that's all! xaláaṣ!
all right ṭáyyib
to be allowed *to*
  are you allowed to go? gayízlak (*or* yigúzlak) tirúuḥ?
alms ḥásana, ḥasanáat
to give alms zákka, yizákki
almsdeeds záka
alone li waḥd + *p.s.*; bass
also kamáan; ʕáyḍan; bárḍu(h)
although maʒʕínn
always tamálli, dáyman
a.m. qabl iḍḍúhr; ṣabáaḥan
amber kahramáan*
American ʕamrikáani (*or* ʕamríiki), ʕamrik(an)íyya, ʕamrik(an)iyyíin *or* ʕamrikáan
among fi; min; been
  from among min ḍímn ...
amount máblaɣ, mabáaliɣ
amusement málha, maláahi
and wi
anger záʒal
angry zaʒláan, zaʒláana, zaʒlaníin; munfáʒil, munfáʒila, munfaʒilíin
to be(come) angry (with) zíʒil, yízʒal (min); yíḍib, yíɣḍab
animal bihíima, baháayim; ḥayawáan, ḥayawanáat
ankle káʒab, ʕakʒáab *or* kuʒúub
annual sanáawi, sanawíyya, sanawiyyíin
another (*see* other)
answer gawáab, ʕagwíba; radd*, rudúud
to answer gáawib, yigáawib
to answer back náaqir, yináaqir; radd*, yirúdd (ʒala)
antique ʕantíika, ʕantikáat
any ʕayy
anyone ḥadd; ʕáyyi wáaḥid
anyway ʒala kúlli ḥáal
apparently yíẓhar inn ...
appetite ʃahíyya

apples[1] tiffáaḥ (c.), tiffáaḥa, tiffaḥáat
application ṭálab, ṭalabáat; (putting into practice) taṭbíiq
application-form ʕistimáara*, ʕistimaráat*
to **appoint** ɣáyyin, yiɣáyyin
appointment maɣáad, mawaɣíid; muqábla, muqabláat
to **approach** qárrab*, yiqárrab*
approximately (*see* about)
apricots míʃmiʃ (c.), miʃmíʃa *or* miʃmiʃáaya, miʃmiʃáat
April ʕabríil (*or* ʕibríil)
Arab(ic) ɣárabi*, ɣarabíyya*, ɣárab* the **Arabic alphabet** ʕilḥurúuf ilɣarabíyya
area manṭíqa, manáaṭiq
to **argue** (*with*) gáadil, yigáadil; náakif, yináakif
arguing gidáal
arm diráaɣ
armpit baaṭ, baṭáat
army geeʃ, giyúuʃ
around (*see* about)
to **arrange** ráttib, yiráttib; raṣṣ, yirúṣṣ
arrangement tartíib; niẓáam
to **arrest** qábaḍ, yíqbaḍ (ɣala)
arrival wuṣúul
to **arrive** wíṣil (*or* wáṣal), yíwṣal
art fann, funúun
artisan ɣáamil, ɣummáal; ʕúṣṭa, ʕuṣṭawáat
as zayy
as for . . . ʕámma . . .; min gíhat . . .
as if kaʕínn
ashamed maksúuf, maksúufa, maksufíin
to be **ashamed** xígil, yíxgal
ash-tray ṭaqṭúuqa, ṭaqaṭíiq
to **ask** sáʕal, yísʕal
to **ask for** ṭálab, yúṭlub
asleep náayim, náyma, naymíin
asphalt ʕasfált
assistant muɣáawin (*or* mi-), muɣáwna, muɣawníin; musáaɣid (*or* mi-), musáɣda, musaɣdíin
attractive gamíil, gamíila, gumáal
auction mabíiɣ, mabiɣáat
August ʕaɣúṣṭuṣ

---

[1] Final italic *s* indicates a collective in Arabic.

aunt (paternal) ɣámma, ɣammáat; (maternal) xáala, xaláat
auspicious múfriḥ, mufríḥa, mufriḥíin
autumn xaríif
aviation ṭayaráan*
axe bálṭa, balṭáat

b

baby ṭifl, ʕaṭfáal
back ḍahr, ḍuhúur
to get **back** (*see* **return**)
bad baṭṭáal, baṭṭáala, baṭṭalíin; wíḥiʃ, wíḥʃa, wiḥʃíin
badge ʃáara*, ʃaráat*; niʃáan, nayaʃíin
bag ʃánṭa, ʃúnaṭ
(Qurban) Bairam ɣíid ilfíṭr, ʕil ɣíid iṣṣuɣáyyar*
(Ramadan) Bairam ɣíid iḍḍiḥíyya, ʕil ɣíid ikkibíir
baksheesh baqʃíiʃ
ball kóora*, kúwar* (*or* kíwar*)
bananas mooz (c.), móoza *or* mozáaya, mozáat
to **bandage** rábaṭ, yúrbuṭ
bank bank, binúuk; (river) ḍáffa, ḍifáaf; náḥya, nawáaḥi
bankrupt mifállis, mifallísa, mifallisíin
bar baar*, baráat*
barber ḥalláaq, ḥallaqíin; mizáyyin, mizayyiníin
barefooted ḥáafi, ḥáfya, ḥafyíin
to **bargain** fáaṣil, yifáaṣil
bargaining fiṣáal, fiṣaláat
to **bark** hábhab,[2] yiḥábhab[2]
barrel barmíil, baramíil
base ʕasáas, ʕúsus
to **base** ʕássis, yiʕássis
basic ʕasáasi, ʕasasíyya, ʕasasiyyíin; ʕáṣli, ʕaṣlíyya, ʕaṣliyyíin
basin (metal) ṭiʃt, ʕiṭʃúut *or* ṭuʃúut; (earthenware) magúur, mawagíir
basis ʕasáas, ʕúsus
basket sábat, ʕisbíta
bath ḥammáam, ḥammamáat
to **bathe** ʕistaḥámma, yistaḥámma
bathroom (*as* **bath**)
to be kaan, yikúun; báqa, yíbqa
be a man! xallíik ráagil*!

---

[2] 'Back' *a*'s.

beans faṣúlya (c.), ḥabbáayit f.,
ḥabbáat f.; fuul (c.), ḥábbit or
ḥabbáayit f., ḥabbáat f.
to bear ḥámal, yíḥmil; (give birth)
wíldit, tíwlid
beard daqn (f.), duqúun
to beat ḍárab, yíḍrab; (defeat) ɣálab,
yíɣlib; (carpet) náffaḍ, yináffaḍ
beautiful gamíil, gamíila, gumáal
because li؟ánn; ҳa(la)ʃáan; madáam
to become ṣaar, yiṣíir; báqa, yíbqa
bed siríir, saráayir
Bedouin bádawi, badawíyya, badw;
ҳárabi*, ҳarabíyya*, ҳárab*
bedroom ؟óḍt innóom, ؟úwaḍ
innóom
beer bíira
bees naḥl (c.), náḥla, naḥláat
before qabl; qáblī ma (+ v.)
to beg ʃáḥat, yíʃḥat
beggar ʃaḥḥáat, ʃaḥḥatíin
to begin ؟ibtáda, yibtídi
beginning ؟ibtída (or ؟ibtidáa؟)
Behera (province) ؟ilbiḥéera
behind wára*
to believe sáddaq, yisáddaq
believing tasdíiq
bell gáras*, ؟agráas*
belonging to bitáaҳ, bitáҳt, bitúuҳ;
tábaҳ
beside gamb; gáanib
best ؟áḥsan
better ؟áḥsan
you'd better go ؟il؟áḥsan tirúuḥ
between been
bicycle baskalítta (or biskilítta),
baskalittáat; ҳágala, ҳagaláat or
ҳágal
big kibíir, kibíira, kubáar*
bill faṭúura, fawaṭíir; ḥisáab, ḥisabáat
bird ṭeer, ṭuyúur
birth miláad, mawalíid
to bite qáṭam, yúqṭum; ҳaḍḍ, yiҳúḍḍ
bitumen bitumíin
black ؟íswid, sóoda, suud
to be(come) black ؟iswádd, yiswádd
to blame laam, yilúum; (rebuke)
wábbax, yiwábbax
to bless báarik, yibáarik
blessing báraka*, barakáat*
blind ؟áҳma, ҳámya, ҳumy
to block sadd, yisídd
blood damm

blow ḍárba, ḍarbáat
blue ؟ázraq, zárqa, zurq
to blush ؟iḥmárr*, yiḥmárr*
blushing ؟iḥmiráar*
board looḥ, ؟alwáaḥ
to boil ɣála, yíɣli; (of milk) faar*,
yifúur
bones ҳaḍm (c.), ҳáḍma, ҳaḍmáat
book kitáab, kútub
to book ḥágaz, yíḥgiz
bookshop maktába, makáatib
born mawlúud, mawlúuda, mawludíin
to borrow ؟istálaf, yistílif
bottle ؟izáaza, ؟azáayiz
bound (obliged) malzúum, malzúuma, malzumíin
he is (in duty) bound to ... wáagib
ҳaléeh inn ...
box sandúuq, sanadíiq; (small box or
packet) ҳílba, ҳílab
boy wálad, wiláad or ؟awláad
brain muxx, ؟imxáax; dimáaɣ
branch farҳ*, furúuҳ
brass niḥáas; niḥáas áṣfar*
to bray náhhaq, yináhhaq
bread ҳéeʃ
European bread ҳéeʃ afrángi*
local bread ҳéeʃ báladi
breadth ҳurḍ (or ҳarḍ)
to break (tr.) kásar*, yíksar*; (intr.)
؟inkásar,* yinkísir
breakfast fuṭúur
to breakfast fíṭir, yífṭar
bridge kúbri, kabáari; (footbridge)
qanṭára, qanáaṭir
to bring gaab, yigíib; qáddim,
yiqáddim; ḥáḍḍar, yiḥáḍḍar
bring! haat (háati, háatu)!
broad ҳaríid*, ҳaríiḍa*, ҳuráaḍ
broadcasting ؟izáaҳa
broom maknása, makáanis
brother ؟axx, ؟ixwáat; (blood brother)
ʃaqíiq, ʃúqaqa
to be(come) brown ؟iṣmárr*, yiṣmárr*
brush fúrʃa, fúraʃ
to brush másaḥ, yímsaḥ bilfúrʃa
bucket gárdal, garáadil
buffaloes gamúus (c.), gamúusa,
gamusáat, gawamíis
buffet buféeh, bufeháat
bugs baqq (c.), baqqáaya, baqqáat
building bináaya, binayáat; ҳimáara*,
ҳimaráat*

bundle rábṭa, rúbaṭ
to **burn** ḥáraq, yíḥraq
bus Ꞩutubíis, Ꞩutubisáat
business tigáara*
busy maſɣúul, maſɣúula, maſɣulíin
but (wi)láakin; Ꞩinnáma; Ꞩámma
butcher gazzáar, gazzaríin
butter zíbda
button zuráar*, zaráayir*
to **buy** Ꞩiſtára*, yiſtíri
buying ſíra
by bi; (beside) gamb

c

cabbages kurúmb (c.), kurúmba *or* kurumbáaya, kurumbáat
café qáhwa, qaháawi
Cairene máṣri, maṣríyya, maṣriyyíin
Cairo maṣr (f.); Ꞩilqa(a)híra†
to **calculate** ḥásab, yíḥsib
to **call** náada, yináadi; (to name) sámma, yisámmi
called mitsámma, mitsammíya, mitsammiyíin
calm háadi, hádya, hadyíin
camel gámal, gimáal
camp (military) muẓáskar*, muẓaskaráat*
can ṣafíiḥa, ṣafáayiḥ
canal tírẓa, tíraẓ
the **Canal** Ꞩilqanáal†
candle ſámẓa, ſamẓáat
canteen mátẓam, maṭáaẓim
(skull-)cap ṭaqíyya, ṭawáaqi
car ẓarabíyya*, ẓarabiyyáat*
card biṭáaqa, biṭaqáat *or* baṭáayiq
care
    take care! xúd (*or* xálli) báalak!
to **take care** *of* xad, yáaxud (*or* xálla, yixálli) baal + *p.s.* + min . . .
carefree muṭmaꞨínn (*or* miṭ-), muṭmaꞨínna, muṭmaꞨinníin
to be **careful** *of* (as *to* **take care** *of*)
carpenter naggáar*, naggaríin*
carpet siggáada, sagagíid
carrots gázar (c.), gázara* *or* gazaráaya*, gazaráat*
to **carry** ḥámal, yíḥmil; ſaal, yiſíil
cart finṭáaz, fanaṭíiz; ẓarabíyya* kárru*, ẓarabiyyáat* kárru*
cashier ṣarráaf*, ṣarrafíin* *or* ṣayárfa*

cat qúṭṭa, qúṭaṭ
to. **catch** (grasp) mísik, yímsik; (train, &c.) líḥiq, yílḥaq
cauliflowers qarnabíiṭ* (c.), qarnabíiṭa*, qarnabiṭáat*
cause sábab, Ꞩasbáab
ceiling saqf
celebration Ꞩiḥtifáal, Ꞩiḥtifaláat
Centigrade ṣantigráad*
centimetre ṣantimítr, ṣantimitráat
centre wuṣṭ (*or* wiṣṭ), Ꞩawṣáaṭ; márkaz, maráakiz
certain (sure) mutaꞨákkid, mutaꞨakkída, mutaꞨakkidíin
for **certain** min ɣéer ſákk
certainly ḥáaḍir; bi kúlli mamnuníyya; Ꞩummáal[1]
certificate ſaháada, ſahadáat
chair kúrsi, karáasi
chance (opportunity) fúrṣa, fúraṣ; ṣúdfa
    by chance biṣṣúdfa
change (remainder) báaqi; (small coin) fákka
    keep the change! Ꞩilbáaqi ẓalaſáanak!
to **change** ɣáyyar*, yiɣáyyar*; (money) fakk, yifúkk
channel tírẓa, tíraẓ
chapter faṣl, fuṣúul
charcoal faḥm (c.), faḥmáaya,[2] faḥmáat
to **charge** (make pay) dáffaẓ, yidáffaẓ
cheap rixíiṣ, rixíiṣa, ruxáaṣ
to be(*come*) **cheap** ríxiṣ, yírxaṣ
to **cheat** ɣaſſ, yiɣíſſ; ḍíḥik, yídḥak (ẓala)
cheek xadd, xudúud
cheese gíbna
chemical (n.) kimawíyya, kimawiyyáat
chemical (adj.) kimáawi, kimawíyya
chemist kimáawi, kimawíyya, kimawiyyíin
cheque ſiik, ſikáat
chest ṣadr (*or* sidr)
to **chew** máday, yúmduɣ
chicken fárxa, firáax; katkúut, katakíit
chicken-farmer farárgi, farargíyya

---

[1] 'Back' aa.
[2] 'Piece of charcoal'.

child wálad, wiláad *or* Ŝawláad;
ƫáyyil, ƫayyíla, ƫiyáal; ṣábi,
ṣabíyya, ṣubyáan
chilli qárni* fílfil, qurúun fílfil
chin daqn (*f.*), duqúun
china ṣíini
China Ŝiṣṣíin (*f.*)
Chinese ṣíini, ṣiníyya, ṣiniyyíin
choice Ŝixtiyáar*
to choose náqqa, yináqqi; Ŝixtáar*,
yixtáar*
church kaníisa, kanáayis
cigar sigáara* zanúbya, sagáayir z.
cigarette sigáara*, sagáayir
citadel qálƫa
city madíina, múdun
class dáraga*, daragáat*
second-class dáraga-skúndu
clay ṭiin (*c.*), ṭíina *or* ḥíttit ṭ., ṭináat *or*
ḥítat ṭ.
clean niḍíif, niḍíifa, nuḍáaf
to clean náḍḍaf, yináḍḍaf
cleaning tanḍíif
clear ẓáahir, ẓáhra; (sky, &c.) ṣáafi,
ṣáfya; (weather) ṣaḥw, ṣáḥwa
clerk káatib, kátaba
chief clerk baʃkáatib
clever ʃáaṭir, ʃáṭra, ʃuṭṭáar
climate ṭaqs
clock sáaƫa, saƫáat
close (weather) káatim, kátma
to close qáfal, yíqfil
closed maqfúul, maqfúula, maqfulíin
cloth (table-) máfraʃ*, mafáariʃ;
(material) qumáaʃ
to clothe lábbis, yilábbis
clothes (*see* garment) hudúum;
maláabis; (way of dressing)
libs
clouds saḥáab (*c.*), saḥáaba, saḥabáat,
súḥub
club (social) náadi, nawáadi *or*
Ŝandíya
coal (*as* charcoal)
cockerel díik, diyúuk
coffee qáhwa
unsweetened coffee qáhwa sáada
well-sweetened coffee qáhwa
súkkar* ziyáada
cold (*n.*) bard; (weather only) sáqƫa;
(in head) zukáam
he caught cold xád bárd
cold (*adj.*) báarid, bárda, bardíin;

(living beings) bardáan, bardáana,
bardaníin
collar yáaqa, yaqáat
to collect gámaƫ, yígmaƫ; lamm,
yilímm; (*intr.*) Ŝitlámm, yitlámm
collecting gamƫ
collection (group) magmúuƫ, mag-
muƫáat
colour loon, Ŝalwáan
to come geh, yíigi
come on! yálla!¹
come here! taƫáala (taƫáali,
taƫáalu)!
to come out ṭíliƫ, yíṭlaƫ
coming (*n.*) migíyy
coming (*adj.*) gaay (*or* gayy), gáaya (*or*
gáyya), gayíin (*or* gayyíin)
commotion dáwʃa; xáwta
communication muwáʃla, muwaṣaláat *or* muwaṣláat
company ʃírka, ʃarikáat
in comparison *with* binnísba li . . .
compartment (railway) diwáan,
dawawíin
to compel ɣáṣab, yíɣṣib; ḍáyaṭ, yíḍyaṭ
he compelled me to do it ɣáṣab
ƫaláyya-nn aƫmílu(h)
to compensate ƫáwwaḍ, yiƫáwwaḍ
complaint ʃákwa, ʃakáawi
complete káamil, kámla, kamlíin
to complete kámmil, yikámmil
completely xáaliṣ; bilmárra*
completion takmíla
to compress ḍáyaṭ, yíḍyaṭ
condiments faláafil
condition ḥaal, Ŝaḥwáal; (pre-requi-
site) ʃarṭ, ʃurúuṭ; (tenet) farḍ,
faráaŜiḍ* (*or* faráayiḍ*)
on condition that . . . ƫala ʃárṭi
Ŝinn . . .
conduct síira
confectioner ḥalawáani, ḥalawaníyya
conference muŜtámar*, muŜ-
tamaráat*
to confess Ŝiƫtáraf*, yiƫtírif
confession Ŝiƫtiráaf*, Ŝiƫtirafáat*
to confuse láxbaṭ, yiláxbaṭ
to be confused Ŝitláxbaṭ, yitláxbaṭ
congratulations! mabrúuk!*
consultation muʃáwra*, muʃawráat*;
Ŝistiʃáara*, Ŝistiʃaráat*

¹ 'Back' *a*'s.

B 4979   R

container maٵúun, mawaٵíin; sahríig, saharíig
to **continue** Ꜥistamárr*, yistamírr
to **continue to** qáٵad, yúqٵud *or* fíȡil, yífȡal (+*impf.*)
contract ٵaqd, ٵuqúud
to **control** daar*, yidíir; ȥábaṭ, yíȥbuṭ
conversation muɦáwra* (*or* mi-), muɦawráat*
cook ṭabbáax, ṭabbaxíin
to **cook** ṭábax, yúṭbux
cooking ṭabx
to **cool** (*intr.*) bárad, yíbrad; (weather) ṭárra, yiṭárri
cooler (*n.*) mubarrída (*or* mi-), mubarridáat
copper niɦáas; niɦáas áɦmar*
to **copy** náqal, yínqil
copying naql
corner rukn, Ꜥarkáan*
correct ṣaɦíiɦ, ṣaɦíiɦa
to **correct** ṣáɦɦaɦ, yiṣáɦɦaɦ
to **cost** kállif, yikállif; (make lose) xáṣṣar, yixáṣṣar
   how much does this cost? dí-b káam?
cost of living maٵíiʃa, maٵáayiʃ
cotton quṭn, Ꜥaqṭáan
council máglis, magáalis
to **count** ٵadd, yiٵídd
to **count on** Ꜥiٵtámad, yiٵtímid (ٵala)
counting tiٵdáad
country bálad (*f.*), biláad; quṭr†, Ꜥaqṭáar†; (nation) dáwla, dúwal; (native land) wáṭan, Ꜥawṭáan; (countryside) ꜤilꜤaryáaf; barr*
course (instructional) birnáamig, baráamig
of **course** maٵlúum, mafhúum, ṭábٵan, &c.
cousin (paternal) Ꜥibnī ٵamm + *p.s.*; (maternal) Ꜥibnī xaal + *p.s.*
cover ɣáṭa, ɣuṭyáan; kiis, kiyáas
crab Ꜥábu galámbu
cream qíʃṭa, qíʃaṭ
crescent hiláal
criminal múgrim, mugríma, mugrimíin; ʃáqi, ʃaqíyya, Ꜥaʃqíya
crops ziráaٵa,[1] ziraٵáat[1]
to **cross** ٵádda, yiٵáddi

crow ɣuráab*, ɣiríba (*or* Ꜥiɣríba) *or* ɣirbáan
crowd záɦma
to **crowd** záaɦim, yizáaɦim
crown taag, tigáan
crude
   crude oil Ꜥizzéet ilxáam
cruel ȥáalim, ȥálma, ȥalmíin
cruelty ȥulm
to **cry** (weep) báka, yíbki; ٵáyyaṭ, yiٵáyyaṭ
cucumbers xiyáar* (*c.*), xiyáara* *or* xiyaráaya*, xiyaráat*
to **cultivate** záraٵ, yízraٵ
cultivation ziráaٵa[2] (*v.n.*)
cunning makkáar*, makkáara*, makkaríin*
cup fingáal (*or* fingáan), fanagíil (*or* fanagíin)
cupboard duláab, dawalíib
to **curse** sabb, yisíbb
curtain sitáara*, satáayir
cushion mixádda, mixaddáat
custom ٵáada, ٵadáat
customer zibúun, zibúuna, zabáayin
Customs (*or* **Customs building**) gúmruk, gamáarik
   to **pass through the Customs** marr*, yimurr bilgumruk
to **cut** qáṭaٵ, yíqṭaٵ; (hair) ɦálaq, yíɦlaq; (with scissors *or* shears) qaṣṣ, yiqúṣṣ; (slice) xáraṭ, yúxruṭ

d

to **damage** tálaf, yítlif
damp raṭb, ráṭba
dampness ruṭúuba
dancing raqṣ
danger xáṭar, Ꜥaxṭáar
to **get dark** dállim, yidállim
   it's getting dark Ꜥiddínya bitdállim[3]
darkness ḍaláam; ḍálma
date taríix, tawaríix
dawn fagr
day yoom, Ꜥayyáam *or* Ꜥiyyáam
   the day after tomorrow báٵdi búkra*

---

[1] 'Back' or 'front' *aa*

[2] 'Back' or 'front' *aa*.
[3] Pronounced *biḍḍ-*

in two days' time báɣdi báɣdi
búkra*
the other day, some days ago
díik (or dáak) innaháar*
these days liyyámdi
dead máyyit, mayyíta, mayyitíin or
ʕamwáat
deaf ʕáṭraʃ, ṭárʃa, ṭurʃ
dear ɣáali, ɣálya, ɣalyíin
(it's) too dear for me ɣáali ɣaláyya
to be(come) dear ɣíli, yíɣla
dearness ɣála
death moot
debt súlfa, súlaf; sálaf
December disímbir
declaration taṣríiḥ, taṣaríiḥ
to decorate záyyin, yizáyyin
decoration zíina; naqʃ
to decrease náqqaṣ, yináqqaṣ; qall,
yiqíll
to deduct xáṣam, yíxṣim
deed fiɣl, ʕafɣáal
degree dáraga*, daragáat*
to delay ʕáxxar*, yiʕáxxar*; ɣáttal,
yiɣáttal
delicate (fine) daqíiq
to be delighted ɣáqtat, yizáqtat;
ʕistábʃar*, yistábʃar*
to deliver sállim, yisállim; wáṣṣal,
yiwáṣṣal
the Delta ʕilwágh ilbáḥari
dentist ḥakíim ilʕasnáan (or lisnáan)
department qálamt, ʕaqláamt;
qismt, ʕaqsáamt; maṣláḥa,
maṣáaliḥ
departure (train, aircraft, &c.) qiyáam
deputy wakíil, wakíila, wúkala
to descend nízil, yínzil
desert ṣáḥra*, ṣaḥáara*
of the desert ṣaḥráawi*, ṣaḥrawíyya*,
ṣaḥrawiyyíin*
to deserve ʕistaḥáqq, yistaḥáqq
to desist (from) káffa, yikáffi (ɣan);
báttal, yibáttal
desk máktab, makáatib
in detail bittafṣíil
dialect láhga, lahgáat
diary mufakkíra* (or mifakkára*),
mufakkiráat*
to dictate (letter) málla, yimálli
to die maat, yimúut
he died of laughing máat ɣala
rúuḥu middíḥk

diesel díizil
to differ ʕixtálaf, yixtílif
difference farq, furúuq
different muxtálif, muxtálifa, muxtalifíin
difficult ṣaɣb, ṣáɣba, ṣaɣbíin
difficulty ṣuɣúuba, ṣuɣubáat; (problem) muʃkíla, maʃáakil
to dig ḥáfar*, yúḥfur
digging ḥafr*
to dine ʕitɣáʃʃa, yitɣáʃʃa
dining-table ṣúfra*, ṣúfar*
dinner ɣáʃa
to direct daar*, yidíir
direction (management) ʕidáara*
under the direction of tábaɣ
director mudíir, mudiríin
dirt(iness) wasáaxa
dirty wísix, wísxa, wisxíin
disagreeable báayix, báyxa, bayxíin
to discharge (see dismiss)
to discover káʃaf, yíkʃif; ʕiktáʃaf,
yiktíʃif
to discuss náaqiʃ, yináaqiʃ
discussion mináqʃa, minaqʃáat
disease márad, ʕamráad
dish ṣaḥn, ṣuḥúun
to dismiss ráfad, yírfid
dispensary ʕagzaxáana, ʕagzaxanáat
to disperse faḍḍ, yifúḍḍ
disposition níyya
dispute miɣáksa (or mu-), miɣaksáat
distance masáafa, masafáat; buɣd
at a distance of ... ɣala búɣd ...
distant biɣíid, biɣíida, buɣáad
distillation taqtíir
to distribute wázzaɣ, yiwázzaɣ; fárraq,
yifárraq
distribution tawzíiɣ
to divide qásam (or qísim), yíqsim;
qássim, yiqássim
to divorce tállaq, yitállaq
to do ɣámal, yíɣmil
doctor ḥakíim, ḥúkama; duktúur,
dakátra; tabíib, ʕatibbáaʕ
dog kalb, kiláab
doing ɣámal
donkey ḥumáar*, ḥimíir
door baab, ʕabwáab or bibáan
dossier duséeh, duseháat
dot núqta, núqat
doubt ʃakk, ʃukúuk
doubtless ma fíiʃ ʃákk; min ɣéer ʃákk

down(stairs) taht
dozen dásta, dísat
draft (letter) miswádda, miswaddáat
dragoman targumáan*, tarágma
drain mígra, magáari; máṣraf, maṣáarif
drapery kíswa, kasáawi
drawer durg, ʕadráag*
dress (lady's) fustáan, fasatíin
dressed láabis, lábsa, labsíin
to **drill** (well) ḥáfar*, yúḥfur
drilling ḥafr*
to **drink** ʃírib, yíʃrab*
drinking ʃurb
to **drive** saaq, yisúuq
driver sawwáaq, sawwaqíin
drum (oil) barmíil, baramíil
drunk sakráan*, sakráana*, sakraníin*
dry náaʃif, náʃfa, naʃfíin or nawáaʃif
to **dry** náʃʃif, yináʃʃif
dumb ʕáxraṣ, xárṣa, xurṣ
to **be(come) dumb** xíriṣ (or xúruṣ), yíxraṣ
durable matíin, matíina, mutáan
during (fi) múddit . . .; ʕasnáaʕ
 I was in Cairo during Ramadan kúntī-f máṣrī múddit ramaḍáan*
dust turáab*; yuráab*
duty-slip taṣríiḥ, taṣaríiḥ

e

each
 how much are they each? bi káam ilwáaḥid?[1]
 like each other záyyī báʕḍ
 next to each other gámbī báʕḍ
ear widn (f.), widáan
early bádri
earth ʕarḍ (f.)
easiness sahúula
east ʃarq
 the Middle East ʕiʃʃárqt ilʕáwṣaṭ
 the Near East ʕiʃʃárqt ilʕádna
eastern(er) ʃárqi, ʃarqíyya, ʃarqiyyíin
easy sahl, sáhla, sahlíin
to be **easy-going** ʕitsáahil, yitsáahil
to **eat** kal, yáakul
economic ʕiqtiṣáadit, ʕiqtiṣadíyyat
economics ʕiqtiṣáadt

economist ʕiqtiṣáadit, ʕiqtiṣadíyyat, ʕiqtiṣadiyyíint
to be **edible** ʕittáakil, yittáakil
effendi ʕafándi, ʕafandíyya
eggs beeḍ (c.), béeḍa, bedáat
 scrambled eggs béeḍ maḍrúub
Egypt maṣr; ʕilqúṭrt ilmáṣri
 Upper Egypt ʕiṣṣaʕíid (or ʕiṣṣiʕíid)
 Lower Egypt ʕilwágh ilbáḥari
Egyptian máṣri, maṣríyya, maṣriyyíin
 Upper Egyptian ṣaʕíidi (or ṣiʕíidi), ṣaʕidíyya, ṣaʕáyda
eight táman, tamánya
eighteen tamanṭáaʃar*
eighth táamin, támna; (fraction) tumn, ʕatmáan or ʕitmáan
eighty tamaníin
either ... or ya ... ya
election ʕintixáab, ʕintixabáat
electrician kahrabáaʕi*, kahrabaʕiyyíin*
electricity kahrába*
elephant fiil, ʕafyáal
eleven ḥiḍáaʃar*
embarrassed maksúuf, maksúufa, maksufíin
embarrassment kusúuf
to **employ** ʕistáxdim, yistáxdim
employee mustáxdim, mustaxdíma, mustaxdimíin; muwáẓẓaf, muwaẓẓáfa, muwaẓẓafíin
empty fáaḍi, fáḍya, faḍyíin; fáariy, fáryа, faryíin
to **empty** fáḍḍa, yifáḍḍi; fárray, yifárray; (intr.) fíḍi, yífḍa; xíli, yíxla
to **end** (intr.) ʕintáha, yintíhi (see also **finish**)
end ʕintiháaʕ (or ʕintíha)
engine (train) wabúur, waburáat*; ʕídda, ʕídad
engineer mihándis (or mu-), mihandisíin
 civil engineer miʕmáari, miʕmariyyíin
engineering (n.) handása
engineering (adj.) handási, handasíyya
 civil engineering ʕilhandásalmadaníyya
 electrical engineering ʕilkahrába
 mechanical engineering ʕilmikaníika

England ʕingiltíra*
English(man) ʕingilíizi, ʕingilizíyya,
ʕingiliziyyíin, ʕingilíiz
to enjoin wáṣṣa, yiwáṣṣi (ɤala)
to enjoy ʕitmáttaɤ, yitmáttaɤ (bi)
enough kifáaya
more than enough kifáaya wi-
zyáada
to be enough káfa, yíkfi; káffa, yikáffi
to have enough ʃíbiɤ, yíʃbaɤ; ʕistákfa,
yistákfa
to enter dáxal, yúdxul; xaʃʃ, yixúʃʃ
entry (entering) duxúul
no entry! mamnúuɤ idduxúul!
envelope ẓarf, ẓurúuf
to equal sáawa, yisáawi
era ɤaṣr, ɤuṣúur
eraser ʕastíika, ʕastikáat
essential ḍarúuri, ḍaruríyya; láazim,
lázma
etcetera wi hakáza; wi ɤeer + p.s.
Europe ʕurúbba
European rúumi, rumíyya, rumiyyíin
or ʕarwáam*; ʕurúbbi, ʕurubíyya,
ʕurubbiyyíin
even ḥátta
evening máɤrib; mísa
in the evening billéel; filmáɤrib
Friday evening yóom iggúmɤa
billéel
good evening mísa-lxéer or misáaʕ
ilxéer
every kull
everyone kúllï wáaḥid; (vocative) (ya)
gamáaɤa
everything kúllï ʃéeʕ
everywhere fi kúllï ḥítta, fi kúllï
makáan
there are people everywhere
ʕiddínya malyáana náas
evil ʃarr*, ʃurúur; suuʕ
exactly! tamáam, maẓbúuṭ, ṣaḥíiḥ,
bizẓábṭ, &c.
to exaggerate báaliɤ, yibáaliɤ
example másal, ʕamsíla
for example másalan; zayy
examination ʕimtiḥáan, ʕimtiḥanáat
to examine (e.g. medically) káʃaf,
yíkʃif; (inspect) fáttiʃ, yifáttiʃ
except ʕílla
to excuse sámaḥ, yísmaḥ (li)
excuse me! ʕismáḥli; ʕastáʕzin
to expect ʕintáẓar, yintíẓir

expectancy ʕintiẓáar
to expel ṭáraḍ, yúṭruḍ
expense maṣrúuf, maṣrufáat or
maṣaríif
experience xíbra
experienced mitmárran* (or muta-),
mitmarrána*, mitmarraníin*
expert xabíir, xúbara*
to explain fáhhim, yifáhhim; ɤárraf*,
yiɤárraf*
to explode ʕinfágar*, yinfígir
explosion ʕinfigáar*, ʕinfigaráat*
extent qadd
to what extent? qáddï ʕéeh?
to extinguish ṭáfa, yíṭfi
to extract ʕistáxrag*, yistáxrag*;
nátag, yíntig
extremely xáaliṣ; lilɤáaya
eye ɤeen (f.), ɤiyúun

f

face wiʃʃ, wuʃúuʃ; wagh, wugúuh;
xílqa, xílaq
to facilitate sáhhil, yisáhhil
facility tashíil, tashiláat
facing (adj.) quddamáani, quddamaníyya, quddamaniyyíin
in fact filwáaqiɤ†; law géet lilḥáqq
the fact is that... ʕilḥaqíiqa-nn...;
ʕilwáaqiɤ inn...; ʕaṣl...
factory máṣnaɤ, maṣáaniɤ
Fahrenheit fihranháyt*
faith ʕimáan
to have faith in ʕáamin, yiʕáamin (bi)
to fall wíqiɤ, yúqaɤ
family (n.) ɤéela, ɤeláat; ʕúsra*,
ʕúsar*
family (adj.) ɤa(a)ʕíli (or ɤáyli),
ɤaʕilíyya
fan marwáḥa*, maráawiḥ*
far biɤíid, biɤíida, buɤáad
as far as (up to) liɤáayit (+ n.),
liḥádd (+ n.)
as far as he can ɤala qáddï ma
yíqdar*
fare ʕúgrit irrukúub
farm ɤízba, ɤízab
fashion móoḍa, moḍáat
fast (adj.) saríiɤ, saríiɤa, sariɤíin
fast (adv.) bi súrɤa; bilɤágal
as fast as possible bi ʕásraɤ ma
yúmkin

to **fast** ṣaam, yiṣúum
fasting ṣoom
fat simíin, simíina, sumáan
fate qádar†*
father ʕabb, ʕabbaháat
fatigue táɣab
Fayoum ʕilfayyúum
from **Fayoum** fayyúumi, fayyumíyya
fear xoof
to **fear** xaaf, yixáaf
feast (festival) ɣiid, ʕaɣyáad
to (*celebrate*) **feast** ɣáyyid, yiɣáyyid
feather ríiʃa, ríyaʃ
February fibráayir
fee maṣrúuf, maṣrufáat *or* maṣaríif
fetch! haat (háati, háatu)!
fever suxuníyya
few qalíil, qalíila, quláal; ʃuwáyya
field ɣeeṭ, ɣeṭáan; ḥaqlṭ, ḥuqúulṭ
fifteen xamasṭáaʃar*
fifth xáamis, xámsa; (fraction) xums, ʕaxmáas *or* ʕixmáas
fifty xamsíin
figs tiin (*c.*), tíina, tináat
file (office-) duséeh, dusaháat; miláff, milaffáat
to **fill** mála, yímla
finally filʕáaxir; ʕaxíiran
to **find** wágad, yíwgid; láqa, yílqa; láaqa, yiláaqi; káʃaf, yíkʃif
fine mixálfa, mixalfáat
finger ṣubáaɣ (*or* ṣáabiɣ), ṣawáabiɣ
to **finish** (*intr.*) kímil, yíkmal; ʕintáha, yintíhi; (complete) kámmil, yikámmil; (use up) xállaṣ, yixállaṣ; (finish with) xíliṣ, yíxlaṣ (min)
to *be* **finished** xíliṣ, yíxlaṣ
fire naar*, niráan*
to **fire** (rifle) fárraɣ, yifárraɣ
firefighting maṭáafi
fire-station (*or* **fire-service**) maṭáafi-lḥaríiq
firm (*as* **company**)
first ʕáwwil; ʕawwaláani, ʕawwalaníyya, ʕawwalaniyyíin
fish sámak (*c.*), sámaka, samakáat, ʕasmáak
to **fish** ʕiṣṭáad, yiṣṭáad sámak
fishmonger sammáak, sammakíin
fit (**for**) ṣáaliḥ, ṣálḥa, ṣalḥíin (li)
to **fit** geh, yiigi ɣala qadd . . .
fitter barráad*, barradíin*
five xámas, xámsa

flag ɣálam, ʕaɣláam
to **flare** *up* ʕitʃáɣlil, yitʃáɣlil
flat (apartment) ʃáqqa, ʃúqaq
to **float** ṭáfa, yíṭfa
floor ʕarḍ (*f.*); (story) door, ʕadwáar*
flowers ẓahr (*c.*), ẓáhra*, ẓahráat*, ẓuhúur
flower-vase zuhríyya, zuhriyyáat
fly (*-ies*) dibbáan (*c.*), dibbáana, dibbanáat
to **fly** ṭaar, yiṭíir
to *make* **fly** ṭáyyar*, yiṭáyyar*
to **follow** tábaɣ, yítbaɣ
to *be* **fond** *of* ḥabb, yiḥíbb
food ʕakl; (cooked) ṭabíix
foot qádam, ʕiqdáam; rigl (*f.*)
   on foot (*see* **walking**)
footbridge qanṭára, qanáaṭir
for li; ɣa(la)ʃáan; liʕánn; (since) min, baqa + *p.s.*, li + *p.s.* (*see* **ago**); (during) múddit . . .
   I've been waiting for you for two hours ʕana mistanníik baqáali saɣtéen
   I stayed in Cairo for a week qaɣádti[1]-f máṣri múddit usbúuɣ
to **forbid** mánaɣ, yímnaɣ
forehead qóora*, qúwar* *or* qoráat*
foreign(er) ʕagnábi, ʕagnabíyya, ʕagáanib; ʕafrángi*, ʕafrangíyya*, ʕafráng*
to **forget** nísi, yínsa
to **forgive** sáamiḥ, yisáamiḥ
fork ʃóoka, ʃúwak
former sáabiq, sábqa, sabqíin
formerly (of old) zamáan
forty ʕarbiɣíin
to **forward** bállaɣ, yibállaɣ
foundation ʕasáas, ʕúsus
four ʕárbaɣ*, ʕarbáɣa*
fourteen ʕarbaɣṭáaʃar*
fourth ráabiɣ*, rábɣa*; (fraction) rubɣ, ʕarbáaɣ *or* ʕirbáaɣ
fox táɣlab, taɣáalib
France faránsa*
to **frank** xátam (*or* xítim), yíxtim
frankly bi kúllī ṣaráaḥa*
frankness ṣaráaḥa*
free ḥurr, ḥúrra*, ʕaḥráar*; (unoccupied) fáaḍi, fáḍya, fadyíin; (gratis) baláaʃ; maggáanan

---

[1] Pronounced *qaɣátti*.

freedom ḥurríyya
French(man) faransáawi*, faransawíyya*, faransawiyyíin*
fresh ṭáaẓa
freshness (weather) ṭaráawa
Friday yóom iggúmʕa
friend ṣáaḥib, ʕaṣḥáab; ḥabíib, ḥabíiba, ḥabáayib
to **frighten** xáwwif, yixáwwif; xaḍḍ, yixáḍḍ
from min; ʕan
in **front** of quddáam
frontier ḥadd, ḥudúud
fruit fákha, fawáakih
fruiterer fakaháani, fakahaníyya
to **fry** qála, yíqli
full malyáan, malyáana, malyaníin
  full of water malyáan máyya
fully bittafṣíil
to **furnish** fáraʃ, yífriʃ
furnishing farʃ
furniture mubílya, mubilyáat; farʃ
in (the) **future** filmustáqbal

g

game líʕba, ʕalʕáab
ganger ráyyis*, rúyasa
garden ginéena, ganáayin
garlic toom (c.), tomáaya, tomáat
garment hídma, hudúum; málbas, maláabis
gas ɣaaz
gate baab, ʕabwáab or bibáan
gazelle ɣazáal, ɣizláan
general (adj.) ʕa(a)mm,¹ ʕá(a)mma¹
generally (see **usually**)
generosity káram*
generous karíim, karíima, kúrama*
gentleman xawáaga, xawagáat
to **get** gaab, yigíib; (prepare) ḥáḍḍar, yiḥáḍḍar
gharry ḥanṭúur, ḥanaṭíir
gharry-driver ʕarbági*, ʕarbagíyya*
gift hadíyya, hadáaya
girl bint, banáat
to **give** ʕídda, yíddi
to **give up** (renounce) báṭṭal, yibáṭṭal; ʕitxálla, yitxálla (ʕan)
Giza ʕilgíiza (or ʕigg-)
glance láḥẓa, laḥaẓáat

glass (drinking-) kubbáaya, kubbayáat: (substance) ʕizáaz
pane of glass lóoḥ ʕizáaz, ʕalwáaḥ ʕizáaz
gloves (pair) guwánti, guwantiyyáat
to **go** raaḥ*, yirúuḥ; sáafir, yisáafir; míʃi, yímʃi; ṭíliʕ, yíṭlaʕ
let's go! yálla² bíina!
to **go away** ɣaab, yiɣíib
to **go around** (encircle) daar*, yidúur; (look over) ʕitfárrag*, yitfárrag*
to **go home** ráwwaḥ*, yiráwwaḥ*
to **go in** dáxal, yúdxul; xaʃʃ, yixúʃʃ
to **go out** ṭíliʕ, yíṭlaʕ; xárag*, yúxrug
going ráayiḥ, ráyḥa, rayḥíin
God ʕalláah²
god ʕiláah
gold dáhab
golf gulf
good (adj.) kuwáyyis, kuwayyísa, kuwayyisíin; ṭáyyib, ṭayyíba, ṭayyibíin
good (n.) xeer
goodbye maʕa-ssaláama; fi ḥífẓilláah, &c.
goods biḍáaʕa, baḍáayiʕ
government ḥukúuma, ḥukumáat
governmental ḥukúumi, ḥukumíyya, ḥukumiyyíin
governor miḥáafiẓ (or mu-), miḥafẓíin
governorate miḥáfẓa (or mu-), miḥafẓáat
grandfather gidd, gudúud
grandmother gídda, giddáat
grapes ʕínab (c.), ḥabbáayit ʕ., ḥabbáat ʕ.
grass ḥaʃíiʃ
grateful mamnúun, mamnúuna, mamnuníin
gratitude mamnuníyya
gravy máraqa, maraqáat
grease ʃaḥm, ʃuḥumáat
to **grease** ʃáḥḥim, yiʃáḥḥim
greasing taʃḥíim
Greece ʕilyunáan (f.)
greed ṭámaʕ
greedy ṭammáaʕ, ṭammáaʕa, ṭammaʕíin
Greek yunáani, yunaníyya, yunaniyyíin

¹ See Part I, Appendix B, note (c).

² 'Back' a's.

green ʔáxḍar, xáḍra, xuḍr
greengrocer xúḍari, xuḍaríyya
grocer baqqáal, baqqalíin
to grow (up) kíbir, yíkbar*
guest ḍeef, ḍiyúuf (or ḍuyúuf); mádʕi, madʕíyya, madʕiyyíin; maʕzúum, maʕzúuma, maʕzumíin or maʕazíim
to guide dall, yidíll
gulf xalíig, xulgáan

h

habit ʕáada, ʕadáat
hair ʃaʕr* (c.), ʃáʕra*, ʃaʕráat*
half nuṣṣ, ʔanṣáaṣ or ʔinṣáaṣ
hall ṣáala, ṣaláat
hammer ʃakúuʃ, ʃawakíiʃ
hand ʔiid or yadd (f.), ʔayáadi
handful ḥábba, ḥabbáat
handkerchief mandíil, manadíil
handle (as hand)
to hang ʕállaq, yiʕállaq
hanger (clothes-) ʃammáaʕa, ʃammaʕáat
hanging mitʕállaq, mitʕalláqa, mitʕallaqíin
to happen ḥáṣal, yíḥṣal
happy mabṣúuṭ, mabṣúuṭa, mabṣuṭíin
harbour míina, mawáani
hardworking ʃayyáal, ʃayyáala, ʃayyalíin
harvest gámʕ ilmaḥṣúul
hashish ḥaʃíiʃ
hashish-addict ḥaʃʃáaʃ, ḥaʃʃaʃíin
hat burnéeṭa (or barníiṭa*), baraníiṭ*
to have ʕand + p.s./n.
to have to láazim (+ impf.)
hawker sarríiḥ, sarríiḥa
haze ʃabbúura*
he húwwa
head (n.) raas* (f.), ruus; (chief) raʔíis*, rúʔasa
head (adj.) raʔíisi*, raʔisíyya*, raʔisiyíin*
headlight fanúus, fawaníis
headman ʕúmda, ʕúmad
health ṣíḥḥa
to hear símiʕ, yísmaʕ
heart qalb, qulúub
heat ḥarr*; ḥaráara*; suxuníyya
to heat sáxxan, yisáxxan; (intr.) síxin (or súxun), yísxan

heavy tiqíil, tiqíila, tuqáal
help(ing) misáʕda
to help sáaʕid, yisáaʕid
here hína
here is/are ʔahó(h), ʔahé(h), ʔahúm; ʔáadi
high ʕáali, ʕálya, ʕalyíin
hill gábal, gibáal
hire ʔúgra*
historical taríixi, tarixíyya, tarixiyíin; ʔásari, ʔasaríyya
history taríix
to hit ḍárab, yíḍrab
hitting ḍarb
to hold mísik, yímsik
hole xúfra*, xúfar*
holiday fúsḥa
holy muqáddas,† muqaddásaṭ, muqaddasíin†
home beet, biyúut; mánzil, manáazil; maḥáll, maḥalláat
honey ʕásal
to honour ʃárraf*, yiʃárraf*
hookah góoza, gíwaz
to hope ʔitʕáʃʃim, yitʕáʃʃim
  I hope that ... ʔin ʃáaʔ alláah¹ ... or ʔinʃálla¹ ...
horse ḥuṣáan, ḥiṣína
horseman fáaris, firsáan
horses xeel (f.)
hot suxn, súxna, suxníin; ḥarr*, ḥárra*
hotel lukánḍa, lukanḍáat
hour sáaʕa, saʕáat
house beet, biyúut; daar*, duur
how ʔizzáay; ʔizzáyy
  how are you? ʔizzáyy ilḥáal?, ʔizzáyyak?, &c.
  how much, many kaam; káam wáaḥid; qáddī ʔéeh
  for how long qáddī ʔéeh
humidity ruṭúuba
hundred míyya
  three hundred, four hundred, &c. tultumíyya, rubʕumíyya, &c.
hunger gúuʕa
hungry gaʕáan, gaʕáana, gaʕaníin or gawáaʕa
to hunt ʔiṣṭáad, yiṣṭáad
in a hurry mustáʕgil (or mi-), mustaʕgíla, mustaʕgilíin

¹ 'Back a's.

to **hurry** Ꜥistáƹgil, yistáƹgil; síriƹ, yísriƹ; ʃáhhil, yiʃáhhil
to **hurt** (injure) gáraḥ, yígraḥ; (*intr.*) wágaƹ, yíwgaƹ
husband gooz, Ꜥigwáaz
hyena ḍabƹ, ḍubúƹa

i

I Ꜥána
ice talg
iced mutállag (*or* mitállig), mutallága
idea fikr, Ꜥafkáar*; xáaṭir, xawáaṭir
if Ꜥiza (kaan), Ꜥin (kaan), law (kaan)
ignorant gáahil, gáhla, gahlíin
ill ƹayyáan, ƹayyáana, ƹayyaníin; maríiḍ*, maríiḍa*, márḍa*
illegible ɣáamiḍ, ɣámḍa
ill-mannered qalíil ilꜥádab, qalílt ilꜥádab, quláal ilꜥádab
illness máraḍ, Ꜥamráaḍ
immediately ƹala ṭúul
important muhímm, muhímma, muhimmíin
  more important Ꜥahámm
imported mustáwrad*, mustawráda*
to **imprison** ḥábas, yíḥbis
to **improve** ḥássin, yiḥássin; (*intr.*) Ꜥitḥássin, yitḥássin
improvement taḥsíin
in fi; (at home) mawgúud, mawgúuda, mawgudíin
  in five minutes baƹdī xámas daqáayiq
increase ziyáada
to **increase** záwwid, yizáwwid
to **incur** (debt) xad, yáaxud (sálaf)
independence Ꜥistiqláal
Indian híndi, hindíyya, hanádwa
individual (*adj.*) fárdi, fardíyya
industrial ṣináaƹi (*or* ṣanáyƹi), ṣinaƹíyya, ṣinaƹiyyíin
industry ṣináaƹa, ṣinaƹáat
inevitable ḍarúuri, ḍaruríyya
to **infect** ƹáda, yíƹdi
infectious múƹdi, muƹdíya, muƹdiyíin
influence nufúuz
to **inform** xábbar*, yixábbar*
information xábar*, Ꜥaxbáar*
to **inhabit** síkin (*or* sákan), yúskun
inhabitant sáakin, sákna, sukkáan

to **injure** gáraḥ, yígraḥ; ƹáwwar*, yiƹáwwar*
injury Ꜥiṣáaba, Ꜥiṣabáat
ink ḥibr
inlaid muṭáƹƹam (*or* mi-), muṭaƹƹáma, muṭaƹƹamíin
inner guwwáani, guwwaníyya, guwwaniyyíin
to **inquire** Ꜥistáfham (*or* Ꜥistáfhim), yistáfham; Ꜥistáƹlim, yistáƹlim
inquiry Ꜥistiƹláam, Ꜥistiƹlamáat
insect ḥáʃara*, ḥaʃaráat*
inside gúwwa; dáaxil
to **inspect** fáttiʃ, yifáttiʃ
inspector mufáttiʃ, mufattiʃíin
instead of bádal min (+ *n.*); bádal ma (+ *v.*)
instruction taƹlíim, taƹlimáat
to **insure** Ꜥámmin, yiꜤámmin (ƹala)
intelligence faṭáara; ƹaql, ƹuqúul; muxx, Ꜥimxáax
intelligent ʃáaṭir, ʃáṭra, ʃuṭṭáar; ƹáaqil, ƹáqla, ƹaqlíin
intending (to) náawi, náwya, nawyíin
intention qaṣd
interesting muhímm, muhímma, muhimmíin
interpreter targumáan*, tarágma
to **interrupt** (*see* delay)
to **investigate** báḥas, yíbḥas
investigation taḥqíiq; baḥs
to **invite** ƹázam, yíƹzim
iron ḥadíid; (hand-) mákwa, makáawi
to **iron** káwa, yíkwi
ironing kawy *or* kayy
to **irrigate** ráwa, yírwi
irrigated rayy*, ráyya*
irrigation rayy*
Islam Ꜥisláam
Islamic Ꜥisláami, Ꜥislamíyya, Ꜥislamiyyíin
Israel ꜤisraꜤíil* (*f.*)
Israeli ꜤisraꜤíili*, ꜤisraꜤilíyya*, ꜤisraꜤiliyyíin*
it húwwa (*m.*), híyya (*f.*)
  it's dark Ꜥiddínya ḍálma
Italy Ꜥiṭálya
Italian ṭalyáani (*or* ṭul-), ṭalyaníyya, ṭaláyna
itinerant mutagáwwil (*or* mitg-) mutagawwíla, mutagawwilíin
ivory ƹaag; sínn ilfíil

j

jackal diib, diyáaba
jacket jakétta,[1] jakettáat
jam mirábba*, mirabbáat*
January yanáayir
Jew(ish) yahúudi, yahudíyya, yahúud
job ʃuɣl, ʕaʃɣáal; ʃúɣla, ʃúɣal
joke núkta, núkat *or* nikáat
journal gurnáal,[2] garaníil*
journey ríħla, riħláat; sáfar*, ʕasfáar*
judgement ħukm
jug ʕabríiq, ʕabaríiq
July yúlya
June yúnya
just (*adv*.) bass; ya dóobak
just as (in the way that) záyyi ma (+ *v*.)

k

to be **keen** *to* bidd + *p.s.* + *v*.
kerosine gaaz
key muftáaħ, mafatíiħ
to **kill** qátal (*or* qítil), yíqtil
kilogram kíilu (*or* kéelu), kiluwáat
kilometre kíilu (*or* kéelu), kiluwáat; kilumítr, kilumitráat
kind (*n*.) nooʕ, ʕanwáaʕ; ʃakl, ʕaʃkáal
king málik, mulúuk
kiosk kuʃk, ʕikʃáak
kitchen máṭbax, maṭáabix
knife sikkíina, sakakíin; muus, ʕamwáas
to **knock** xábbaṭ, yixábbaṭ; daqq, yidúqq
to **know** ʕírif, yíʕraf*
the **Koran** ʕilqurʕáant

l

laboratory máʕmal, maʕáamil
ladder síllim, saláalim
lady sitt, sittáat
lame ʕáʕrag*, ʕárga*, ʕurg
lamp fanúus, fawaníis; lámba,[3] lambáat[3]
land ʕarḍ (*f*.), ʕaráaḍi; (opposed to sea) barr*

language lúɣa, luɣáat
large kibíir, kibíira, kubáar*
last ʕáaxir; ʕaxráani, ʕaxraníyya, ʕaxraniyyíin; ʕaxíir, ʕaxíira
at last ʕaxíiran
last week ʕilʕusbúuʕ illi fáat
late mitʕáxxar*, mitʕaxxára*, mitʕaxxaríin*; wáxri, waxríyya, waxriyyíin
later baʕdéen
to **laugh** ḍíħik, yíḍḥak
laughter ḍiħk
laundryman makwági, makwagíyya
lavatory kabinéeh, kabineháat; béet irráaḥa*
law qanúunt, qawaníint
lazy kasláan, kasláana, kaslaníin *or* kasáala; múhmil, muhmíla, muhmilíin
lead (metal) ruṣáaṣ
leaf (palm) garíida, garáayid
to **learn** ʕitʕállim, yitʕállim; záakir, yizáakir; (by heart) ħáfaḍ (*or* ħáfaẓ), yíħfaḍ (*or* yíħfaẓ)
least ʕaqáll
at least ʕalʕaqáll
leave ʕagáaza, ʕagazáat
on leave fi ʕagáaza
sick leave ʕagáaza maraḍíyya
to **leave** saab, yisíib; xálla, yixálli; (set off) sáafir, yisáafir
Lebanon libnáan (*f*.)
lecture muħáḍra, muħaḍráat
left ʃimáal
leg rigl (*f*.)
lemons lamúun (*c*.), lamúuna, lamunáat
to **lend** sállif, yisállif
length ṭuul, ʕaṭwáal
to **lengthen** ṭáwwil, yiṭáwwil
lengthwise bi ṭúul; miṭáwla
to **lessen** (*tr. and intr*.) qall, yiqíll; náqqaṣ, yináqqaṣ
lesson dars, durúus
to **let** xálla, yixálli
let's go! yálla[4] bíina!
letter gawáab, gawabáat; (of alphabet) ħarf*, ħurúuf
letter-box sandúuq búṣṭa, sanadíiq búṣṭa
lettuces xaṣṣ (*c*.), xaṣṣáaya, xaṣṣáat

---

[1] See Introduction, p. 8.
[2] 'Back' *aa*.
[3] 'Back' *a*'s.

[4] 'Back' *a*'s.

liar kaddáab (*or* kazzáab), kaddáaba, kaddabíin
library maktába, maktabáat
to **lie** (prevaricate) kídib (*or* kízib), yíkdib
lies (*as* **lying**)
life ḥayáah (*f.*); ɣumr
lift ʕaṣanṣéer, ʕaṣanṣeráat*
to **lift** ráfaɣ*, yírfaɣ
light (*n.*) nuur, ʕanwáar*; (bulb) lámba,[1] lambáat[1]
put on the light! wállaɣ innúur!
light (*adj.*) xafíif, xafíifa, xufáaf
to **light** wállaɣ, yiwállaɣ
lighter (cigarette) walláaɣa, wallaɣáat; (boat) maɣúun, mawaɣíin
lighting ʕináara*
like zayy
to **like** ḥabb, yiḥíbb
  which one did you like? ʕanhú-lli ɣágabak?
to **like** *to* ḥabb, yiḥíbb
likely min ilmuḥtámal
limit ḥadd, ḥudúud
to **limit** ḥáddid, yiḥáddid
line ṣaff, ṣufúuf; (of writing) ṣaṭr, ṣuṭúur; xaṭṭ, xuṭúuṭ
lion sabɣ, subúɣa; ʕásad, ʕusúud *or* ʕusúda
(*in*) **liquid** (*form*) sáaʕil (*or* sáayil), sa(a)ʕíila (*or* sayla), sawáaʕil (*or* sawáayil)
to **listen** símiɣ, yísmaɣ
little (*adj.*) ṣuɣáyyar*, ṣuɣayyára*, ṣuɣayyaríin*; baṣíiṭ, baṣíiṭa, buṣáaṭ
a **little** ʃuwáyya; qalíil, qalíila, quláal
to **live** ɣaaʃ, yiɣíiʃ; (inhabit) síkin (*or* sákan), yúskun
load ḥiml, ʕiḥmáal
to **load** ḥámmil, yiḥámmil; ʃáḥan, yíʃḥin
loading ʃaḥn
loaf riɣíif, ʕarɣíifa
loan salafíyya, salafiyyáat
local
  local cheese gíbna báladi
  local customs ɣadáat ilḥáyyi da
lock qifl, ʕiqfáal
to **lock** qáfal, yíqfil
locomotive wabúur, waburáat*
London lándan[1]

[1] 'Back' *a*'s.

long ṭawíil, ṭawíila, ṭuwáal
to **look (at)** baṣṣ, yibúṣṣ (li)
  you look ill báayin ɣaléek taɣbáan
  it looks as if . . . yíẕhar inn . . .
to **look after** (see *take care of*)
to **look for** dáwwar*, yidáwwar* (ɣala)
to **look round** ʕitfárrag*, yitfárrag*
lorry lúuri, luriyyáat
to **lose** ḍáyyaɣ, yiḍáyyaɣ
  I've lost it (*f.*) ráaḥit mínni
to **lose one's temper** (see *angry*)
to **lose one's way** ḍall, yiḍíll
loss xuṣáara*, xasáayir
lost táayih, táyha, tayhíin
to **be(come) lost** taah, yitúuh; ḍaaɣ, yiḍíiɣ
a **lot (of)** (see *much*)
lounge ʕóḍt iggulúus
lover ḥabíib, ḥabíiba, ḥabáayib
low wáaṭi, wáṭya, waṭyíin
lower taḥtáani, taḥtaníyya, taḥtaniyyíin; (comparative of wáaṭi) ʕáwṭa
to **lower** názzil, yinázzil
to **lubricate** záyyit, yizáyyit
lubrication tazyíit
luck baxt, ḥaẕẕ
lucky
  you are lucky ɣándak báxt (*or* ḥáẕẕ)
luggage ɣafʃ
lunch ɣáda
to **lunch** ʕitɣádda, yitɣádda
Luxor lúqṣur
lying kidb (*or* kizb)

m

macaroni makaróona*
machine mákana, makanáat
mad magnúun, magnúuna, maganíin
to **madden** gánnin, yigánnin
made (of) maṣnúuɣ, maṣnúuɣa *or* maɣmúul, maɣmúula (min)
magazine magálla, magalláat
majority ʕaɣlabíyya; ʕáɣlab
to **make** ɣámal, yíɣmil; (manufacture) ṣánaɣ, yíṣnaɣ
  to make a scene ɣámal, yíɣmil dáwʃa
Mamur maʕmúur, maʕamíir
man ráagil*, riggáala

manager mudíir, mudiríin
mangoes mánga (c.), mangáaya, mangáat
manœuvre munáwra*, munawráat*
to **manufacture** ṣánaɛ, yíṣnaɛ
many kitíir, kitíira, kutáar*; ziyáada
map xaríiṭa*, xaráayiṭ*
March máaris
market suuq, ʕaswáaq
married mitgáwwiz (or migg-), mitgawwíza, mitgawwizíin
to be **married** ʕitgáwwiz (or ʕigg-), yitgáwwiz
mat kilíim, ʕiklíma
matches kabríit
material (cloth) qumáaʃ
raw materials ʕilmawá(a)dd ilxáam
mathematics riyáaḍa
matter mawḍúuɛ, mawaḍíiɛ; masʕála, masáaʕil
it doesn't matter ma ɛaléhʃ; ma-yhímmiʃ
no matter! ma-yhímmiʃ !
personal matter masʕála fardíyya
what's the matter? máalak?; gára* (or yígra*) ʕéeh?
what's the matter with you? (rebuke) wi baɛdéen wayyáak baqa?
May máayu
meal ʕakl
I **mean** (that is to say) yáɛni
meaning máɛna, maɛáani
means wáṣṭa, waṣáayiṭ
by means of bi wáṣṭit . . .
measles ḥáṣba
meat láḥma or laḥm (c.), ḥíttit láḥma, ḥítat láḥm, liḥúum
Mecca mákka
mechanic mikaníiki, mikaːnikíyya
medal niʃáan, nayaʃíin
medical ṭíbbi, ṭibbíyya
medicine dáwa (m.), ʕadwíya; (medical science) ṭibb
to prescribe medicine for dáawa, yidáawi
Medina madíina
medium mutawáṣṣiṭ (or mitwáṣṣaṭ), mutawaṣṣíṭa, mutawaṣṣiṭíin
to **meet** qáabil, yiqáabil; láqa, yílqa; ṣáadif, yiṣáadif; (intr.) ʕitqáabil, yitqáabil
meeting muqábla, muqabláat
member ɛuḍw, ʕaɛḍáaʕ

to **mention** ẕákar, yúẕkur gaab, yigíib síira (ɛan)
merchandise biḍáaɛa, baḍáayiɛ
merchant táagir, tuggáar*
mercy ráḥma*
messenger (office-) farráaʃ*, farraʃíin*
metal máɛdan, maɛáadin
meter (taxi-) ɛaddáad, ɛaddadáat
method ṭaríiqa, ṭúruq; wasíila, wasáaʕil
metre mitr, ʕamtáar* or ʕimtáar*
middle wuṣṭ (or wiṣṭ)
midnight núṣṣ illéel
to **migrate** ráḥal*, yírḥal
mildness (weather) ʕiɛtidáal
mile miil, ʕamyáal
milk lában
milleme mallíim, malalíim
million milyóon (or mal-), malayíin
mind dimáaɣ; ɛaql, ɛuqúul; xáaṭir, xawáaṭir
do you mind if . . .? ɛándak máaniɛ inn . . .?
minister wazíir, wúzara*
prime minister raʕíis* ilwizáara
ministry wizáara
mint niɛnáaɛ
minute (n.) daqíiqa, daqáayiq
mirror miráaya, mirayáat
miser(ly) baxíil, baxíila, búxala
to **miss**
he missed the train ʕilqáṭrɪ fáatu(h)
missing (short) náaqiṣ, náqṣa, naqṣíin; (lost) táayih, táyha, tayhíin
mist ʃabbúura*
to make a **mistake** yíliṭ, yíɣlaṭ
mistaken ɣalṭáan, ɣalṭáana, ɣalṭaníin
misunderstanding súuʕ ittafáahum
modern ɛáṣri, ɛaṣríyya, ɛaṣriyyíin
moment láḥẓa, laḥaẓáat
Monday yóom litnéen
money filúus (f.)
month ʃahr*, ʃuhúur or ʕáʃhur
last month ʕiʃʃáhr illi fáat
next month ʕiʃʃáhr iggáay
monthly (adj.) ʃáhri, ʃahríyya, ʃahriyyíin
monthly (adverb) ʃahríyyan
(ancient) **monument** ʕásar*, ʕasáar*
moon qámar*
more ʕáktar*; ʕázyad
more than that ʕáktar min kída

morning ṣubḥ; qabl iḍḍúhr
  this morning Ṣiṣṣúbḥ
  good morning ṣabáaḥ ilxéer,
    ṣabáaḥ innúur, &c.
mosque gáamiȝ, gawáamiȝ
mosquitoes namúus (c.), namúusa,
  namusáat; baȝúuḍ (c.), baȝúuḍa,
  baȝuḍáat
mosquito-net namusíyya, namusiyyáat
mother Ṣumm, Ṣummaháat
motor-cycle mutsíkl (or mutusíkl),
  mutsikláat
to mount ríkib, yírkab
mountain gábal, gibáal
mouse faar*, firáan
moustache ʃánab, Ṣaʃnáab
mouth buqq
to move ḥárrak*, yiḥárrak*
much kitíir, kitíira, kutáar*
mud ẓábaṭ; ṭiin
to muddle láxbaṭ, yiláxbaṭ
muddling (n.) laxbáṭa
Mudir mudíir, mudiríin
multiplication ḍarb
to multiply ḍárab, yíḍrab
muscle ȝáṣab, Ṣáȝṣáab
museum Ṣantikxáana, Ṣantikxanáat
Muslim múslim, muslíma, muslimíin
must láazim . . .; la búdd . . .; (it is my
  duty to) wáagib ȝaláyya-nn . . .
  they must have gone zamánhum
  míʃyu
mustard muṣṭárḍa
mutton ḍáani
  leg of mutton fáxda (or fáxdit)
  ḍáani

n

nail muṣmáar, maṣamíir; (finger, toe)
  ḍáafir or ḍufr, ḍawáafir
name Ṣism, Ṣasáami
narrow dáyyaq, dayyáqa, dayyaqíin
nation dáwla, dúwal
national Ṣáhli, Ṣahlíyya, Ṣahliyyíin;
  wáṭani, waṭaníyya, waṭaniyyíin
naughty ʃáqi, ʃaqíyya, Ṣaʃqíya
navy baḥríyya
near quráyyib*, qurayyíba*, quray-
  yibíin*
necessary láazim, lázma; ḍarúuri,
  ḍaruríyya

neck ráqaba
need luzúum; Ṣiḥtiyáag, Ṣiḥtiyagáat
  in need of miḥtáag, miḥtáaga, miḥtagíin (li)
  to need Ṣiḥtáag, yiḥtáag (li); yílzam
  the room needs cleaning ṢilṢóoḍa
  miḥtáaga littandíif
  I need a pound yilzámni-gnéeh
needle Ṣíbra, Ṣíbar or Ṣúbar*
neighbour gaar*, giráan
neither . . . nor la . . . wala
net ʃábaka, ʃabakáat or Ṣiʃbíka
never Ṣábadan; ȝumr + p.s. + ma . . .
  I've never seen him ȝúmri ma
  ʃuftúuʃ
nevertheless Ṣinnáma; maȝa záalik
new gidíid, gidíida, gudáad
news xábar*, Ṣaxbáar*
newspaper garíida, garáayid; gurnáal,[1] garaníil*
next gaay (or gayy), gáaya (or gáyya),
  gayíin (or gayyíin); táani, tánya,
  tanyíin
  next month Ṣiʃʃáhr* iggáay
  the next house Ṣilbéet ittáani
next to gamb
nice kuwáyyis, kuwayyísa, kuwayyisíin; laṭíif, laṭíifa, luṭáaf; ẓaríif,
  ẓaríifa, ẓuráaf
niceness luṭf
night leel; léela, layáali
  at night billéel
  tonight Ṣilléela; Ṣilleláadi
Nile Ṣinníil
of the Nile níili, nilíyya
nilometer miqyáasṭ inníil
nine tísaȝ, tísȝa
nineteen tisaȝṭáaʃar*
ninety tisȝíin
ninth táasiȝ, tásȝa; (fraction) tusȝ,
  Ṣatsáaȝ or Ṣitsáaȝ
no laṢ
noble ʃaríif, ʃaríifa, Ṣaʃráaf* or ʃúrafa*
noise dáwʃa; xáwta
noisy dawʃági, dawʃagíyya
nomad ráaḥil*, rúḥḥal
nomadic mitnáqqil, mitnaqqíla, mitnaqqilíin
nonsense kaláam fáariy
noon ḍuhr
north (of) ʃamáal

---

[1] 'Back' aa.

northern(er) báhari, baharíyya, bahariyyíin
nose munxáar*, manaxíir; Sanf, Sunúuf
to **notice** láhaz̧, yílhaz̧
November nufímbir
now dilwáqti
nowadays liyyámdi; Silyoméen dóol
Nubian núubi, nubíyya, nubiyyíin
number nímra, nímar; z̧ádad, Saz̧dáad

O

objection
    there's no objection ma fíiʃ máaniz̧
to **obtain** háşşal, yiháşşal
occasion márra*, marráat*
October Suktóobar*
of bitáaz̧, bitáz̧t, bitúuz̧; min
office máktab, makáatib; diwáan, dawawíin
officer z̧áabiţ (*or* ḑáabit), z̧ubbáaţ
official (*adj.*) rásmi, rasmíyya, rasmiyyíin
to **ogle** báşbaş, yibáşbaş
oil zeet, ziyúut
    fuel oil mazúut
    lubricating oil zéet iʃʃáhm
to **oil** záyyit, yizáyyit
oiling tazyíit
oke wíqqa, wíqaq
old kibíir, kibíira, kubáar*; z̧agúuz, z̧agúuza, z̧agáayiz; (ancient) qadíim, qadíima, qudáam
on z̧ála
once márra* wáhda
    at **once** z̧ala ţúul; háalan
one wáahid, wáhda
    I haven't a single one ma z̧andíiʃ wála wáahid
one-eyed Sáz̧war*, z̧óora*, z̧uur
onions báşal (*c.*), báşala *or* başaláaya, başaláat
only bass; ya dóobak; şirf, şírfa; ma . . . yeer
open maftúuh, maftúuha, maftuhíin
to **open** fátah, yíftah; (*intr.*) Sinfátah, yinfítih; (of flower, eye, &c.) fáttah, yifáttah
operation z̧amalíyya, z̧amaliyyáat
opinion raSy*; fikr, Safkáar*

opportunity fúrşa, fúraş
opposite quşáad
or wálla; Saw
oranges burtuqáan (*c.*), burtuqáana, burtuqanáat
order Samr*, Sawáamir
to **order** Sámar*, yúSmur
    in **order** *to* z̧a(la)ʃáan
organization (organizing) niz̧áam
origin Saşl, Suşúul
ornament zíina, zináat
other táani, tánya, tanyíin; Sáaxar*, Súxra*; (*see also* **each**)
    another one wáahid táani
    another (*sc.* different) **ship** márkib yérha
otherwise waSílla; Sáhsan
outer barráani*, barraníyya*, barraniyyíin
outside bárra* (min); xáarig
oven furn, Safráan*
overcoat bálţu, baláaţi
to **overturn** qálab (*or* qílib), yíqlib
owner şáahib, Saşháab

P

packet z̧ílba, z̧ílab
paint búuya, buyáat
to **paint** dáhan, yídhin; (cream *or* white) báyyaḑ, yibáyyaḑ
painting dáháan; tabyíiḑ; (picture) şúura*, şúwar*
palace qaşr, quşúur
palm-trees naxl (*c.*), náxla, naxláat, naxíil
paper wáraq (*c.*), wáraqa, waraqáat, Sawráaq; (newspaper) garíida, garáayid
parasol ʃamsíyya, ʃamáasi
parcel ţard, ţurúud
part qism, Saqsáam; (of body) z̧uḑw, Saz̧dáaS; (car, &c.) guzS, SagzáaS
partner ʃaríik, ʃúraka*
party háfla, hafaláat
pasha báaʃa, baʃawáat
to **pass (by)** faat, yifúut; marr*, yimúrr
past máaḑi, máḑya, maḑyíin
patience şabr
pavement raşíif, Sarşífa; tilitwáar*, tilitwaráat*

keep on the pavement! xallíik ɣarraṣíif!

pay Ṣúgra*; mahíyya, maháaya

to pay dáfaɣ, yídfaɣ; (debt) sadd, yisídd

payment (paying) dafɣ

peace ṣulḫ; (tranquillity) saláam

peaches xoox (c.), xóoxa, xoxáat

peanuts fúul sudáani

pears kommítra (c.), kommitráaya, kommitráat

peas bisílla (c.), ḥabbáayit b., ḥabbáat bisílla

peasant falláaḥ, falláaḥa, fallaḥíin

pedlar sarríiḥ, sarríiḥa

pen qálam, Ṣiqláam (ḫíbr)

pencil qálam, Ṣiqláam (ruṣáaṣ)

penknife muus, Ṣamwáas

penniless mifállis, mifallísa, mifallisíin

pension maɣáaʃ, maɣaʃáat

people naas; gamáaɣa; (race) Ṣahl, Ṣaháali

pepper fílfil

pepper-plants fílfil (c.), filfíla, filfiláat

percentage nísba, nísab

ninety per cent. tisɣíin filmíyya

perhaps yímkin

period múdda, múdad

permission Ṣizn

to ask permission ṢistáṢzin, yistáṢzin

Persian ɣágami, ɣagamíyya, ɣágam

person ʃaxṣ, Ṣaʃxáaṣ

personal ʃáxṣi, ʃaxṣíyya

petition ɣardiḥáal, ɣardiḥaláat; ɣaríiḍa*, ɣaráayiḍ*

petrol banzíin

petroleum (n.) bitróol

petroleum (adj.) bitróoli, bitrolíyya

Pharaonic farɣúuni, farɣuníyya, faráɣna*

photograph ṣúura*, ṣúwar*

to photograph ṣáwwar*, yiṣáwwar*

piastre qirʃ, qurúuʃ; qírʃi sáaɣ

half-piastre qírʃi taɣríifa; qírʃ ábyaḍ

pickles mixállil (c.), mixallíla, mixalliláat

pickpocket naʃʃáal, naʃʃalíin

picture ṣúura*, ṣúwar*

piece ḥítta, ḥítat; lúqma, lúqam

pig xanzíir, xanazíir; ḥallúuf, ḥalalíif

pilgrim ḥagg, ḥuggáag (or ḥiggáag)

pilgrimage ḥigg (or ḥagg)

to make the pilgrimage ḥagg, yiḥígg

the pilgrimage-month Ṣilḥígga (or Ṣilḥúgga)

pillow mixádda, mixaddáat

pillow-case bayáaḍa, bayaḍáat

pin dabbúus, dababíis

pipe masúura*, mawasíir; (smoking) bíiba, bibáat

pity

what a pity! ya-xṣáara!

place maḥáll, maḥalláat; makáan, Ṣamáakin; máṭraḥ, maṭáariḥ

plant (industrial) giháaz, gihazáat or Ṣaghíza; (horticultural) nabáat (c.), nabáata, nabatáat

to plant záraɣ, yízraɣ

plastic(s) bilástik

plate ṭábaq, Ṣaṭbáaq; ṣaḥn, ṣuḥúun

plated máṭli, maṭliyya, maṭliyyíin

to play líɣib, yílɣab

pleasant laṭíif, laṭíifa, luṭáaf

please min fáḍlak; wi-ḥyáatak

please do! Ṣitfáḍḍal!

to please ráḍa, yírḍi; Ṣárḍa, yírḍi; ɣágab, yíɣgib (see like)

pleased mabṣúuṭ, mabṣúuṭa, mabṣuṭíin; ráaḍi, ráḍya, raḍyíin

to be pleased Ṣinbáṣaṭ[1], yinbíṣiṭ[1]; ríḍi, yírḍa

pleasure surúur; fúsḥa

pocket geeb, giyúub

police bulíiṣ

policeman ɣaskári (bulíiṣ), ɣasáakir; ʃawíiʃ, ʃawiʃíyya

police-station karakóona*, karakonáat*

policy siyáasa

to polish (metal) báyyaḍ, yibáyyaḍ

polite muṢáddab, muṢaddába, muṢaddabíin

politeness Ṣádab

political siyáasi, siyasíyya, siyasiyyíin

politics siyáasa

poor faqíir, faqíira, fúqara*; maskíin, maskíina, masakíin

pork (see pig)

port míina, mawáani

porter ʃayyáal, ʃayyalíin

portion naṣíib; qism, Ṣaqsáam

[1] Pronounced Ṣimb-

Port Said bursaɣíid
position márkaz, maráakiz
possession maal, ʕamwáal; milk, ʕamláak
possible múmkin
 to be **possible** ṣaḥḥ, yiṣáḥḥ
post baríid; búṣṭa
postal-order ʕíznī baríid, ʕuzunáat baríid
postman buṣṭági, buṣṭagíyya; sáaɣi, suɣáah
post-office máktab ilbúṣṭa
pot ḫálla, ḫílal
potatoes baṭáaṭiṣ (c.), baṭaṭṣáaya, baṭaṭṣáat
poulterer farárgi, farargíyya
pound ginéeh, ginɛháat
to **pour** ṣabb, yiṣúbb; kabb, yikúbb
prawns gambári (c.), gambaríyya, gambariyyáat
to **pray** ṣálla, yiṣálli
prayer ṣála, ṣalawáat
to **precede** sábaq, yísbaq
preceding sáabiq, sábqa, sabqíin
to **prefer** fáḍḍal, yifáḍḍal
 I **prefer** **football** *to* **tennis** ʕilkóora* ɣánd(i)-aḥámmī mittínis
pregnancy ḥaml
to be **pregnant** ḥámalit, tíḥmil
to **prepare** gáhhiz, yigáhhiz; ḥáḍḍar, yiḥáḍḍar
prepared (*see* **ready**)
presence wugúud
present (*n.*) hadíyya, hadáaya
present (*adj.*) mawgúud, mawgúuda, mawgudíin; ḥáaḍir, ḥáḍra, ḥaḍríin
at **present** filwáqt ilḥáaḍir
to be **present** *at* ḥáḍar, yíḥḍar
to **press** (compress) ḍáɣaṭ, yíḍɣaṭ; (switch, button) daqq, yidúqq
pretty gamíil, gamíila, gumáal
to **prevent** mánaɣ, yímnaɣ
prevention manɣ
price siɣr, ʕaṣɣáar*; táman, ṣatmáan
price-list tasɣíira
primus-stove wabúur, wabɣáat*
prince ʕamíir, ʕúmara*
prison sign, sugúun
private xa(a)ṣṣ,[1] xá(a)ṣṣa;[1] ʃáxṣi, ʃaxṣíyya
 private car ɣarabíyya* malláaki

problem muʃkíla, maʃáakil
procès-verbal máḥḍar, maḥáaḍir
product má(a)dda[1], mawá(a)dd[1]
petroleum products ʕilmuntagáat ilbitrolíyya
production ʕintáag; ʕistixráag*
professor ʕustáaz, ʕasádza
to make a **profit** kísib, yíksab
profiteer miɣlawáani, miɣlawaníyya, miɣlawaniyyíin
programme birnáamig, baráamig
to **progress** ʕitqáddim, yitqáddim; ʕitqáwwa, yitqáwwa; (be promoted) ʕitráqqa, yitráqqa
to **promise** wáɣad, yíwɣid; ʕídda, yíddi kílma
promotion tarqíya
pronunciation nuṭq; lafẓ
properly bizzábṭ
property maal; milk, ʕamláak
prophet nábi, ʕanbíya; rasúul*, rúsul
proverb másal, ʕamsáal
province mudiríyya, mudiriyyáat
public ɣa(a)mm,[1] ɣá(a)mma; ɣumúumi, ɣumumíyya, ɣumumiyyíin
to **pull** garr*, yigúrr; ʃadd, yiʃídd
pump búmba, bumbáat
purpose ɣáaya, ɣayáat; ɣárad, ʕaɣráad; qaṣd
purse kiis, kiyáas; maḥfáẓa, maḥáafiẓ
to **push** zaqq, yizúqq
to **put** ḥaṭṭ, yiḥúṭṭ
pyramid háram* *or* ʕahráam*, ʕahramáat*

q

quarrel xináaqa, xinaqáat; dáwʃa
to **quarrel** xáaniq, yixáaniq; ɣáakis, yiɣáakis
quarter rubɣ, ʕarbáaɣ *or* ʕirbáaɣ; (of town) ḥayy, ʕaḥyáaʕ
queen málika, malikáat
question suʕáal, ʕasʕíla
quick(ly) (*see* **fast**)
quiet sáakit, sákta, saktíin
to be(come) **quiet** síkit (*or* sákat), yúskut
quite (rather) ʃuwáyya; (completely) xáaliṣ; (exactly) bizzábṭ

[1] See Part I, Appendix B, note (c).

r

rabbit Sárnab, Saráanib
radishes figl (*c.*), fígla, figláat
rag xírqa, xíraq
railway Sissíkka-lḥadíid
rain máṭar
raincoat bálṭu, baláaṭi
rank (taxi-) máwqif, mawáaqif; (*see
    also* **degree**)
rate Súgra*
rather Sáḥsan; (somewhat) ʃuwáyya
razor múus ḥiláaqa, Samwáas ḥ.
to **read** qára*, yíqra*
readiness Sistiẓdáad
reading qiráaya, qirayáat
ready gáahiz, gáhza, gahzíin; musta-
    ẓídd (*or* mi-), mustaẓídda, musta-
    ẓiddíin
to be **ready** Sistaẓádd, yistaẓídd
rearmost warráani*, warraníyya*,
    warraniyyíin*
rebuking tawbíix
receipt waṣl (ittasgíil), wuṣuláat;
    ḥáfẓa, ḥawáafiẓ
to **receive** Sistálam, yistílim; (pay)
    qábaḍ, yíqbaḍ
to **reckon** ḥásab, yíḥsib
record (dossier) duséeh, duseháat;
    (gramophone) Suṣṭuwáana, Suṣ-
    ṭuwanáat
to **record** sággil, yisággil
to **recover** xaff, yixíff; ʃáfa, yíʃfi; ṭaab,
    yiṭíib
red Sáḥmar*, ḥámra*, ḥumr
to be(come) **red** Siḥmárr*, yiḥmárr*
to **reduce** (decrease) náqqaṣ, yináq-
    qaṣ; (bring down (price)) názzil,
    yinázzil
to **refine** (oil) kárrar*, yikárrar*
refinery (oil) zetíyya
refining takríir
refrigerator talláaga, tallagáat
regards
    give my regards to . . . sallímli
    ẓala . . .
to **register** sággil, yisággil; (letter)
    ṣóogar*, yiṣóogar*
registration tasgíil
regulation taẓlíim, taẓlimáat
relation ẓaláaqat, ẓalaqáat†
    industrial relations Silẓalaqáat
    iṣṣinaẓíyya

public relations Silẓalaqáat
    ilẓá(a)mma
relative qaríib, qaráayib*
religion diin (*or* diyáana), Sadwáan
    (*or* diyanáat)
religious díini, diníyya, diniyyíin
to **rely on** Siẓtámad, yiẓtímid (ẓala);
    Sittákal, yittíkil (ẓala)
to **remain** báqa, yíbqa; fíḍil, yífḍal
remainder baqíyya
remaining báaqi, báqya, baqyíin;
    fáaḍil, fáḍla, faḍlíin
remains (meal, &c.) fáḍla
to **remember** Siftákar*, yiftíkir
    **do you remember when he came
    last year?** Sinta fáakir (*or* tiftíkir)
    lamma géh issána-lli fáatit?
    remember me to . . . sallímli
    ẓala . . .
to **remind** fákkar*, yifákkar*
reminding tafkíir
to **remove** wádda, yiwáddi; ʃaal,
    yiʃíil
renewal tagdíid
    subject to renewal qáabil littag-
    díid
to **repeat** kárrar*, yikárrar*
repetition takríir
report taqríir, taqaríir; máḥḍar,
    maḥáaḍir
reputation síira
request ṭálab, ṭalabáat
to **request** ṭálab, yúṭlub
research baḥs
to **resign** Sistaqáal, yistaqíil
responsibility masSulíyya, masSuliy-
    yáat; Sixtiṣáaṣ, Sixtiṣaṣáat
responsible (for) masSúul, masSúula,
    masSulíin (ẓan)
rest ráaḥa*; (remainder) baqíyya
to **rest** Sistaráyyaḥ, yistaráyyaḥ
restaurant máṭẓam, maṭáaẓim
result natíiga, natáayig *or* natáaSig
to **retire** Siṭḥáal, yiṭḥáal (ẓalmaẓáaʃ)
retirement Siḥáala, Siḥaláat
to **return** (give *or* bring back) radd*,
    yirúdd; rággaẓ, yirággaẓ; (go *or*
    come back) rígiẓ, yírgaẓ
returning radd*; rugúuẓ
to **revere** Siḥtáram*, yiḥtírim
rice ruzz
rich ɣáni, ɣaníyya, Saɣníya
to **ride** ríkib, yírkab

riding rukúub (*v.n.*); ráakib, rákba, rakbíin (*a.p.*)
right ḥaqq, ḥuqúuq; yimíin
  you are right ẓándak ḥáqq
  on the right ẓalyimíin
ring xáatim, xawáatim
to ring (bell) daqq, yidúqq; (phone) ḍárab, yíḍrab
ripe mistíwi, mistiwíyya, mistiwiyyíin
to ripen ṭaab, yiṭíib
to rise (get up) qaam, yiqúum; (milk) faar*, yifúur
rivalry mináfsa
river nahr*, Ɂanháar*
road síkka, síkak; ṭaríiq (*m. or f.*), ṭúruq
rock ṣaxr, ṣuxúur
Roman rumáani, rumaníyya, rumaniyyíin
Rome rúuma
roof ṣatḥ, ṣuṭúuḥ
room Ɂóoḍa, Ɂúwaḍ (*or* Ɂíwaḍ); (space) máṭraḥ
rosary síbḥa, síbaḥ
rough háayig, háyga, haygíin
row (line) ṣaff, ṣufúuf
rubber kawítʃ; (eraser) Ɂastíika, Ɂasatíik
rude ʃáqi, ʃaqíyya, ʃaʃqíya (*see also* ill-mannered)
ruler maṣṭára, maṣáaṭir
to run gára (*or* gíri), yígri

S

safe (*n.*) xazáana, xazáayin *or* xazanáat
safety wiqáayaṭ; saláama
sailing-boat fulúuka, faláayik
sailor baḥḥáar*, baḥḥáara*
sake
  for your sake ẓa(la)ʃan xáṭrak
Sakkaara saqqáara*
salad ṣálaṭa
salary mahíyya, maháaya *or* mahiyyáat
sale (selling) beeẓ; (auction) mabíiẓ, mabiẓáat
  for sale lilbéeẓ
salt malḥ
same
  the same side náfs innáḥya
sand raml*, rimáal

sandstorm zawbáẓa, zawáabiẓ
sandy rámli*, ramlíyya*
sardines sardíin (*c.*), sardíina, sardináat
Saturday yóom issábt
saucepan kasaróona*, kasaronáat*
to save wáffar*, yiwáffar*; (money) ḥáwwiʃ, yiḥáwwiʃ
to say qaal, yiqúul
saying (saw) másal, Ɂamsáal
scales mizáan, mawazíin
school madrása, madáaris
  secondary school madrása sanawíyya
  primary school madrása-btida-Ɂíyya
scissors maqáṣṣ, maqaṣṣáat
to scratch xárbiʃ, yixárbiʃ
screw barríima, barrimáat
screwdriver mifákk, mifakkáat
scribe ẓardiḥálgi, ẓardiḥalgíyya
sea baḥr*, biḥáar*
  the Red Sea Ɂilbáḥr ilɁáḥmar* (*or* láḥmar*)
  the Mediterranean Sea Ɂilbáḥr ilɁábyaḍ ilmutawáṣṣiṭ
sea-shells ṣádaf (*c.*), ṣádafa, ṣadafáat
season faṣl, fuṣúul
second (numeral) táani, tánya
second (time) sánya, sawáani
to second (support) sánna, yisánni
second-hand mistáẓmil, mistaẓmíla, mistaẓmilíin
secretariat sikirtárya (*or* sikirtaríyya)
secretary sikirtéer, sikirtéera*, sikirteriyyíin
section qismṭ, Ɂaqsáamṭ
to see ʃaaf, yiʃúuf
seed ḥábba *or* ḥabbáaya, ḥabbáat
self
  herself nafsáha
  he talks to himself biykállim rúuḥu(h)
  he came himself huwwa géh bi záatu(h)
to be self-opinionated Ɂitkábbar*, yitkábbar*
to sell baaẓ, yibíiẓ
seller bayyáaẓ, bayyáaẓa, bayyaẓíin
to send báẓat, yíbẓat
sense (meaning) máẓna, maẓáani
  it doesn't make sense da malúuʃ máẓna

to **separate** fáraz, yífriz; fáṣal, yífṣil

September sibtímbir

sergeant ʃawíiʃ, ʃawiʃíyya

servant xaddáam, xaddáama, xaddamíin

to **serve** xádam, yíxdim

service xídma, xadamáat

I am at your service ʕána-f xidmítak

settee kánaba, kanabáat; ʃizlóon, ʃizlonáat

seven sábaʕ, sábʕa

seventeen sabaʕtáaʃar*

seventh sáabiʕ, sábʕa; (fraction) subʕ, ʕasbáaʕ *or* ʕisbáaʕ

seventy sabʕíin

shade ḍall

shape ʃakl, ʕaʃkáal

sharp ḥáami, ḥámya, ḥamyíin

6 o'clock sharp ʕissáaʕa sítta bizzábṭ

to **shave** ḥálaq, yíḥlaq

shaving ḥiláaqa

she híyya

sheep náʕga, naʕgáat *or* niʕáag; xarúuf*, xirfáan

sheet bayáaḍa, bayaḍáat; miláaya, milayáat

sheikh ʃeex, ʃiyúux

shelf raff*, rufúuf

to **shine** lámaʕ, yílmaʕ

ship márkib (*f.*), maráakib

shirt qamíiṣ, qumṣáan

shoelaces rubáaṭ (iggázma)

shoemaker gazmági, gazmagíyya

shoes (pair) gázma, gízam

shop dukkáan, dakakíin

to **shop** báḍḍaʕ, yibáḍḍaʕ

shopkeeper bayyáaʕ, bayyaʕíin; ṣáaḥib dukkáan

shore sáaḥil, sawáaḥil

short quṣáyyar*, quṣayyára*, quṣayyaríin*

shorthand ʕixtizáal

shoulder kitf, ʕaktáaf *or* ʕiktífa

to **shout** záʕʕaq, yizáʕʕaq; (shout at) ʃáxaṭ, yíʃxaṭ (fi)

to **show** wárra, yiwárri; dall, yidíll; (show round) fárrag*, yifárrag*

side gamb, ʕignáab; (road, &c.) gíha, giháat

side-street ḥáara*, ḥawáari

sign ʕiʃáara*, ʕiʃaráat*

to **sign** máḍa, yímḍi; (contract) sáadiq, yisáadiq

sight (view) mánzar, manáaẓir

silent sáakit, sákta, saktíin

to **be**(*come*) **silent** síkit (*or* sákat), yúskut

silk ḥaríir

silly ɣaʃíim, ɣaʃíima, ɣuʃm

silver fáḍḍa

silvered mifáḍḍaḍ, mifaḍḍáḍa, mifaḍḍaḍíin

silver-plated máṭli bilfáḍḍa, maṭlíyya b., maṭliyyíin b.

similar záyyi báʕḍ

simultaneously sáwa; fi wáqti wáaḥid

Sinai ʕissíina

since (because) madáam; (time) min

to **sing** ɣánna, yiɣánni

single *one* fárda, fírad

I haven't a single one ma ʕandíiʃ wála wáaḥid

sister ʕuxt, ʕixwáat

to **sit** qáʕad, yúqʕud

sitting quʕáad

sitting-room ʕóḍt iggulúus

six sitt, sítta

sixteen siṭṭáaʃar*

sixth sáatit, sátta; sáadis, sádsa; (fraction) suds, ʕasdáas *or* ʕisdáas

sixty sittíin

size ḥagm, ʕaḥgáam *or* ḥugúum; maqáas, maqasáat

skill fann, funúun

skilled fánni, fanníyya, fanniyyíin

sky sáma

sleep noom

to **sleep** naam, yináam

sleeve kumm, ʕikmáam

to **slice** xáraṭ, yúxruṭ

to **slip** daas, yidúus

slowly ʕala máhlak; biʃwéeʃ

small ṣuɣáyyar*, ṣuɣayyára*, ṣuɣayyaríin*; quṣáyyar*, quṣayyára*, quṣayyaríin*; baṣíiṭ, baṣíiṭa, buṣáaṭ

to **smash** kássar*, yikássar*

smell ríiḥa, rawáayiḥ*

to **smell** ʃamm, yiʃímm

smoke duxxáan

smoking tadxíin

no smoking! mamnúuʕ ittadxíin!

so kída

not so fast! múʃ bi súrʕa kída!

not so much múʃ qaddï kída
soap ṣabúun (c.), ṣabúuna,[1] ṣabunáat
sociable ʕigtimáaʒi, ʕigtimaʒíyya, ʕigtimaʒiyyíin
social (as **sociable**)
socks (pair) ʃaráab*, ʃarabáat*
soldier ʒaskári, ʒasáakir
solution ḥall, ḥulúul
to **solve** ḥall, yiḥíll
some baʒd; ḥábba
someone ḥadd; wáaḥid
something ḥáaga
sometimes ʕaḥyáanan; marráat*
son ʕibn, ʕabnáaʕ; wálad, wiláad or ʕawláad
song ʕuɣníya (or ʕuɣníyya), ʕaɣáani
soon báʒdï-ʃwáyya; quráyyib* táani; ḥáalan
as **soon** as ʕáwwil ma, ʒándï ma (+ v.)
sorrow ʕásaf
sorry mutaʕássif, mutaʕassífa, mutaʕassifíin; ʕáasif, ʕásfa, ʕasfíin; maʒa-lʕásaf
sort nooʒ, ʕanwáaʒ
to **sort (out)** fáraz, yífriz
soup ʃúrba
south (of) ganúub
southern(er) qíbli, qiblíyya, qibliyyíin
spacious wáasiʒ, wásʒa, wasʒíin
to **speak** ʕitkállim, yitkállim; kállim, yikállim
speak up! (raise your voice) ʕírfaʒ ṣóotak!
speaker (orator) xaṭíib, xúṭaba
special maxṣúuṣ, maxṣúuṣa, maxṣuṣíin; xuṣúuṣi, xuṣuṣíyya, xuṣuṣiyyíin; xa(a)ṣṣ,[2] xá(a)ṣṣa[2]
special to . . . bi xuṣúuṣ . . .
specialist (as **specialized**)
specialized mitxáṣṣaṣ (or muta-), mitxaṣṣáṣa, mitxaṣṣaṣíin
specially xuṣúuṣan
speech kaláam; (oration) xúṭba, xúṭab
speed súrʒa
to **spend** ṣáraf*, yíṣrif
the **Sphinx** ʕábu-lhóol
spider ʒáqrab*, ʒaqáarib
to **spill** dálaq, yúdluq

to **spin** (textiles) ɣázal, yíɣzil
spinning ɣazl
spoon maʒláqa, maʒáaliq
sport riyáaḍa
spring (season) rabííʒ*
square (open space) midáan, mayadíin
to **stack** raṣṣ, yirúṣṣ
stamp ṭáabiʒ, ṭawáabiʒ
  fiscal stamp wáraqit dámɣa
  two-piastre stamps ṭawáabiʒ min ʕábu qirʃéen
to **stamp** xátam (or xítim), yíxtim
stand kúrsi, karáasi; (rank) máwqif, mawáaqif
to **stand (up)** qaam, yiqúum; (tr.) qáwwim, yiqáwwim
standing qiyáam (v.n.); wáaqif, wáqfa, waqfíin (a.p.)
star nígma, nugúum (or ni-)
to **start** ʕibtáda, yibtídi; (car, train, &c.) qáwwim, yiqáwwim
station maḥáṭṭa, maḥaṭṭáat; márkaz, maráakiz
to **stay** báqa, yíbqa; qáʒad, yúqʒud; (at hotel, &c.) nízil, yínzil
to **steal** sáraq, yísraq
steam buxáar*
step qádam, ʕiqdáam; (rung) dáraga*, daragáat*; sillíma, saláalim
still líssa; bárḍu(h)
stockings (pair) ʃaráab*, ʃarabáat*
stomach baṭn (f.), buṭúun
stones ḥágar* (c.), ḥágara*, ḥagaráat*, ḥigáara* or ʕaḥgáar*
stop (bus-) maḥáṭṭa, maḥaṭṭáat; (full-stop) núqṭa, núqaṭ
to **stop** wíqif, yúqaf; (tr.) wáqqaf, yiwáqqaf; (prevent) mánaʒ, yímnaʒ; ḥaaʃ, yiḥúuʃ; (give up) báṭṭal, yibáṭṭal
store máxzan, maxáazin
to **store** xázan, yíxzin; xázzin, yixázzin
storing taxzíin
storm ʒáaṣif, ʒawáaṣif; (sand-) zawbáʒa, zawáabiʒ
story (floor) door, ʕadwáar*
straight away ʒala ṭúul
straight on dúyri
strange(r) ɣaríib, ɣaríiba, ɣúraba*
  how strange! ʃéeʕ ɣaríib!
  the strange thing is that . . . ʕilɣaráaba*-nn . . .

---

[1] 'Cake of soap'.
[2] See Part I, Appendix B, note (c).

strengthening taʃdíid
to **stretch** (*tr.*) madd, yimídd; (*intr.*)
Ɂimtádd, yimtádd
to be **strict** *with* ḫáakim, yiḫáakim
string dubáara*; fátla, fítal
to **strive** Ɂigtáhad, yigtíhid
stroll fúsḥa
to go for a **stroll** Ɂitmáʃʃa, yitmáʃʃa
strong qáwi, qawíyya, qawiyyíin; (of
wind, &c.) ʃidíid, ʃidíida, ʃudáad;
(durable) matíin, matíina, mutáan
stud (*as* button)
student ṭáalib, ṭálaba
to **study** dáras, yídris; qára*, yíqra*;
Ɂitᴢállim, yitᴢállim; záakir,
yizáakir
to **stumble** daas, yidúus
subject (matter) mawḍúuᴢ, mawaḍíiᴢ
to **subtract** ṭáraḫ*, yíṭraḫ*
suddenly biṣṣúdfa
Suez Ɂissuwées (*f.*)
sugar súkkar* (*c.*), ḫíttit s., ḫítat s.
suit bádla, bídal; kíswa, kasáawi
suitable munáasib, munásba, munasbíin
more suitable Ɂánsab
summer ṣeef
to **summer** ṣáyyif, yiṣáyyif
sun ʃams (*f.*)
Sunday yóom ilḫádd
sunny ʃámsi, ʃamsíyya
sunrise ṭulúuᴢ iʃʃáms
sunset ɣurúub iʃʃáms
supervisor múʃrif, muʃrifíin
to **suppose** fáraḍ, yífriḍ
sure mutaɁákkid (*or* mitɁ-), mutaɁak-
kída, mutaɁakkidíin
surgery (waiting-room) ᴢiyáada,
ᴢiyadáat
to be **surprised** Ɂistáɣrab*, yistáɣrab*
to **swallow** bálaᴢ, yíblaᴢ
sweat ᴢáraq
to **sweep** kánas (*or* kínis), yíknis
(*or* yúknus)
sweet (*n.*) ḫaláawa, ḫalawiyyáat
sweet (*adj.*) ḫilw, ḫílwa, ḫilwíin
to be(*come*) **sweet** Ɂiḫláww, yiḫláww
to **sweeten** ḫálla, yiḫálli
to **swim** ᴢaam, yiᴢúum
swimming ᴢoom; sibáaḥa
to **swindle** ɣaʃʃ, yiɣíʃʃ
swindler ɣaʃʃáaʃ, ɣaʃʃáaʃa, ɣaʃʃaʃíin;
naṣṣáab, naṣṣáaba, naṣṣabíin

switch kubs, kubsáat
sword seef, siyúuf

t

table ṭarabéezᴀ, ṭarabezᴀáat
to **take** xad, yáaxud
how long did it take you to ...?
qaddi Ɂéeh xadítak ᴢaʃan ...
he took a long time to answer
xád wáqtĭ ṭawíil firrádd*
take care! xúd (*or* xálli) báalak!;
Ɂíwᴢa (Ɂíwᴢi, Ɂíwᴢu); Ɂiyyáak
(Ɂiyyáaki, Ɂiyyáaku)
to **take away** wádda, yiwáddi
to **take down** názzil, yinázzil
to **take off** (aircraft) qaam, yiqúum
to **take out** ṭállaᴢ, yiṭállaᴢ
taking place ḫuṣúul (*v.n.*)
to **talk** Ɂitkállim, yitkállim; kállim,
yikállim; ḫáka, yíḫki
tall ṭawíil, ṭawíila, ṭuwáal
tangerines yusafándi (*c.*), yusafandíyya, yusafandiyyáat
tank (container) tank, tunúuk *or* tankáat; sahríig, saharíig
tap ḫanafíyya, ḫanafiyyáat
tar zift
tarboosh ṭarbúuʃ, ṭarabíiʃ*
tasty lazíiz, lazíiza, luzáaz
taxi táksi, taksiyyáat; taks, taksáat
tea ʃaay
to **teach** ᴢállim, yiᴢállim; dárris,
yidárris
teacher muᴢállim, muᴢallíma, muᴢal-
limíin; mudárris, mudarrísa,
mudarrisíin
technical fánni, fanníyya, fanniyyíin
technique fann, funúun
telegram talliɣráaf*, talliɣrafáat*
telephone tilifóon, tilifonáat
telephone operator ᴢáamil ittilifóon
to **telephone (to)** ḍárab, yíḍrab
tilifóon (li)
to **tell** qaal, yiqúul; (relate) ḫáka,
yíḫki
to **tell the truth** sádaq, yísdaq
temperature ḫaráara*; dáragit*
ilḫaráara*
ten ᴢáʃar*, ᴢáʃara*
tennis tínis

tenth ɣáaʃir, ɣáʃra; (fraction) ɣuʃr, Saɣʃáar* *or* Siɣʃáar*
testimony ʃaháada, ʃahadáat
to thank ʃákar*, yúʃkur
    thank you Saʃkúrak*, káttar* xéerak, maɣa-ʃʃúkr, &c.
thanks ʃukr
that/those da, di (díyya, díyyat), dool; dúkha, díkha, dúkham
that (*relative*) Silli
that (*conjunction*) Sinn
theft sírqa
then filwaqtída; báqa; Summáal[1]
    let's see how clever you are, then! Samm-aʃúuf ʃaṭártak baqa!
there hináak
there is/are fiih; Sahó(h), Sahé(h), Sahúm; Sáadi
    there isn't any more ma ɣátʃi fíih
therefore ɣala kída
these (*see* this)
they húmma
thief ḥaráami*, ḥaramíyya*
thigh fáxda, Sifxáad
thin rufáyyaɣ, rufayyáɣa, rufayyaɣiin
thing ḥáaga, ḥagáat; ʃeeS, Sáʃya
to think Siftákar*, yiftíkir; ɣann, yizúnn; (ponder) fákkar*, yifákkar*
thinking tafkíir
third táalit, tálta; (fraction) tilt, Satláat *or* Sitláat
thirst ɣáṭaʃ
thirsty ɣaṭʃáan (*or* ɣatʃáan), ɣaṭʃáana, ɣatʃaníin
thirteen talaṭṭáaʃar*
thirty talatíin
this/these da, di (díyya, díyyat), dool
    like this zayyï kída
those (*see* that)
thought fikr, Safkáar*
thousand Salf, Saláaf
thread fátla, fítal
three tálat, taláata
to throw ráma, yírmi
Thursday yóom ilxamíis
ticket tazkára*, tazáakir
ticket-clerk tazkárgi, tazkargíyya
tie (neck-) garafíṭṭa*, garafiṭṭáat*
to tie rábaṭ*, yúrbuṭ

        [1] 'Back' *aa.*

tight dáyyaq, dayyáqa, dayyaqíin
tiles baláaṭ (*c.*), baláaṭa, balaṭáat
    tiled floor baláaṭ
time waqt, Sawqáat; márra*, marráat*
    what time is it? Sissáaɣa káam?
    at that time saɣítha
    for some time min múdda
    on time filmaɣáad
    a long time ago (min) zamáan
    I've known him for a long time Sana ɣárfu min zamáan
tip baqʃíiʃ
tired taɣbáan, taɣbáana, taɣbaníin
to be (*come*) tired tíɣib, yítɣab; (be tired of) zíhiq, yízhaq
tiresome mútɣib, mutɣíba, mutɣibíin
tiring (*as* tiresome)
to li; liḥádd
toast tust
tobacco duxxáan
today Sinnahárḍa
together wayya báɣḍ
tomatoes qúuṭa (*c.*), quṭáaya, quṭáat *or* quṭayáat
tomb máɣbad, maɣáabid; ṭúrba, ṭúrab
tomorrow búkra*
    the day after tomorrow báɣdï búkra
too (*see* very)
    too difficult for ... ṣaɣbï ɣala ...
tooth sinn, Sasnáan
on top *of* fooq
total (arithmetic) náatig, nawáatig
to tour Sitfárrag*, yitfárrag*
tourist sawwáaḥ, sawwáaḥa, sawwaḥíin
towel fúuṭa, fúwaṭ
town bálad (*f.*), biláad; madíina, múdun; bándar*, banáadir
town-council baladíyya, baladiyyáat
townsman mádani, madaníyya, madaniyyíin
toy líɣba, líɣab
trace Sásar*, Sasáar*
tractor garráara*, garraráat*
trade (occupation) míhna, míhan
tradesman táagir, tuggáar*
trade-union niqáabaṭ, niqabáat†
traffic murúur
train qaṭr, quṭuráat* *or* qúṭura*
training tadríib

tram(way) turmáay,[1] turmayáat
to **transfer** ḥáwwil, yiḥáwwil; náqal,
 yínqil
to **translate** tárgim, yitárgim
transport naql
to **transport** náqal, yínqil
to **travel** sáafir, yisáafir
tray ṣaníyya (*or* ṣi-), ṣawáani
treatment (medical) tadáawi
trees ʃágar* (*c.*), ʃágara*, ʃagaráat*,
 ʕaʃgáar*
tribe qabíila, qabáayil; bádana,
 badanáat
trick ḥíila, ḥíyal
trickster ḥíyali, ḥiyalíyya, ḥiyaliyyíin
tricky (*as* trickster)
trifling baṣíiṭ, baṣíiṭa, buṣáaṭ
troublemaking dawʃági, dawʃagíyya
trousers banṭalóon, banṭalonáat
trustworthy ʕamíin, ʕamíina, ʕúmana
truth ḥaqq
to **try** ḥáawil, yiḥáawil
Tuesday yóom ittaláat
Turk(ish) túrki, turkíyya, ʕatráak* *or*
 tarákwa*
turkey díik rúumi
turn door, ʕadwáar*
 in turn biddóor
to **turn** (take turning) ḥáwwid,
 yiḥáwwid
turning taḥwíida, taḥawíid
twenty ʒiʃríin
two ʕitnéen
to **type** kátab, yíktib ʒalʕáala-lkátba
typewriter ʕáala kátba, ʕaláat kátba
tyre kawítʃ, kawitʃáat

u

umbrella ʃamsíyya, ʃamáasi
uncle (paternal) ʒamm, ʕaʒmáam;
 (maternal) xaal, xiláan
uncouth qabíiḥ, qabíiḥa, qabáayiḥ *or*
 qúbaḥa
under(neath) taḥt
underpants libáas, libísa (*or* ʕilbísa)
 or libasáat
to **understand** fíhim, yífham
understanding ʒaql; tafáahum
to **come to an understanding** ʕitfáahim, yitfáahim

¹ 'Back' *aa.*

to **undo** fakk, yifúkk; ḥall, yiḥíll
unemployed baṭṭáal, baṭṭáala, baṭṭalíin
union ʕittiḥáad, ʕittiḥadáat: (*see also*
 trade-union)
university gámʒa, gamʒáʕt
unlikely múʃ min ilmuḥtámal; múʃ
 manzúur; ma-yṣáḥḥiʃ
unoccupied fáaḍi, fáḍya, faḍyíin
to *be*(*come*) **unoccupied** fíḍi, yífḍa
unsweetened sáada
until liɣáayit ma (+ *v.*), liḥáddï ma
 (+ *v.*)
unwell taʒbáan, taʒbáana, taʒbaníin
up(stairs) fooq
upper foqáani, foqaníyya, foqaniyyíin
uproar héeṣa; zambaléeṭa
use ʕistiʒmáal, ʕistiʒmaláat; (consumption) ʕistihláak; (advantage)
 fáyda, fawáayid
 it's no use ma fíiʃ fáyda; ma yinfáʒʃ
 it's no longer any use ma ʒátʃï
 fíih fáyda mínnu(h)
to **use** ʕistáʒmil, yistáʒmil; (consume)
 ʕistáhlik, yistáhlik
useful mufíid, mufíida
to *be* **useful** náfaʒ, yínfaʒ
usually filʒáada; ʒadátan

v

value fíyya, fiyyáat
veal bitíllu *or* láḥma-btíllu
vegetable xúḍra, xuḍáar
vehicle ʒarabíyya*, ʒarabiyyáat*;
 sayyáara*, sayyaráat*
to **ventilate** háwwa, yiháwwi
ventilation tahwíya
to **verify** ḥáqqaq, yiḥáqqaq
very qáwi; gíddan; xáaliṣ
village bálad (*f.*), biláad; qáryat,
 qúrat*
vinegar xall
visit ziyaara*, ziyaráat*
to **visit** zaar, yizúur
visitor záayir, záyra, zuwwáar*
voice ṣoot, ʕaṣwáat
vulgar báladi, baladíyya

w

wage(s) mahíyya, maháaya *or* mahiyyáat; ʕúgra*
 a low wage ʕúgra baṣíiṭa

to **wait** ʔistánna, yistánna
waiter ṣufrági*, ṣufragíyya*
to **wake** ṣáḥḥa, yiṣáḥḥi
to **walk** míʃi, yímʃi
to go for a **walk** ʔitmáʃʃa, yitmáʃʃa
walking maʃy (*v.n.*); máaʃi (ʕala riglééh), máʃya, maʃyíin (*a.p.*)
wall ḥeeṭ, ḥeṭáan
wallet maḥfáẓa, maḥáafiẓ
to **wander about** laff, yilíff
to **want** to nifs (*or* nafs) + *p.s.* + *impf.*; bidd + *p.s.* + *impf.*
  the shoes want cleaning ʔiggázma miḥtáaga littandíif
wanting to ʕáawiz (*or* ʕáayiz), ʕáwza (*or* ʕáyza), ʕawzíin (*or* ʕayzíin)
war ḥarb*, ḥurúub
to **wash** ɣásal, yíɣsil
washing ɣasíil
to **waste** ḍáyyaʕ, yiḍáyyaʕ
watch sáaʕa, saʕáat
watchman ɣafíir, ɣúfara*
water máyya¹
to **water** ráwa, yírwi
way (road) síkka, síkak; ṭaríiq, ṭúruq; (method) ṭaríiqa, ṭúruq
we ʔíḥna
wearing libs (*v.n.*); láabis, lábsa, labsíin (*a.p.*)
weather ṭaqs; gaww
weaving nasíig
Wednesday yóom lárbaʕ*
week ʔusbúuʕ (*or* ʔisbúuʕ), ʔasabíiʕ
to **weigh** wázan, yíwzin
to **welcome** ráḥḥab*, yiráḥḥab* (bi)
welfare tarfíih*
well (*n.*) biir, ʔabáar* *or* ʔabyáar*
well (*adj.*) mabṣúuṭ, mabṣúuṭa, mabṣuṭíin; fi xéer
well (*adverb*) kuwáyyis
well-made mútqan, mutqána
west ɣarb*
western(er) ɣárbi, ɣarbíyya, ɣarbiyíin
wet mablúul, mablúula, mablulíin
to **wet** ball, yibíll
what (exclamative) déhda!; yáa saláam!; (interrogative) ʔeeh
wheat qamḥ
wheel ʕágala, ʕagaláat *or* ʕágal
  spare wheel ʔistíbna, ʔistibnáat

steering-wheel ʕágalit issiwáaqa
when lámma; wáqtï ma, sáaʕit ma, ʕándï ma (+ *v.*); (interrogative) ʔímta
whence (interrogative) minéen
whenever kúllï ma
where (interrogative) feen
which (relative) ʔílli; (interrogative) ʔayy; ʔánhu, ʔánhi, ʔánhum
to **whisper** wáʃwiʃ, yiwáʃwiʃ
whistle ṣuffáara*, ṣafafíir
white ʔábyaḍ, béeḍa, biiḍ
to **be(come) white** ʔibyáḍḍ, yibyáḍḍ
who (relative) ʔílli; (interrogative) miin
wholesome ṣáaliḥ, ṣálḥa, ṣalḥíin
why (interrogative) leeh
wide wáasiʕ, wásʕa, wasʕíin; ʕaríiḍ*, ʕaríiḍa*, ʕuráaḍ
widespread muntáʃir, muntáʃira*, muntaʃiríin
width ʕurḍ (*or* ʕarḍ)
wife sitt, sittáat; mára*
  my wife ʔissíttï-btáʕti²
willy-nilly ɣáṣbin ʕan + *p.s.*
wind riiḥ, ʔaryáaḥ
to **wind (round)** laff, yilíff
window ʃibbáak, ʃababíik
wine xámra*
winter ʃíta
to **wipe** másaḥ, yímsaḥ
wire silk, ʔasláak *or* sulúuk
wireless (set) rádyu, radyuháat
with bi; wáyya; máʕa; ʕand
without bidúun; min ɣéer; baláaʃ; min ɣéer ma (+ *v.*)
witness ʃáahid, ʃáhda, ʃahdíin
to **witness** (see) ʃaaf, yiʃúuf; (bear witness) ʃíhid, yíʃhad
wolf diib, diyáaba
woman sitt, sittáat; mára*
wonderful múdhiʃ, mudhíʃa, mudhiʃíin; ʕaẓíim, ʕaẓíima, ʕúẓama *or* ʕuẓamáaʔ
wood xáʃab (*c.*), xáʃaba *or* xaʃabáaya, xaʃabáat
wooden xáʃabi, xaʃabíyya
word kílma, kilmáat
work ʃuɣl, ʔaʃɣáal; ʕámal, ʔaʕmáal
to **work** (*intr.*) ʔiʃtáɣal, yiʃtáɣal; (*tr.*) ʃáɣɣal, yiʃáɣɣal

---

¹ 'Back' *a* in first syllable.

² Cf. *sitti* 'my grandmother'.

workman ɣáamil, ɣummáal
workshop wárʃa, wíraʃ
world dínya
worrying ʃáaɣil, ʃáɣla, ʃaɣlíin
to **wound** gáraḥ, yígraḥ; (draw blood)
   xárʃim, yixárʃim
to **wrap (up)** laff, yilíff
to **write** kátab, yíktib
writing kitáaba (*v.n.*); (calligraphy)
   xatt

y

year sána, siníin, sanawáat; ɣaam,
   ɣaɣwáam
   this year ʕissána *or* ʕissanáadi
   last year ʕissána-lli fáatit

yellow ʕáṣfar*, ṣúfra*, ṣufr
yes ʕáywa; náɣam
yesterday ʕimbáariḥ
   the day before yesterday ʕáwwil
   imbáariḥ
(not) yet líssa; liḥáddi dilwáqti; (*see
   also* **nevertheless**)
you ʕínta (*m.s.*), ʕínti (*f.s.*), ʕíntu
   (*pl.*)
young ṣuɣáyyar*, ṣuɣayyára*, ṣuɣayyaríin*

z

Zamalek ʕizzamáalik
zone mantíqa, manáatiq
zoo ginént ilḥayawanáat

PART IV

KEY TO EXERCISES

Note. For use of round and square brackets see introductory note to Part II

Lesson 1

A

1. A good servant.
2. The cupboard drawer.
3. The company manager.
4. The work is heavy.
5. The manager's house is (a) big (one).
6. She's the messenger's daughter.

B

1. ṭaríiq wíḥiʃ.
2. sandúuq sagáayir.
3. garáayid innahárḍa.
4. ʕittáman ɣáali qáwi.
5. báab ilmáktab maftúuḥ.
6. midáan báab ilḥadíid.

Lesson 2

A

1. It's like spring today.
2. The coat's on the hanger behind the door.
3. The broadcasting station is in 'Ilwi Street in Cairo.
4. The boy's shirt has been at the laundry since yesterday.
5. Bring the file on the desk!
6. The bar's downstairs and the library on the upper floor.

B

1. ʕilfilúus fi géeb ilbanṭalóon.
2. ʕilmaṭáar bárra-lmadíina.
3. ʕilmilayáat gamb ilfúwaṭ fi duláab ilhudúum.
4. háat báltu-ssíttĭ min wára-lbáab.
5. huwwa táḥtĭ maʕa-lmudíir.
6. húmma foq báʕḍĭ fiddúrg.

Lesson 3

A

1. The boy's head is hot.
2. The inspector's car is (a) very nice (one).
3. The elder girl is off-colour today.
4. The service-station is on the right.
5. The kitchen floor's very dirty.
6. The Sheikh's flat is pleasant and roomy.

B

1. ʒílbit sagáayir kibíira.
2. ṣawáabiʒ ilʕíid iʃʃimáal.
3. hiyya bínti gamíila xáaliṣ.
4. maḥáṭṭit ilʕutubíis qurayyíba qáwi milbéet.
5. híyya taʒbáana-ʃwayya-nnahárḍa.
6. ʕizzamáalik biʒíida-ʃwayya ʒan wúṣṭ ilmadíina.

Lesson 4

A

1. The driver's waiting (*lit.* standing) near the station.
2. The Zoo(logical Garden) (*lit.* garden of the animals) is in Giza.
3. The fitters are [present] in the workshop.
4. The workmen want a rise (*lit.* increase in the rate).
5. The waiters are busy at the moment.
6. The police are dressed alike.

B

1. min (múddit) saʒtéen.
2. ʒadáthum zayyï báʒḍ.
3. ʕaɣlabíyyit ilmaṣriyyíin muslimíin.
4. humma rayḥíin baʒd idḍúhr.
5. da súuq ʒaʃan issawwaḥíin báss.
6. ʕana ʒárfa kúll ittuggáar miɣlawaniyyíin.

Lesson 5

A

1. Petroleum products are (of) various (kinds).
2. Do you understand me (*lit.* my speech) properly?
3. They've come to an agreement [with each other].
4. Our house is rather a long way from here.
5. My brother's in front of you.
6. Heᵢ's got the money.

B

1. ʕiḥna rayḥíin béthum ʒaʃan ilʒáʃa.
2. ʒandúhum itnéen xaddamíin nubiyyíin.
3. humma ʒarfíin abúuya min zamáan.
4. ʒándu lilbéeʒ ḥagáat gamíila gíddan maṣnúuʒa minniḥáas ilʕáṣfar.
5. féen ʒílbit ikkabríit bitáʒti? dí-btaʒtak ínta.
6. fíih ḥagáat laṭíifa qáwi fissúuq, bássi ɣálya.

Lesson 6

A

1. His eyes are (feeling) rather sore today.
2. Their maid went to the market two hours ago (*lit.* is in the market since two hours).
3. I owe Muhammad five pounds.
4. Have you an envelope, 'Adil?
5. Have you any lighter fluid, please?
6. There's (some) excellent news in the paper(s) today.

B

1. humma rayḥíin maſyíin.
2. taҳáala-mҳáaya lilৎóoḍa-btáҳti (or liḥadd ilৎóoḍa, &c.). ৎana ҳándi ḥáaga lák (or ҳalaſáanak).
3. ৎana muſ fáahim ilmasৎaláadi. ṣáҳba ҳaláyya qáwi.
4. ৎana ҳándi maҳáad maҳa ḥakíim ilৎasnáan (or lisnáan) búkra baҳd idḍúhr.
5. fíih taҳlimáat tánya xáṣṣa bissáfar?
6. fih wáaḥid bárra ҳandu ſákwa.

Lesson 7

A

1. She went out without a hat.
2. I fell down and hurt my leg.
3. He's just stopped [now] in front of the house.
4. He drank the whole dose (lit. medicine) at once (lit. one time).
5. Mahmoud has sent us a nice present.
6. I wrote a couple of letters yesterday to my relatives in England.

B

1. ṭálab minni-flúus ҳaſan ৎúgrit irrukúub lilbéet.
2. sáҳti wíqfit w-ana muſ wáaxid báali.
3. ৎiḥna-smíҳna dilwáqti báss innŭhum wíṣlu.
4. fátaḥu-lbáab wi dáxalu ҳala ṭúul.
5. zíҳil mínni-w ҳamálli dáwſa.
6. qábaḍ filúusu min yoméen báss, wi maҳa záalik ṣaráfha kulláha.

Lesson 8

A

1. Do (it) as per my letter (lit. as I wrote you).
2. Write us an application and send it by post.
3. We're going to (Professor) Mahmoud's farewell party tonight.
4. Are you (fem.) going to wear your new dress for the party tomorrow?
5. We Egyptians drink very strong tea.
6. Ask the chief clerk where the manager is, Abdu.

B

1. báayin ҳaléeh taҳbáan innaharḍa. ৎisৎálu máalu(h).
2. ৎíqfil iſſababíik. ৎiddínya malyáana-tráab (or fíih turáab fi kúllï ḥítta).
3. m-aҳráſſ aҳmil éeh. ৎaktíblu (not ḥaktiblu) walla ৎéeh?
4. ҳawiz áfṭar búkra bádri liৎánni ráayiḥ issuwées.
5. ৎuskútu-w ſúufu ſuҳlŭkum, wi ৎáwwil ḥáaga-ɣsílu-lҳarabíyya!
6. ৎismáҳi, ৎana ҳáwzik tiҳmilíih zayyï kída.

Lesson 9

A

1. The staff leave [their work] early during Ramadan.
2. We've guests for lunch tomorrow.
3. I've known him for a very long time.
4. They're going to stay at the Misr Hotel in Suez.
5. There's a holiday next Tuesday for the feast.
6. I want to cash a cheque for ten pounds.

B
1. ʕistáxgil ʃuwayya! ḥanúxrug baxdï xáʃar daqáayiq.
2. biyíṣrif filúus kitíir xalmaláahi.
3. biyiwṣálu xadátan qablï kída. nídrab lúhum tilifóon?
4. ʕitnéen xasáakir bulíiṣ kanu ḥadríin saxítha.
5. ʕilbáḥrï kan háadi-ṣṣúbḥ lakin dilwáqti háayig.
6. ʕana ḥaqsímha bénku xaʃan ma-ykúnʃï fih dáwʃa.

Lesson 10

A
1. The [telephone] operator was out when the telephone rang.
2. The carpenter was making the desk but then gave up.
3. He wanted to give me six piastres for the book.
4. Come here, Ahmad, I want you!
5. Be careful, there are a lot of pickpockets there.
6. This is the latest fashion (just) arrived from France.

B
1. ʕáaxir márra ʃúftu kan biyúṭbux ilyáda.
2. síbtu náayim wi-rgíxtï laqéetu líssa náayim.
3. huwwa kan líssa xáarig w-íḥna daxlíin.
4. dóol dáyman biyáxdu waqtï ṭawíil firrádd.
5. ʕana maʃyúul qáwi dilwaqti. tiqdar tíigi táani baxdï sáaxa?
6. ʕiḥna gaxaníin xáaliṣ liʕannína kalna ʕáklï baṣíiṭ filfuṭúur.

Lesson 11

A
1. I believe he's coming [to me] tomorrow.
2. I think we can finish tonight.
3. Do you mind if I come with you?
4. What's the matter with you today? You look ill.
5. Would you please take a letter of mine (lit. for me) with you to give [it] to my father.
6. He promised [me] to return me the book when he's finished with it.

B
1. min fadlúku-smaḥúlna,[1] ʕilwáqtï mitʕáxxar w-iḥna taxbaníin ʃuwayya.
2. ʕana ṭalábtï qáhwa lakin inta gibtíli ʃáay.
3. ʕáqdar astilífha mínnak? ḥaruddäháalak baxdï yoméen.
4. ʕana mitʕássif (or mutaʕássif), ʕaftíkir innu míʃi.
5. ʕazúnnï múʃ min ilmuḥtámal (or múʃ manzúur) innu ḥayíigi hína qabli búkra.
6. biyqúulu ʕinnï lintixabáat ḥatkúun baxdï ʃahréen.

Lesson 12

A
1. I shan't be able to see you tomorrow.
2. We haven't got enough cigarettes (for) this evening.
3. He hasn't come yet, perhaps something's happened to him on the way.
4. I haven't the time to go and meet him at the station.
5. He doesn't listen to me when I give him advice.
6. They're not used to drinking wine.

---

[1] Pronounced smaḥúnna.

B

1. múʃ min ixtiṣáaṣi. di tábaɛ qísm ilḥisabáat.
2. ʕana m-aɛráfʃi ʕáyyï ḥáaga ɛan ilmawḍúɛda.
3. da-btáaɛak, múʃ bitáaɛi.
4. ma ɛátʃï fih fáyda mínnu(h).
5. ma ɛandïnáaʃ (or ma fíiʃ ɛandïna) béed̩ kifáaya lilfuṭúur.
6. ʕiggázma di múʃ (or ma gátʃ) ɛala qáddi. dayyáqa-ʃwayya.

Lesson 13

A

1. Don't go to the fruiterer's today. We don't want anything.
2. Don't leave the window open again, I tell you.
3. He can neither read nor write Arabic.
4. I wish he hadn't gone.
5. No, really (lit. by God), I couldn't eat (lit. I haven't any appetite).
6. It's neither [very] bad nor good but between the two.

B

1. ma tinsáaʃ tifáaṣil maɛa-lbayyáaɛ, waʕílla ḥayíd̩ḥak ɛaléek (lit. laugh at you, here = deceive) min ɣéer ʃakk.
2. wi-ḥyátku-skútu-ʃwayya (ya gamáaɛa)! miʃ qáadir ásmaɛ ḥáaga mittilifóon.
3. ma tuqṭumháaʃ wala tumduɣháaʃ, ʕiblázha¹ ɛala ṭúul!
4. ʕana ma ʃúftiʃ irragílda qablï kída? ma kánʃï-byiʃtáyal ɛandïna?
5. ɛúmru ma gábli síira ɛán da (or kída). miʃ ɛáarif leh láʕ.
6. síbtï sagáyri filbéet. ma-mɛíiʃ wála wáḥda.

Lesson 14

A

1. Do you want coffee with or without sugar (lit. unsweetened or with sugar)?
2. Have you ever been there before? It's a very nice place.
3. Is there in your opinion any difference between the speech of Cairo and Alexandria?
4. Can you change me a pound please?
5. Is there a speed-limit [for cars] in Cairo?
6. Have you had any [former] experience of cooking?

B

1. ʕiggawáab xíliṣ. ʕagíibu ɛaʃan timd̩íih?
2. ʕinta fáaḍi walla maʃɣúul dilwaqti?
3. fíih máwqif taksiyyáat quráyyib min hína (or fi ʕáyyï ḥitta hina-qráyyib)?
4. da ɛaʃáani? mutaʃákkir qáwi, lakin ínta mutaʕákkid innak muʃ ɛáwzu(h)?
5. mantaʃ gáay maɛáana? di masáafa baṣíiṭa, muʃ kída?
6. rayḥin nílɛab walla láʕ? law (or ʕin) géet lilḥáqq, ʕinta muʃ ɛáayiz, muʃ kída?

Lesson 15

A

1. Who told you I'm not going?
2. What's that crowd over there? What's going on?
3. Where've you been? I haven't seen you for a long time.
4. Good morning, do sit down, what can I do for you?

¹ May be pronounced ʕibláḥḥa.

5. Hey, you standing over there! Why aren't you working?
6. How far (*lit.* to what extent the distance) is it from (*lit.* between) Cairo to Suez?

B

1. Sarmíiha walla Séeh?
2. míin illi kátab ittaqríir da? da malúuʃ máɣna xáaliṣ.
3. bitqulúuha-zzáay bilɣárabi?
4. Séeh Sanwáaɣ illáḥma-lmawgúuda-nnahárḍa fissúuq?
5. huwwa ḥáṭṭ ikkitáab ill-ana-ddetúulu féen?
6. qaddï Séeh yikallífni lamm-ánzil fi lukánḍa?

Lesson 16

A

1. (The cost of) living is very high nowadays.
2. He's (*lit.* that's) a clever man, he's bound to get on.
3. They are Nubians (*lit.* Nubian people), they've a [special] language of their own.
4. You can have (*lit.* take) that little book for nothing.
5. There's my teacher just arrived!
6. There goes the whistle! Let's go!

B

1. Séeh máɣna-kkilmáadi?
2. Sana ʃúft irráagil dá fissuwées ilSusbúuɣ illi fáat.
3. Sahum hináak (ahúm) qaɣdíin gambï báɣd!
4. Saxíiran ad-ínta géet! Sinta ɣaṭṭaltíni-ktíir.
5. Sahe laqétha! kanit fiddúrgï da taḥt ilwáraq.
6. xúd, Sadi-gnéeh! w-ibqa raggaɣúuli (*or* wi tíbqa-traggaɣúuli) baɣdéen.

Lesson 17

A

1. The hard worker makes money (*lit.* He who works a lot, earns a lot).
2. Have you seen what they're saying in the papers [my friend]?
3. Do you remember what (*lit.* the story that) I told you yesterday?
4. Give me one of yours.
5. This kind of work needs a lot of thought.
6. Hey, the man over there! Come here please!

B

1. xúd ill-inta ɣáyzu(h).
2. ɣandína ʃúylï-ktíir lazim niɣmílu(h).
3. Silɣarabíyya-ll-ana ṭalabtǎha mawgúuda?
4. míin illi wáaqif hináak gamb ilbáab?
5. Sáadi-rragil ill-ínta ɣáwzu(h), Saho-hnáak (aho) gamb ittáksi!
6. Saftíkir innak ɣáarif ill-ana ḥaqulúulak.

Lesson 18

A

1. His house is No. 15, 'Abdu Basha Street.
2. Give me ten two-piastre stamps.

3. This suit costs (*lit.* is at) nineteen pounds. It's a little dear but the material's good (*lit.* strong).
4. He's in charge of sixteen men.
5. Any one of them earns at least five pounds a week.
6. It's a bad road. Don't drive at more than 40 k.p.h.

B

1. húmma-f ʕagáaza luhum (*or* min) tálat ʕasabíiʒ.
2. ʕilʒáqdĭ-btáaʒi-b múddit xámas siníin qáabil littagdíid.
3. ʕiʃʃírka-btíddi ʃaráat lílli-byixdímu fíiha min ʒáʃar siníin li talatíin sána.
4. huwwa-byídfaʒ arbáʒa-gnéeh fiʃʃáhr ʒaʃan yisídd issálaf (*or* issúlfa) illi ʒaléeh.
5. húwwa filʕáwwil ʈálab mínni tamanʈáaʃar ginéeh filbadláadi-wlakin filʕáaxir iʃtarétha-b xamasʈáaʃar.
6. ʕírgaʒ (*or* taʒáala táani) baʒdĭ ʒáʃar daqáayiq walla rúbʒĭ sáaʒa.

Lesson 19
A

1. The phone number is Cairo 234.
2. I'm (*lit.* I my life is) thirty-six and my son is nine [years old].
3. He went to Port Said three months ago.
4. There are five million acres fit for cultivation in Egypt.
5. That merchant's very rich, he's got millions.
6. There are about eleven thousand students in Cairo University.

B

1. ʕiddíini min fáḍlak máṣr xumsumíyya taláata-w sittíin.
2. ras ɣáarib ʒala búʒdĭ míyya-w xamsíin míil ganúub issuwées.
3. dáragit ilḥaráara káanit imbáariḥ taláata w-arbiʒíin ṣantigráad, yaʒni taqríiban míyya-w tísʒa fihranháyt.
4. huwwa ḥayitḥáal ʒalmaʒáaʃ fi sanat ʕálfĭ tusʒumíyya-tnéen wi sittíin.
5. ʕana ʕammíntĭ ʒala ḥayáati-b ʕálfĭ-gnéeh.
6. di ʃírka-kbíira, ma-btistaxdímʃĭ wáaḥid walla-tnéen, wiláakin miyyáat.

Lesson 20.
A

1. The size of the carpet is three metres by two and a half.
2. I was married three years ago last month.
3. Government departments begin [their] work at half-past eight.
4. Four eighths are the same as (*or* equal) a half or eight sixteenths.
5. The plane is taking off next Wednesday at a quarter to ten in the evening.
6. A flat of that size would cost [one] hundreds to furnish [it].

B

1. ʕana mawlúud fi wáaḥid wi ʒiʃríin sibtímbir sanat ʕálfĭ tusʒumíyya wáaḥid wi ʒiʃríin.
2. ṣaḥḥíini-ssaʒa sítta-w núṣṣĭ bizzábṭ, w-ibqa hátli mayya súxna ʒaʃan ilḥiláaqa.
3. ʕana ráayiḥ issúuq. ḥárgaʒ baʒdĭ núṣṣĭ sáaʒa.
4. maʒáaʃu ḥaykúun tiltéen mahiyyítu lamma yitḥáal ʒalmaʒáaʃ.

5. ʒaʃan tiḥáwwil iṣṣantigráad lilfihranháyt, tíḍrab fi wáaḥid w-árbaʒt ixmáas wi-tḍíif¹ itnéen wi talatíin.

6. ʒaʃan tiḥáwwil ilfihranháyt liṣṣantigráad, tíṭraḥ itnéen wi talatíin wi tíqsim ʒala tísʒa ʒala xámsa (*or* ʒala tísaʒt ixmáas).

Lesson 21

A

1. I've lost (*lit.* has gone from me) my wallet and [lost] all my pay.
2. When you arrive, go straight in, don't knock on the door.
3. When you answer the telephone, don't say 'Who is it?' but give (*lit.* say) your name first [It's better].
4. He rang the bell but the current was off (*lit.* cut).
5. [I say, everybody = ya gamáaʒa] I left my watch on the desk yesterday. Has anybody seen it?
6. The book's missing! I put it here yesterday, I'm sure of it (*lit.* there's no doubt).

B

1. Ṣéeh Ṣánsab wáqtï Ṣáqdar aʃufhum fíih?
2. qúlha ʒala máhlak ʒaʃan áfham.
3. fih ṭayyáara ḥatqúum issáaʒa tísʒa-w núṣṣ, wi ḥatíwṣal rúuma-ssáaʒ-arbáʒa.
4. biyḥíbbu-ssiyáasa qáwi-w biyḍayyáʒu waqtǔhum filkaláam fíiha.
5. w-inta náazil fúut ʒaṣṣarráaf.
6. Ṣúskut, ma-trúddïʃ ʒaláyya (*or* ma-tnaqirníiʃ)! rúuḥ ʃuf ʃúylak!

Lesson 22

A

1. I'm telling you to go now before the butcher closes.
2. Don't forget you're coming to have dinner with us tomorrow.
3. I went to see him yesterday and found him very ill.
4. If you don't drink the medicine, you won't get better.
5. How many years have you been in Egypt?
6. What's the matter with you, shouting at each other (like that)?

B

1. m-aftikírʃ innak ḥatilqáaha ṣáʒba.
2. Ṣiddíini-ttaṣríiḥ amdíilak ʒaléeh (*or* amdíih).
3. Ṣíkwi-lfustánda táani! Ṣinta ma ʒamaltúuʃ (*or* kawatúuʃ) kuwáyyis.
4. Ṣana m-aqdárʃ áqra ʒárabi-lḥaddï dilwáqti, yaʒni lamma-ykúun maktúub bilḥurúuf ilʒarabíyya.
5. baqáalu filmustáʃfa múdda lakin ḥáltu-btitḥássin.
6. maʒa-lṢáṣaf, nisíit agíibu(h). láazim síbtu filbéet.

Lesson 23

A

1. The traffic held me up and I couldn't arrive on time.
2. I saw (*lit.* met) the manager and told him the whole story.
3. I bought it for only five piastres.

¹ Pronounced ḍḍiif. The verb Ṣaḍáaf, yuḍíif is learned and an example of a derived form with the prefix Ṣa-. See Lesson 25, 4.

4. Go and take this note to the Efendi in the office next door (*lit.* next to me).
5. Porter, can you please show me to the platform?
6. He was sunburned (*lit.* his face was browned) when he came back from the seaside.

B
1. Sittadxíin yáali-w battáal ɛaṣṣíḥḥa. léeh ma-tḥawílʃí-tbattálu(h)?
2. názzil ilḥagátdi millúuri-w ḥuttǎha filmáxzan.
3. sallímli ɛalɛéela w-inʃáaS alláah aʃúufak quráyyib táani.
4. huwwa muʃ ɛáwzak tisáɛdu(h).
5. tiftíkir innu ḥaywarriháali?
6. Sizzáay tintízir innǔhum yiʃtáɣalu-b Súgra baṣíita zayyǐdi?

Lesson 24
A
1. He was caught and put in prison.
2. You must be photographed for an identity card.
3. It (*lit.* the world) gets dark early in winter and we must soon finish therefore.
4. When you speak about anyone, take care and don't exaggerate (*lit.* don't be eloquent in the speech).
5. The letter you were asking about has been found.
6. You don't find a thing like this easily (*lit.* a thing . . . is not found . . .).

B
1. xádtǐ qaddǐ Séeh ɛaʃan titɛállim iʃʃuɣláadi?
2. huwwa biyqúul innu-tnáqal lakin aftíkir innu-tráfad.
3. bititɛáʃʃu-ssaɛa káam filɛáada (*or* ɛadátan).
4. fíih ḥáddǐ mínku-byitkállim ingilíizi?
5. yalla bíina nitmáʃʃa! niqdar nitkállim w-íḥna maʃyíin.
6. tiḥíbbǐ nitqáabil yom lárbaɛ iṣṣúbḥ ɛaʃan nináaqiʃ ilmasSála bittafṣíil?

Lesson 25
A
1. Wait! I want to talk to you for a minute (*lit.* little).
2. We must get ready to go (*lit.* for the journey), we haven't got a lot of time.
3. Nobody is to use my office while I'm away.
4. The coffee's been spilt on the table. Bring a rag and wipe it up!
5. I was delighted to hear that his health has improved.
6. The dog's barking, it looks as if a stranger is about (*lit.* there is a stranger come).

B
1. Sistaqáal ɛaʃan ṣiḥḥítu taɛbáana.
2. nistannáak qaddǐ Séeh?
3. Siḥna-bnitɛízim kulli yóom gúmɛa billéel ɛandǐ gamáaɛa-ṣḥábna.
4. kúllǐ gawáab biyinxítim qáblǐ ma yitbíɛit ɛaʃan ma ḥáddiʃ yistáɛmil wáraqit ilbúṣta táani.
5. xálli-rriggáala yistarayyáḥu! Siddínya ḥárrǐ-w húmma-ʃtáɣalu-ktíir.
6. tárgim iggawábda-l lingilíizi-w raggaɛúuli-b Sásraɛ ma yúmkin.

Lesson 26

A

1. I can't come out now. I must finish this job before anything else (*lit.* before everything).
2. I propose to spend the summer in Alexandria this year.
3. Why have you (pl.) stopped work? What are you thinking of [doing]?
4. No one can go in without a ticket.
5. I can only give you five pounds.
6. We must be very careful.

B

1. ҁayiz áḥgiz makanéen fi Ҁáwwil ṭayyáara-tqúum yóom iggúmҁa-ggáaya.
2. múmkin tiwarríini ḥáaga tánya? dí muʃ ill-ana ҁáwzu bizҙábṭ.
3. yilzámak sikkíina ḥámya qáwi ҁaʃan tíqṭaҙ iddubáara di.
4. Ҁana muʃ ҁáawiz aʃtíri ḥáaga, múmkin báss atfárrag?
5. Ҁana Ҁáasif ma kanʃí mumkínn-agi-mbáariḥ liҁanni kan lazímn-azҙúur[1] axúuya filmustáʃfa.
6. nifs-atҙállim baҙḍ ilҙadáat min ҁadáat ilḥáyyï da. Ҁaҙmil éeh ҁaʃan atҙallímha.

Lesson 27

A

1. They missed (*lit.* weren't able to catch) the train and arrived late.
2. I've sent him to look for the messenger.
3. Instead of spending your money on cigarettes (*lit.* smoke), use (*lit.* put) it for something else.
4. Let's go for a walk, I want to stretch my legs (*lit.* get my blood flowing).
5. The ganger will tell you everything (*lit.* go to the ganger who will, &c.). I know nothing about it (*lit.* I haven't any news).
6. Leave him (alone), he's better on his own.

B

1. Ҁiḥna ya dóobak (or Ҁáwwil ma) ibtadéena niʃtáyal gum ҁaṭṭalúuna.
2. ma tuqҙúdʃi (or tifḍálʃí) titkállim kitíir! ʃuf ʃúylak!
3. da-kfáaya! ma niqdárʃí nistáҙmil Ҁáktar min kída Ҁábadan.
4. ṭáyyib, Ҁismaḥúuli, láazim aráwwaḥ dilwaqti.
5. yalla bíina (or ma[2] tíigi-nrúuḥ) niṣṭáad sámak yom ilḥádd.
6. Ҁilҁáḥsan tirúuḥ filmáyrib lamma-ddínya-ṭṭárri.[3]

Lesson 28

A

1. Excuse me, may I take a cigarette?
2. Ask him if he can come tomorrow or not?
3. If you work well, I'll increase your pay (*lit.* for you the pay).
4. Go and make me a cup of coffee.
5. Go in and see whether he's inside or not (*lit.* see him inside or not).
6. If you (pl.) finish early, you can go home.

[1] See Introduction, B (ii).
[2] See Lesson 13, 3, note (iii).
[3] Pronounced *ṭṭárri.*

B

1. law kunna-mʃíina sáaɣit ma qultǐlak, kan zamánna- (or kunna-wṣílna-) hnáak dilwáqti.
2. law kúntǐ ṭalabtǎha mínnu kan iddaháalak.
3. da ɣáali gíddan. Ṣiza nazzílt ittáman ʃuwayya, yímkin aʃtíri.
4. ma-yhímmiʃ (iza) gúm walla ma gúuʃ.
5. ṢisṢálu-za kan miggáwwiz wi ɣándu Ṣawláad.
6. ya réet kunt áɣraf innúhum ḫayíigu walla láṢ.

Lesson 29

A

1. Your (pl.) work today is much better than [that of] yesterday.
2. It's a lot hotter today than yesterday.
3. Life in Port Said is quieter and cheaper than in Cairo.
4. The best thing you've done today was to come early.
5. This tomato is still a bit green, it isn't ripe.
6. The Egyptian flag [its colour] is green with a crescent and three stars in the middle (lit. and in its middle, &c.).

B

1. Ṣilkaláam Ṣáshal milɣámal.
2. tiftíkir issáfar bilqáṭr (Ṣ)ásraɣ milɣarabíyya?
3. Ṣan-afáḍḍal asáafir biṭṭayyáara liṢannǎh-ásraɣ¹ min Ṣáyyǐ ḫáaga tánya.
4. ma-tzaɣɣáqʃǐ² kida, húww-an-áṭraʃ!
5. miʃ ḫárr innahárda zayy imbáariḫ.
6. ɣándak Ṣóoḍ-árxaṣ mill-ána fíiha dilwáqti?

Lesson 30

A

1. Our flat's on the sixth floor, (so) take the lift.
2. My son came [out] fifth in this year's examination.
3. Take the first [turning] on your right and then the third on your left.
4. I am paid (lit. receive my pay) on the last day of the month.
5. Leave (pl.) the first eleven chapters and begin from Chapter 12.
6. The party is on the seventeenth of next month.

B

1. di Ṣáaxir márr-aqúllak.
2. féen liṭnáaʃar ginéeh ill-ána salliftúhúmlak min zamáan?
3. dí muʃ Ṣáwwil márra-tqúlli ɣaláada.
4. tiftíkir aqúllu Ṣéeh lamm-aʃúufu marra tánya?
5. tárgim ittalatíin ṣáṭr ilṢawwalaniyyíin li lingilíizi.
6. xúd ittáalit min ɣaʃʃimáal wi baɣdéen ímʃi ɣala ṭúul, ḫatilqáah baɣdǐ mitéen Ṣaw tultumíit mítr.

Lesson 31

A

1. There may be lemons in the market tomorrow.
2. An oke of oranges today costs (lit. is at) five piastres.
3. I need a pound of meat a day.

¹ = liṢinnǎha + Ṣasraɣ.
² Pronounced dz-.

4. Could I have (*lit.* give me) another lump of sugar please?
5. An oke of bananas works out at ten average-sized fruits.
6. We need two loaves of European bread daily.

B

1. ḫatíᵹmil iʃʃúrba-zzáay min ɣéer láḥma walla-xḍáar?
2. ʃana m-adfáᵹʃ ittáman da filbaṭáaṭiṣ.
3. bi káam ilwáḥda milburtuqánda wi-b káam ilwíqqa?
4. xámas ṣawáabiᵹ móoz yíigu núṣṣi wíqqa taqríiban.
5. fárdit ʃaráabi táyha. ʃísʃal ilmakwági-za kanit (líssa) ᵹándu(h).
6. ʃiza baṣṣéet táḥt ilwáraq da, ʃaftíkir ḥatilqáaha.

Lesson 32

A

1. There isn't any more fruit (*lit.* fruits) in the market. It's completely sold out (*lit.* finished).
2. There aren't enough windows in the room for ventilation.
3. You must study the examples thoroughly in order to understand.
4. Don't be late tomorrow, we've guests coming.
5. Go on to the station ahead of me with the bags, I'll catch you up shortly.
6. I haven't seen him for six months. Where has he gone?

B

1. ᵹawiz atfárrag ᵹala sanadíiq sagáayir rixíiṣa-ʃwayya.
2. ʃana ᵹándi-ʃwayyit sanadíiq gamíila qáwi-mṭaᵹᵹáma bilᵹáag (*or* sínn ilfíil).
3. la búddi taxud báalak mizzawáabiᵹ illi bitqúum fiṣṣáḥra liyyámdi.
4. dá ᵹaʃan ilʃayníya báss, múʃ lilfúqara-lli zayyi ḥalátna.
5. tíqdar tiqúlli ᵹala ʃasáami ʃagzáaʃ ilᵹarabíyya?
6. ʃamráaḍ ilᵹiyúun muntáʃira qáwi-f máṣr, ᵹaʃan kída-ktíir middakátra-lmaṣriyyíin mutaxaṣṣaṣíin f-amráaḍ ilᵹiyúun.

Lesson 33

A

1. I've been waiting two hours for you.
2. He's promised me to come.
3. I found him asleep and couldn't wake him up.
4. Don't leave the door open when you go out.
5. He's been sentenced to three months' imprisonment for theft.
6. I'm looking for the silver-plated spoons. Where are they?

B

1. huwwa qáaᵹid hináak baqáalu sáaᵹa.
2. fíih sanadíiq búṣṭa maxṣúuṣa maktúub ᵹaléeha 'mustáᵹgil'.
3. ʃana miʃ ᵹáarif izzáay afahhimháalak.
4. ʃilmudárris mistaᵹíddi-ysáᵹdak ᵹala qáddi ma yíqdar.
5. ʃahóh, xúdu(h)! ʃinta miḥtáglu ʃáktar mínni, lakin xúd (*or* xálli) báalak mínnu(h) (*or* iwᵹáalu(h)).
6. miʃ ᵹáarif yikun féen! ʃúftu mitᵹállaq wara-lbáab innahárḍa-ṣṣúbḥ.

Lesson 34

A

1. Don't (fem.) worry (*lit.* be afraid)! I've marked our bags, they won't get lost.

2. Aren't you going to do as I tell you!
3. You're right. I'd forgotten I had an appointment with you.
4. I thought I'd finish today, but I wasn't able to.
5. Thank you, (but) I can't eat again. I had lunch an hour ago.
6. I handed it to him in front of 'Atif Efendi.

B

1. Ṣana ma kúntiʃ ẓáarif innída kan ittartíib.
2. min húwwa-lli ʃúftu fáayit dilwaqti?
3. Ṣana qáaẓid hína min (or baqáali) núṣṣi sáaẓa.
4. ráayiḥ féen? míin illi middíik Ṣizni tímʃi?
5. w-íḥna maʃyíin ʃúftu biṣṣúdfa wáaqif figgíha-ttánya miʃʃáariẓ.
6. ʃuftu láabis maláabis Ṣurubbíyya díik innaháar. ẓadátan ma-byilbisháaʃ, miʃ kída?

Lesson 35
A

1. He took a long time to make it as nice as that.
2. Don't be too hard on the workmen, otherwise they will become discontented.
3. Do you mind my sitting here (or is there any objection, &c.)?
4. Show me a small shaving-mirror.
5. I hear (lit. heard) that you have met each other for the first time.
6. I don't like him coming here a lot. Tell him not to come again.

B

1. bénhum wi ben báẓdi-mnáfsa-kbíira qáwi fiʃʃúyl.
2. ma fiʃ máẓna-l lintiẓáar. zamánhum (or láazim yikúunu) míʃyu.
3. xallíik dáyman ẓarraṣíif! Ṣilmáʃyï-f wuṣt iʃʃáariẓ xáṭar ẓaléek.
4. huwwa miẓtímid ẓala-msaẓdíthum lúh.
5. ẓamálha biṭṭaríiqa díyya-ywáffar wáqtï-ktíir.
6. ma fiʃ fáyda milgidáal. ṢilṢóoda miḥtáaga littabyíiḍ ḍarúuri.